PSYCHIATRY AND THE HUMAN CONDITION

Psychiatry
and the
Human Condition

By

IAGO GALDSTON, M.D.

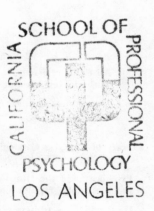

BRUNNER/MAZEL, *Publishers* • New York

Published by
BRUNNER/MAZEL, INC.
64 University Place, New York, N.Y. 10003

Library of Congress Cataloging in Publication Data
Galdston, Iago, 1895

  Psychiatry and the Human Condition.
  Includes bibliographies and index.

  1. Psychiatry—Addresses, essays, lectures, I. Title. [DNLM: 1. Psychiatry—Collected
works. WM7 G149p]
RC458.G32   616.8'9'008   75-15857
ISBN 0-87630-105-7

TO THE MEMORIES OF

A. A. BRILL

JOHN C. WHITEHORN

AUBREY LEWIS

Introduction

To assemble in one book psychiatric essays and studies spread over a period of some thirty years is a bold but well-justified exercise, claiming convenience and historical interest, rather than apodictic truth. As Sir Thomas Browne wrote, *"If there be any singularity therein correspondent unto the private conceptions of any man, it doth not advantage them; or if dissentaneous thereunto, it no way overthrows them. . . . It was set down many years past, and was the sense of my conceptions at that time, not an immutable law unto my advancing judgment at all times; and there-fore there might be many things therein plausible unto my passed ap-prehension, which are not agreeable unto my present self. . . . Lastly, all that is contained therein is in submission unto maturer discernments; and as I have declared, shall no further father them than the best and learned judgments shall authorise them."*

This unassuming deference to the mature judgment of himself and others has a parallel in a number of passages in Dr. Galdston's book, such as the modest assertion regarding gifted persons, *"mavericks."* "Nothing in the present-day training or education of the psychiatrist, psychoanalyst, or other, prepares or qualifies the psychiatrist to deal with the primary, basic abnormality of the maverick—his giftedness—his *'divine madness.'* At best the psychiatrist can deal only with the consequent or secondary problems and even there not much better than symptomatically."

In this collection of papers, a scholarly mind is brought to bear on a remarkable range of topics, from Paracelsus to the dynamics of cure. At first blush it might seem that apart from articles dealing with psycho-analysis and existentialism, there is little to connect many of the articles with one another—those on gambling, for example, with those on de-personalization, or those on social medicine with "Job on the meaning of life." But this would be a hasty and mistaken judgment. There is a common theme running through the superficially disparate papers which stamps them as the product of a humanist, a reflective historian preoccupied with the ethical and social bearing of his profession. In its scope and concern for the preservation of human values it belongs among the *Literae Humaniores*. Dr. Galdston's opinions, expressed with much felicity of language, attest his courage in questioning received beliefs; his affirmations are an intellectual challenge, his negations a temperate examination of the untenable. He holds that it is the duty of man to guard and cherish, and if possible advance his cultural heritage.

The spirit of this injunction permeates the whole of Dr. Galdston's book.

Sir AUBREY LEWIS

December, 1974.

Contents

Part I:
PSYCHOPATHOLOGY AND PSYCHOTHERAPY

1

The Anatomy of a Psychosis

AMONG THE MANY NOTABLE ACHIEVEMENTS of modern psychiatry there is one which is but seldom found in the lists. This achievement is the emendation of a gross error which first intruded into the thoughts of thinking men at the time of the intellectual renaissance, i.e., in the 17th Century. This error, involving the relationship of man to his universe, has persisted for long, and is far from obliterated even today.

Medieval science was aptly described as the study of the universe with man left out. Modern science, and particularly the biological sciences, can be described in like terms as the study of man with his universe left out. These summary descriptions are perhaps too terse to be equitable, but they are at least founded on valid facts.

In the Intellectual Renaissance man, the individual, was rediscovered. Its newborn science studied man intensively. But it did so in a manner which tore him from his social matrix, and by a method which further dismembered him. In the following centuries man was, so to say, torn into finer and ever finer shreds, and these *parts of parts* were studied scrupulously. All this was done according to the Méthode formulated by René Descartes, and in the conviction that only the summation of the knowledge of the parts can yield a complete knowledge of the whole.

This error modern psychiatry has tended to correct in an effective measure. The credit for this achievement belongs, not as one might at first think, to Koffka and the Gestalt School, but rather to Freud and his co-workers.

For it was Freud who most effectively demonstrated that man is greater than the sum of his anatomical and physiological parts. In his postulations on the id, the ego, and the superego, and in his theories on the

3

etiology of the neuroses, Freud affirms that to be understood, man must be studied in his social setting, as he lives and functions within the social matrix.

Jung has developed these thoughts even further. Freud views man as the creature of his contemporary and immediate milieu, deriving the content and character of his superego from the parent or parent substitute. Jung has shown man to be a creature who carries within himself the dynamic psychological derivatives of countless ages. He maintains not only that man shares in the collective unconscious of the human race, but that the ego ideal draws a substantial portion of its content from the collective and archaic ideals of the human race.

These theories of Freud and of Jung are common knowledge to all who are versed in the literature of psychiatry and psychoanalysis, and it were needless to cite them but for the fact that their implications and revolutionary effects are not fully appreciated. These are more than theories on the origin of the superego or on the genesis of the neurosis. They are affirmations that nothing but the study of the whole man can give us an effective understanding of man. The current interest in psychosomatic medicine reflects in a measure the impact of these teachings of Freud and his followers upon clinical medicine. But all who have followed medical literature during the last quarter century have witnessed how the exponents of the medicine of the mortuary, and of the special laboratory, have been compelled grudgingly but surely to acknowledge that theirs is but a fractionalized knowledge of man, which, to be effective, must be integrated by a discipline which is in so many respects the very antithesis of their own. I need not dilate on how much good has come to us from the labors of those who held that a knowledge of the whole can be gained only by a study of its parts. We owe to them all of what is aptly called the preclinical sciences of medicine. To the *Etiological School* so graphically described and so passionately defended by von Behring we owe our knowledge of the specific factors in pathology. Knowledge of the whole man were indeed a meager knowledge without those elements contributed by what I have termed the students of fractionalized man. I want rather to turn to the other side of the medal, to the "harm that good men do." I want to dwell on the handicap which, it seems to me, psychiatry has suffered in its all too exclusive devotion to the study of the whole man. However, before elaborating on this theme, I want to set it on the record that I bring no charges and no accusations, but rather only submit for your thinking a number of questions which have troubled my mind.

There is no dearth of theories and observations on the etiology of psychoneurosis, particularly in psychoanalytical literature. The genetics of the psychosis are less adequately postulated. We do indeed confess that we know very little of the etiology of the major psychoses. But even where we do have theoretical formulations on the etiology of given psychopathies, these are most often vague, and their vagueness, I am persuaded, is due to the extensiveness of the base of their derivation which most often takes in nothing less than "the whole man." I would not have you believe that I question for a moment but that in every etiology the whole man is involved, in a simple infection no less than in a psychopathy. I am convinced, however, that it is possible and would be profitable to study psychopathies as singular phenomena manifest among complexities of phenomena, to regard them in other words as of, but apart from, the total man. Psychopathies are phenomena. They are manifestations of the dynamic interrelation of psychological forces. They have patterns of their own, structures, and histories, even as a vortex does, seen within a flowing stream of water.

It is the dynamics of the psychopathies that to my mind need study so that we might gain some idea as to their structure, their evolution, their issue. This type of study is seldom to be found in psychiatric literature. More common is the study of the total personality.

Let me illustrate what I mean by drawing on clinical medicine for an example, even though I am fully aware of the risk involved. One can study the case of a man with tuberculosis and give a complete record of his history from primary infection to the terminal stages. Such a study would constitute the record of a man suffering from tuberculosis. But one can also study, as my friend Alan Krause did so brilliantly, "the tubercle" and gain thereby a most illuminating insight into the anatomy, if you please, the dynamics, the alternate and ultimate destinies of the pathologic entity, the tubercle. In such a study the tubercle is dealt with as a singular phenomenon manifest in a complex of phenomena. Such a study affords one a very clear idea of the dynamics of that pathologic entity, and enables us better to trace and relate its effects on the complex of phenomena that is the patient. The dynamics of pathologic entities and phenomena have been similarly and profitably studied in many other fields, in endocrinology, in nutritional deficiencies, in the degenerative changes. Professor Lewis contributed brilliantly to our understanding of angina pectoris by his studies on the effects of ischaemia on muscle tissues. It is to be granted that the patho-dynamics of the psychopathies are qualitatively different from those witnessed in other types of disease, but the difference is not so great as to invalidate the comparison.

It should therefore be possible, and I am certain it would be profitable, to study the patho-dynamics of the psychopathies in ways similar to those in which we have studied the patho-dynamics of other types of diseases: in diphtheria, for example, or in diabetes. To be able to do this effectively it may be necessary for us to study our patients "fractionally"—to regard the psychopathy as if it were, as indeed it often is, the resultant of some foreign body—toxic or otherwise—or of some hyper- or hyposecretion of a hormone, or of some nutritional or other deficiency. In other words, we may be required to abstract the psychopathy from the total personality and study it as a singular phenomenon.

I am aware that not a few psychiatrists agree with this point of view; at least I am tempted to read as much into their words, and I am persuaded that our experience with the neuropsychiatric casualties of the war will compel us to recognize its validity.

In support of and in illustration of the thesis which I have attempted to advance I submit the case of a patient who has been under my care for some time. The analysis, to follow my own precept, will be largely devoted to his psychosis, though to illuminate its dynamics it will of course be necessary to draw upon certain data of the patient's life and experience.

The patient is a young man, in his early thirties, unmarried, living with his younger brother and widowed mother. His complaint given in his own words is as follows:

This is a short account of what I remember of the events leading to my illness and my resignation from. . . .
I had become greatly dissatisfied with my situation in that organization, and gradually, day by day, I became increasingly convinced that some person or persons unknown were endeavoring to make an unsatisfactory position still more unsatisfactory and to block my legitimate aspirations in every possible direction. More and more I became preoccupied with this state of affairs: trying to set some clear idea of what was going on, trying to anticipate plots and circumvent snares. I became an insomniac, and day after day I would go to work after but three or four hours sleep. Night after night I would lay awake smoking. With these ever persistent thought waves pursuing me, I could find no relaxation. Whenever I hazarded a suggestion, at random, in my work, it seemed to me that a pattern of behavior in accordance with that suggestion would ensue. This procedure, I postulated, was followed to keep me from gaining any insight into what was going on. Finally, from the accidental behavior

of various colleagues, both within and without the organization, I became convinced that I was being spied upon systematically, even to the extent of listening to my telephone conversations; and I was filled with great anger and indignation. In order to terminate this almost insupportable situation, I resigned from my position. At the time, as I recall, I was some twelve to fourteen pounds under my normal weight, my physical endurance was considerably reduced, and, at times, I would feel somewhat vertiginous. I thought that if matters went on in this fashion much longer, I would have a nervous breakdown.

This "short account" is to be supplemented with the following data. After resigning from his position in business, the patient withdrew more and more from the outside world. He remained in his home, talked little and seemed always "absent-minded." He had numerous paranoic ideas, to the effect that he was on a black-list, that derogatory statements about him were published in the press, that electrical currents were directed at him through the floor of the bathroom. He would not answer the telephone, fearing plots against him.

The diagnosis was schizophrenia, with paranoid ideas. The patient was mildly psychotic. Now if, instead of having a psychosis, the patient had a myocardial insufficiency, we would naturally be prompted to seek its origin and to define its dynamics. We would in the parlance of the day want to know "how did he get that way." For though heart failure is a rather definite clinical entity with a distinctive symptomatology it may be due to any one or even to several varying conditions such as rheumatic fever, lues, essential hypertension, or arteriosclerosis. This patient, however, did not suffer with a myocardial insufficiency but rather with a psychosis. Still, may we not similarly seek to determine "how did he get that way?" In this case, at least, I am convinced that the dynamics of the psychosis can be traced almost as clearly as those of a case of myocardial insufficiency giving a history of rheumatic fever.

I first saw the patient when he was sent to me primarily for diagnosis. My notes thereon read "schizoid personality, mild paranoid schizophrenia, well oriented, fairly good insight. Prognosis—on treatment—fair." In discussing the case with the patient's younger brother, I advised institutional treatments. He answered that their mother would not consent. I then advised trying treatment by a private psychiatrist. That appeared rather difficult because of the expense involved. The patient was not able to attend any public clinics, and so the matter of treatment was left to the future.

It was almost a year later that the patient asked that I should treat him. Despite the obvious difficulties involved in the situation, I was glad to take him on, anticipating quite correctly that he would prove an interesting case. When treatment was initiated, the patient was 33 years of age. The essential facts about him are as follows: He is a college graduate and a lawyer. He is the older of two sons. His father, who died in 1938 of heart disease, was a Jew. His mother is a Christian. The patient has no definite religious convictions, but is not inclined to consider himself a Jew. Physically the patient is of somewhat slender build, 5' 9" in height, and weighing 135 pounds. He never weighed more than 146 pounds. His complexion is fair, pale. His eyes are rather large, presbyopic and markedly astigmatic. His reactions are outwardly slow and most negativistic. Though he has experienced no serious physical illness, he is inclined to be hypochondriacal. In posture, sitting or standing, he appears to hug himself. His fingers are moderately long but shapeless, and his fingernails are stumpy. His smile is striking. It is a broad grin involving his entire face, including his eyes. His lips draw back to reveal a large mouth and much of the gums.

It was not difficult, despite the paucity of details, to construct the genetic pattern of the patient's difficulties. Constitutionally he is of the type which Abraham Myerson has so aptly named anhedonic. The "fire of life never glowed brightly within him." His libidinal drive is not strong. He is, however, endowed with an uncommonly good brain. He went to a private boarding school for his primary education, then to one of our best Eastern colleges, and studied law in a leading university. His scholastic record was excellent. Before deciding on law, he majored in chemistry, and thought too of studying medicine. He was a voracious reader and is well versed in literature.

His home background was quite uncommon. His father was an aggressive, somewhat choleric man. His mother was rather passive. The financial status of the family was fair. There were, however, some periods of financial strain. But the family was without a permanent home and lived most of the time in hotels. The patient thus never had the advantages of a home circle, nor did he ever acquire an appreciable number of playmates or acquaintances. Though he professes to be attached to his family, the patient reveals no strong affection for his father, and little more for his mother or brother. He was a precocious child, largely left to his own devices and ways. In his younger years, that is, between the ages of 7 and 12, he was somewhat aggressive, and got into a number of fistfights. However, when faced with the reaction of his school mates, who considered him "too rough," he decided to change, and became more seclusive. While in prep school the patient took part in athletics, favoring soccer and track. He earned his athletic letter. When the patient was 16 years of age, he suffered a spell of illness, probably a schizoid depression, which baffled his family and his physician, and necessitated his withdrawal from school for a period of three months. His complaint was great fatigue and somnolence. During this period the patient remained at home, spending much time in bed, and seeing no one but his family. He did, however, continue his studies. He returned to school and was able to pass all his examinations, including the college boards. That summer he went abroad, travelling with another boy through France and England.

Intensely unhappy in the last years of his prep school, the patient found college life and work more acceptable. However, he did not mix well with his classmates but remained rather aloof. He became interested in the Literary Circle of the college, but did not succeed in gaining acceptance. He wrote some poetry dealing mainly with "mild" love themes, and with nature. He was also interested in drama. At college he majored in chemistry and took courses in advanced mathematics and art. He graduated with distinction and directly began the study of law. His experiences in law school were not unlike those in college. He graduated from law school, passed the bar examinations, attempted for a while to develop a practice, and failing in this, looked for and found a position paying a modest salary. He worked at this job until his illness compelled him to resign.

The erotic life of the patient was singularly poor. He has had no sexual contacts, masturbated little, and had comparatively infrequent nocturnal emissions. He had but one so-called love affair at the age of 27 which ended unhappily and contributed to his last illness. The patient became interested in a young woman working in his office. He courted her for a period of 7 months. His courtship consisted in taking the girl to lunch, to the movies, and for walks and bus rides. He never caressed her, nor made any erotic advances. He described the girl as physically very attractive, "slim, with a boyish figure, looking like 17, though she was 22 years of age." The difficulty in his relations with the girl was ascribed by the patient to their difference in temperaments. "She wanted me to sweep her off her feet all at once" was the way he phrased it. He considered her simple and naive. He said he wanted her to pursue him, and when she failed to do so, they drifted apart. He later learned that she had married and was about to have a child. This upset him.

I now turn to the dynamics of the patient's psychosis, leaving the other pertinent facts of the patient's experiences to be brought out in the process of this consideration.

The patient came for treatment quite willingly, and alone, but he proved rather difficult at first. He was taciturn, very slow in his responses, and productive of very little. Left to himself, he would say nothing; prodded, he could think of little to say. According to his version, his life was uneventful. His account of his illness was that he just "ran down and got sick." He thought that if he could only "build himself up" he would get well again. At first he said little about his delusions, only that people had watched him when he was in the public library. Of this experience he spoke in an uncertain vein, granting only now and then that perhaps he had "imagined it."

I saw the patient but once each week, for one hour. Progress was very slow at first, and it required much effort to gain even an outline of the patient's history. But the rigid, aloof attitude of the patient and his negativism after a little time gave way to a more responsive participation in the treatment.

I observed early that the only ready avenue of approach to the patient was through his intellectual feelings. This was in agreement with Oberndorf's observations on the "factually minded patient." He was therefore given large doses of explanation and interpretation, and many of his own reported experiences were discussed with him on a purely intellectual plane, and quite abstractly. These discussions at first seemed too desultory to be therapeutically effective, but a number of episodes soon revealed that they had a thawing effect upon the patient's resistance, not only in the transference situation but in relation to his own mentations on his problem. He made progress in an episodic rather than continuous manner. The psychodynamics of his therapeutic progress patently followed their own innate pattern and neither the patient's intent nor conscious effort could direct them. He was, so to say, no less the "victim" of his cure than he was of his psychopathy. This is reflected in the eruptive way in which he brought forth the most pertinent of materials. When asked to tell of his early erotic experiences, he first maintained that he had had none. Then he told that he had once been invited by a boy companion to peep through a knot hole at some women who were undressing in a seashore cabin. The patient refused to look. When I asked him why he refused, the patient offered a number of irrelevant reasons. I suggested that possibly he was afraid to look. The patient denied this with some vehemence and then as proof of the fact that he was not afraid, he volunteered the following information: "I once made an assault on school property," he said. Asked to explain, he told that he had obtained a brace and bit and had drilled a hole through a wall in one of the school buildings. The wall was that of a washroom (not a toilet) which was used by the janitor to rinse his floor mops and the like. Further questioning revealed that this "assault on school property" followed on the peeping episode. The action was of course completely irrational *to the patient*. He had no idea why he did so senseless a thing. Later in the treatment he came to appreciate the significance of this phantom gesture, and he recognized that it was representative of many similar instances in which he endeavored to resolve a conflict-situation by some innocuous act which was but a phantom token of the required effective action.

The point to be underscored at this stage is that this pertinent revelation came so to say automatically; that it was not volitional, conscious, or deliberate; that it came forth not as a product of insight, but involuntarily as a cough might, or a hiccup; that it was, in other words, relevant and rational in the psychodynamics of the patient, but not in any other relationship. I had merely suggested to the patient that possibly he was afraid to peep. He denied this and attempted to convince me that he was not a coward. In proof of his contention he could have cited any number of instances in which he was brave or courageous. He had many fistfights, had looked at pornographic pictures, had carried a condom to Europe and back. Why did he choose to prove his bravery by the psychologically so pertinent, and otherwise so seemingly unrelated and irrational story of the "assault on school property"? The answer lies in the innate rationale of the psychodynamics of the patient recovering from a psychopathy. It is akin to the rationale of the calcium deposition in a tuberculous lesion of a patient recovering from tuberculosis.

There were many instances of this nature during the treatment of the patient. I will cite two of the more significant ones. At one stage of the treatment I suggested to the patient that he keep a diary. He followed the suggestion, but his entries were stereotyped and insignificant, so that after a while I did not encourage him to read them to me. Then at one session he sounded discouraged. Asked why he felt discouraged, he said he felt he was making no progress, and in evidence of this he cited his inability to keep up his diary. In comment, I suggested that I was in part responsible for this, since I ceased asking him to read his entries to me. I went on to explain that the reason I did so was because his diary notes offered little of value, hence there was no profit in spending time in hearing them. The patient responded by saying that he too recognized that his entries were insignificant, but then he could not make them more revealing because he was secretive. But he could not tell precisely what he held in secret. He had a vague feeling that somewhere there was a closet skeleton—but where or what he could not tell. At this point I suggested that he imagine something about which he might be secretive. I encouraged him to draw upon his fancy. To this suggestion the patient responded by saying that if it were a matter of fancy, he need not create a new one since he had written such a story in college. He then told the plot of his story. It was built on the story of Pygmalion and Galatea, save that Galatea was displaced by Pan. In the patient's story, the sculptor is modeling a statue of Pan. The work is progressing wonderfully. But then the sculptor discovers that he has fallen in love with his model, a young and handsome boy. He is so shocked by this discovery that he promptly destroys the statue of Pan. The sculptor is then relieved of his distasteful passion.

You will of course recognize at once that this story is an epitome of the patient's dilemma, and that it also reveals the way in which the patient attempted to resolve it. But again I want to fix your attention on the manner in which these revelations issued. They seemingly had no issue in anything preceding. They came forth as spontaneously and abruptly as a projectile vomiting might in a cerebral neoplasm. This was not the only story the patient had written in his college days. Nor is he lacking in imagination. Why then did he bring forth this particular story? The answer is, I believe, to be found in the innate psychodynamics of the patient's recovery process. The patient did not, at the time he told this story, have any insight into its significance, nor recognize its pertinence.

In this connection it is of interest to report that the patient has been unable to rewrite the story, the original having been lost. He is resistant to the very suggestion.

The last instance I will cite in illustration of the innate psychodynamics of the patient not only reveals a part of the therapeutic process but also the nexus of his psychopathy. At one session the patient declared that what troubled him most was the question why he had failed. He felt that he should have succeeded, and the lack of success was, to his mind, the chief cause of his difficulties. When asked what he envisaged by success he responded by saying "earning a living." When encouraged to tell what he thought were the reasons for his failure he cited the following items: his Jewishness; the fact that he had no pull or familial prestige; the law school from which he graduated; and being "too much to himself." But then the patient went on to discount each of these reasons, citing others who were Jews, of no better families, and graduates of the same law school who had done well professionally, despite. He then continued by saying that all these reasons proving inadequate, he could not but conclude that his failure was due to "inimical forces."

It was thus that the patient laid bare the "anlage" of his paranoia. The patient also summed up his problem in a phrase which he repeated many times, "I passed all the tests, and yet failed." Passing the tests meant to him literally what the phrase implied: examinations, in school, in college, in law school, and before the bar. The patient had, however, left out of account the most important of all tests, that of the affect and libidinal relations to other human beings.

That score the patient thought he had settled long ago. He did not like the emotions and would have as little of them as he could manage.

Enough of the patient's history has been cited, I believe, to illustrate the thesis of this presentation, and we may now turn to consider more specifically the anatomy of his psychosis. I use the term anatomy in the meaning of "a critical examination of any subject or thing physical or metaphysical" (Funk & Wagnalls). In the vernacular it means the examination of "how he got that way."

The constitutional factors in this case are the first to arrest attention. The patient is asthenic and anhedonistic. I am, however, disinclined to grant the constitutional factor much weight. The patient is within the range of the normal according to all anatomical criteria, and he shows no endocrine deficiency. If he is rather boyish for his 34 years and slight in body, it is, I am persuaded, because he is retarded in his psychological functions. He lives on the level of a boy. Were he to attain the emotional stature of an adult he would "grow up" accordingly. The only constitutional factor I consider to be of significance is his uncommon intellectual competence. This did weigh the issue. But the anatomy of the psychosis can be considered apart from the constitutional factors. In essence the psychodynamics of his psychosis appear to be these. In his early preadolescent years the patient was frustrated and hurt in his affect experiences and contacts. Conditioned against them by experience, he avoided them. But this involved deprivations for which he needed to find compensations. These he found, negatively in rationalized disparagement of the affects, and positively in cultivating his intellectual and literary faculties. The ego strength which the normal individual derives from his libidinal development, the patient sought to gain and did derive from the "power of his intellect." He planned his life on a logical pattern, in which definite consequences were to be drawn from clearly formulated antecedents. This involved anticipating, preparing for, and passing tests. Since the patient does have an uncommonly good brain, he managed to follow his plan for a good many years without encountering serious difficulties. School life even at the college and professional level is still comparatively sheltered. When, however, the patient left school and entered the arena of every-day business life, his troubles began. The success he envisaged and considered his due was not forthcoming. He did not succeed in gaining a practice. The job he took was mediocre; the salary poor; advancement slow. He was deeply upset when a $5.00 raise he asked for was denied him. Then, too, came the episode of his brief and disappointing courtship. By these experiences he was obliged to conclude that he had failed, and being a logical person he sought to find reasons for his failure. He could find none in the pattern of his plans, nor in the way he carried them out. There remained but one way to account for his failure. He was the victim of inimical forces. The times were out of joint—the new boss, his co-workers, were against him. Once persuaded that he had failed, and that his failure was due to external, inimical forces, the patient was well on the road to his schizophrenic paranoic disintegration.

Three factors then are outstanding in this anatomy of the psychosis —first is the rejection of the affect experiences with atrophy of the affect faculties. This led to over-development of and over-investment in the intellectual faculties, which, when "life failed him," in turn led to the development of paranoic delusions.

This is the aetiological pattern of the patient's psychosis. It is moreover the common aetiological pattern of a variety of psychoneurotic conditions, including, as Oberndorf has so ably pointed out, depersonalization. The pathogenic sequence described above does not invariably end in a schizophrenic psychosis. It may give rise to a variety of conditions, some of them of a mild nature. Always, however, there is some degree of paranoid delusion. The individual has failed, more or less, and he is convinced that his failure is due to inimical forces. He may blame his wife, anti-semitism, anti-catholicism, capitalism, his immediate superiors, and an infinite number of other persons and conditions. His basic difficulty, however, lies in his affect functions.

Here we have a nosological complex that may be compared to untreated rickets. The disease begins in infancy: it is due chiefly to the lack of essential nutritional elements. The ricketic individual grows, but in a distorted pattern. The main anatomical effects are to be seen in the skeletal system, but the functional disorders associated with the condition are numerous. The disease is preventable in childhood. It is difficult to deal with it in the adult.

In summary, the main burden of my presentation has been to urge the value and importance of the study of the pathodynamics of the psychopathies. To achieve this, it is necessary to consider the psychopathy as a singular phenomenon manifest among a multitude of phenomena, thus giving us a clear and dynamic psychiatric nosography.

The dynamic pattern revealed constitutes a nosological complex in which deficiency in affect function leads in certain individuals to an over-development of and over-investment in the intellectual function which, when they fail to find an effective position in life, in turn gives rise to paranoic ideas, of differing intensity and complexity.

2

The Psychopathology of Paternal Deprivation

THE RISE AND DECLINE OF FATHERHOOD

MOTHERHOOD IS A PRIMORDIAL INSTITUTION, founded by nature. Fatherhood, in contrast, is of later origin and is essentially a product of socialization. In this affirmation I do not intend to suggest that some time in the past human beings were reproduced parthenogenetically. This is a something prognosticated for the future. In the past, as far back as dependable evidence reaches, it is quite certain that human reproduction was effected only by the sexual conjunction of male and female. However, and this is the point of my initial affirmation, when a birth resulted, the male partner of the sexual conjunction did not always in the past act as father to the child. He was, so to say, there at the beginning but not always at the end or thereafter. It is in this sense that even today we speak of fatherless children, meaning not only those orphaned.

Fatherhood, then, as affirmed, is of comparatively recent origin and is essentially a product of socialization. Paradoxically, it is argued in earnest that fatherhood not only is a product of socialization, but is itself the begetter of social existence, that is, of society and of social ethos.

Since both these postulations are deeply involved in, indeed are basic to, my thesis and exposition, I shall explore them in detail. Fortunately, the subject has been well studied by a number of pre-eminent scholars and I intend to cite them freely.

Johann Jacob Bachofen, in his classical work *Das Mutterrecht*, wrote,

> Woman comes first, but man becomes. Male and female do not appear simultaneously; they are not of the same order. . . . The female is primary, the male is only what comes out of her. . . . In the realm

16

of the physical . . . the masculine principle is of second rank, subordinate to the feminine. . . . The man appears as creature, not as creator; as effect, not cause. The reverse is true of the mother. She comes before the creature, appearing as cause, the prime giver of life, and not as an effect. She is not to be inferred from the creature, but is known in her own right. In a word, woman first exists as a mother, and the man first exists as a son (1).

It is thus that masculinity is initially manifest in the son, and from the son is the father much later inferred. This relationship is the basis of *gynocracy* which long anteceded both matriarchy and patriarchy. In gynocracy the lover of the mother, he of her choice, was the son, not the father, who in that realm was (no pun intended) inconceivable. "The young men," wrote Eric Neumann,

> whom the Mother selects for her lovers may impregnate her, they may even be fertility gods, but the fact remains that they are only phallic consorts of the Great Mother, drones serving the queen bee, who are killed off as soon as they have performed their duty of fecundation. . . . In the earliest fertility cults, the gory fragments of the sacrificed victim were handed round as precious gifts and offered up to the earth, in order to make her fruitful. These human sacrifices for fertility occur all the world over quite independently of one another, in the rites of America and in the Eastern Mediterranean, in Asia and in Northern Europe. Everywhere blood plays a leading part in fertility ritual and human sacrifice. The great terrestrial law that there can be no life without death was early understood, and still earlier represented in ritual, to mean that a strengthening of life can only be bought at the cost of sacrificial death. . . . We misunderstand these rites if we call them cruel. For the early cultures, and even for the victims themselves, this sequence of events was necessary and self-evident (2, 3).

The progression of woman from the *uroboric*—the term is cryptic and means self-begetting—state through the stages of gynocracy and matriarchy to patriarchy took an indeterminate but most certainly a very long time and was effected by the interplay of numerous and complex material and psychological forces. Here we can trace that progression only sketchily, and primarily as it bears on the emergence of fatherhood. Neumann summarizes this progression in terms of the depotentiation of the female, to be seen most clearly in the *status* of woman.

> At first, as the birth-giver, she had complete control over her child; there was no father to contend with, particularly while the connection between the sexual act and birth remained unrecognized. Later,

the father was a stranger, institutionally excluded from exercising authority over the children. [This is during matriarchy.] In the patriarchate, on the other hand, the father who begets the child is its master and woman is only the vessel, the birth-passage, the nurse (4).

The progression of the male from being nothing more than the bearer of a phallus to master of the *oecos* and *pater familias* is the counterpart adventure of the depotentiation of the female. It was effected, according to Neumann by the slow emergence of human consciousness, primarily a potentiate and endowment of the masculine psyche, though also shared but in a lesser measure by the female. The argument runs somewhat as follows: At a certain prehistoric stage in male-female relations, the young man growing conscious of himself repudiates the orgiastic, phallic sexual advances of the Great Mother and compels a new order of relationship. He transmutes the incidental and primal into a more enduring relation, that of the matriarchal family. Gynocracy thus yields to matriarchy. For the male this represents the coming to consciousness of the "higher" masculinity as opposed to the "lower" phallic variety, a progression which persists as a "recapitulation" in the normal ontogeny of "boy to man" (5).

The forces that helped effect this change in male to female relations derive from the banding together of males, first of the young in the "mother-cluster" family groups, and later of the exogamously mated adults living matrilocally, "strangers in the wife's tribe." This banding together in time leads to the creation of male secret and friendly societies.

The male group steadily gains in strength, and political, military and economic considerations. Within these groups the cultivation of friendship is more important than rivalry and more stress is laid on male similarity and on dissimilarity from the female, than on mutual jealousies (6).

A likely contributing dynamic in this development was the slow but consistent increase in human population resulting in closer proximation among males. The lonely and isolated male could do little to change his lot. Coming together with others, his strength and means were multiplied.

The ascendancy of the male did not involve the degradation of the female, but it did involve a radical change in the structure of the family group and in the operations of its members. The family developed a new commitment—it became the nidus of culture. Heretofore chthonic in nature, dedicated to the worship of Dionysus, it now added the counterbalancing devotion to Apollo.

"The matriarchal group with its mass emotionality between mother and children, its strong local ties and its greater inertia, is to a large extent bound to nature and instincts" (7). The masculine group as we have noted is necessarily mobile and enterprising, it is constantly exposed to danger, and hence is stimulated to develop consciousness and awareness. The male thus grows manly and manliness is characterized by physical and "moral" courage, the ability to stay awake, to endure hunger, fatigue and pain, and above all to be brave, that is, to defend the ego against childish fears and unconscious impulses. The criteria of manliness are institutionalized as prerequisites for initiation into men's society. They are further institutionalized and elaborated as human culture. "It is no accident," wrote Neumann,

> that all human culture, and not Western civilization alone, is masculine in character from Greece and the Judeo-Christian sphere of culture, to Islam and India. Woman, too, has a share in this culture, but it is mostly imperceptible and unconscious, though of pertinent significance in scope. The masculine trend is toward greater coordination of spirit, ego, consciousness, and will (8).

It is thus that the male collective became "the source of all the taboos, laws and institutions that are destined to break the dominance of the uroboros and Great Mother. Heaven, the father, and the spirit go hand in hand with masculinity and represent the victory of the patriarchate over the matriarchate" (9).

At this stage we witness the emergence of Fatherhood, not simply as phallic function, but in the "heavenly" sense. Initially credited to the Hero, the demigod among men, the father is conceived

> . . . as a spiritual figure not primarily connected with nature; he belongs to the primordial age, to the dawn of history, and steps out of it to bring culture and salvation to mankind.* He is timeless in the sense that he does not enter into time, but dwells in the background of time, in the primordial time that regulates our earthly chronology. Characteristic, too, is his relation to history and moralities; for as the tribal ancestor he is directly related to the medicine men and elders, the representative of authority, power, wisdom and esoteric knowledge (10).

"In pre-patriarchal conditions, the men and the elders stand for 'heaven' and they transmit the collective cultural heritage of their day and generation." "The fathers" are the representatives of law and order, from the earliest taboos to the most modern juridical systems. They hand down the

---

*As, in mythology, Prometheus did.

highest values of civilization, whereas the mothers control the highest, that is, deepest, values of life and nature. The world of the fathers is thus the world of collective values. It is historical and related to the fluctuating level of consciousness and cultural development within the group. The prevailing system of cultural values, i.e., the canon of values which gives a culture its peculiar physiognomy and its stability has its roots in the fathers, the grown men who represent and reinforce the religious, ethical, political and social structure of the collective.

> The fathers are the guardians of masculinity and the supervisors of all education. That is to say, their existence is not merely symbolical; as pillars of the institution that embody the cultural canon, they preside over the upbringing of each individual and certify his coming of age. It makes no difference how this cultural canon is constituted, whether its laws and taboos be those of a tribe of head hunters or of a Christian nation. Always the fathers see to it that the current values are impressed upon the young people and that only those who have identified themselves with those values are included among the adults. The advocacy of the canon of values inherited from the fathers and enforced by education manifests itself in the psychic structure of the individual as "conscience."
>
> This paternal authority, whose necessity for culture and the development of consciousness is beyond dispute, differs from the maternal authority in that it is essentially relative, being conditioned by its day and generation, and not having the absolute character of maternal authority (11).

This schema of the decline of matriarchy and the supervention of patriarchy, of the regression of the uroboric-primal and the emergence of the masculine-moral, is well epitomized in the two majestic Greek tragedies—the Bacchae of Euripides and the Oresteia of Aeschylus. The Oresteia is in effect a trilogy—Agamemnon, The Choephori and The Eumenides.

The Bacchae mirrors the orgiastic worship of Dionysius with its unbridled lust and sanguinous murders. The shepherd messenger reporting to Pentheus, King of Thebes, what he came upon at the mountain's peak, says in trepidation:

> "I have seen the wild white women there, Oh, King,
> Whose fleet limbs darted arrow-like but now
> From Thebe away, and come to tell thee how
> They work strange deeds and passing marvel."
>
> . . . . . .
>
> "A marvel of swift ranks I saw there rise
> Dames young and old, and gentle maids unwed" (12).

Among the celebrants was Agave, mother of King Pentheus. The shepherd attempted unsuccessfully to seize her. But this only heightened her frenzy and she and the other women turned upon the shepherds, who fearing for their lives, fled, leaving their herds behind them.

> "They," the shepherd told, "swept towards our herds
>   that browse the green
> Hill grass. Great uddered kine then hadst thou seen
> Bellowing in sword-like hands that cleave and tear,
> A live steer riven asunder, and the air
> Tossed with rent ribs or limbs of cloven tread
> And flesh upon the branches, and a red
> Rain from the deep green pines. Yea, bulls of pride
> Horns swift to rage, were fronted and aside
> Flung stumbling, by those multitudinous hands
> Dragged pitilessly. And swifter were the hands
> Of garbed flesh and bone unbound withal
> Than on thy royal eyes the lids may fall." (13)

King Pentheus is deeply stirred by this report:

> "It bursts hard by us," is his comment, "like a smothered fire,
> This frenzy of Bacchic woman! All my land
> Is made their mock. This needs an iron hand!" (14)

King Pentheus, dressed as a woman, goes to spy upon the Bacchae. There Dionysius betrays him. Pentheus is discovered, set upon and torn apart, his own mother leading the frenzied herd. Though Pentheus pleads with her,

> "Have mercy, Mother! Let it not befall
> Through sin of mine, that thou shouldst slay thy son!"
> But she, with lips-a-foam and eyes that run
> Like leaping fire, with thoughts that ne're should be
> On earth, possessed by Bacchios utterly,
> Stays not nor hears. Round his left arm she put
> Both hands, set hard against his side her foot,
> Drew . . . and the shoulder severed! (15)

>   . . . .

> With groans that faded into sobbing breath,
> Dim shrieks, and joy, and triumph-cries of death.
> And here was borne a severed arm, and there
> A hunter's booted foot; white bones lay bare
> With rending; and swift hands insanguined
> Tossed as in sport the flesh of Pentheus dead" (16).

This ghoulish play reaches its crescendo when the mother, Agave, presents the severed, impaled head of her son, King Pentheus, to her own father, the old King Cadmus, as a "trophy of the hunt."

The Bacchae was the last play Euripides wrote before his death (407-406 B.C.). It is believed that while in Macedonia he had himself witnessed the wild and orgiastic worship of Dionysius with its attendant frenzies and ritual mysticism. This play reflects Euripides' deep concern over the moral and religious deterioration suffered by the Athenians during the later stages of the Peloponnesian War.

Euripides' concern with the primal forces that animated the uroboric mother is reflected in another of his plays. *Medea,* wherein the wild-eyed savage murders her children to injure her treacherous husband (Jason). In her is expressed the elemental nature of woman untrammeled by Greek convention (17).

The Oresteia of Aeschylus, and most notably the last in this trilogy of plays—The Eumenides—stands forth as the polar opposite to The Bacchae. The myth-plot of the Oresteia is too well known to call for an ample resume. Because Agamemnon sacrificed his daughter, Iphegenia, to appease the wrath of Artemis and thus release the Greek fleet to sail against Troy, Clytemnestra, the wife of Agamemnon, together with her lover, Aegisthus, murder Agamemnon upon his return from the war in Troy. Subsequently Orestes, the son of Agamemnon and Clytemnestra, distressed by his mother's bloody deed and goaded on by his sister Electra, avenges the murder of his father by killing both his mother and her lover. For this crime he is hounded by the Furies and formally prosecuted before a jury of twelve Athenian citizens.

During the trial, the God Apollo comes to Orestes' aid and argues his case. Orestes admits he murdered his mother and pleads that he did so "by oracles of him who here attests me" intending by this Apollo, and also because "in her combined two stains of sin—slaying her husband she did slay my sire." Against this plea the prosecution argues that Agamemnon was not kin of blood to his wife, whereas Orestes was. "She was not kin by blood to him she slew," says the leader of the twelve Athenian citizens, to which Orestes responds with the questioning plea, "And I, am I by blood my mother's kin?" The leader answers in scorn.

> "O cursed with murder's guilt, how else wert thou
> The burden of her womb? Dost thou forswear
> Thy mother's kinship closest bond of love?" (18)

Orestes, finding this beyond his ken, turns then to Apollo, saying,

> "It is thine hour, Apollo—speak the law."

And Apollo did speak the law, but it was the *new* law, that of patriarchy (19).

> He said, "Mark a soothfast word,
> Not the true parent is the woman's womb
> That bears the child; she doth but nurse the seed
> New-sown; the male is parent; she for him,
> As stranger for a stranger, hoards the germ
> Of life, unless the god its promise blight."

Athena, presiding over the trial, turned for the judgement to the jury, yet not without a singular prejudice, for she avows

> "Mine is the right to add the final vote
> And I award it to Orestes' cause."
>
> . . . .
>
> "I vouch myself the champion of the man,
> Not of the woman, yea, with all my soul—
> In heart, as birth, a father's child alone. . . .
>   And if the votes
> Equal do fall, Orestes shall prevail. . . . (20)

The vote *was* equal and Athena cast the decisive vote. Orestes was freed from guilt of blood.

Yet the Furies, those

> . . . beldames old
> Unto whose grim and wizened maidenhood
> Nor god nor man nor beast can e're draw near

were not content.

They cursed and lamented. They threatened the gods—

> "Woe on you, younger gods! The ancient right
> Ye have o'erriden, rent it from my hands" (21).

And for themselves they wept—

> "Alack, alack, forlorn
> Are we, a bitter injury have borne!
> Alack, O sisters, O dishonored brood
> Of Mother night!" (22)

In the end Athena appeases them by promising them "a holy sanctuary—deep in the heart of this my land" (23). Thus reconciled, the Furies —now Eumenides—that is, gracious goddesses, return to their home below —Night's childless children—to darkness' deep primeval lair, far in Earth's bosom (24).

Even as The Bacchae was the last of the plays composed by Euripides, so too, is the Oresteia trilogy the last work which Aeschylus composed. It gained him first prize in the tragic contest held in 458 B.C. He died while in Sicily in 455 B.C.

At this point we must descend from the lofty realm of the immortal Greek poets to pursue further the more prosaic argument of our presentation.

Precisely when in the long span of time matriarchy yielded to patriarchy and patriarchy became the predominant pattern of the family is undetermined. In effect the question is largely unrealistic. It cannot be answered. For as David Bidney correctly states, "We can never be certain of the actual course of events in prehistoric times, and it is futile, therefore, to engage in a search for 'origins' and 'historic causes' since no decisive evidence is available" (25). But we can witness the stark affirmation of patriarchy in the Judeo-biblical story of the creation of woman. Here woman is not the prior creature but is derivative. "The rib which He had taken from man, Jehovah fashioned into a woman and brought her to man" (26). The creation of Eve appears to be essential to the plot. Without her man would not have been tempted and would not have lost his Garden of Eden.

The temptation and the fall of man has its counterpart in the Greek myth of Epimetheus and Pandora. Here, too, man in the person of Prometheus had offended the gods by stealing fire. In punishment the gods contrived Pandora and placed her among men. She tempted Epimetheus, the brother of Prometheus, and as the phrase runs, he fell for her. He opened the casket she brought as a bridal gift (a picturesque and suggestive Freudian fancy) and as a result, in the words of Hesiod, "Countless plagues (now) wander amongst men: for earth is full of evils and the sea is full," but "Ere this the tribes of men lived on earth remote and free from toil and heavy sickness" (27).

In the Old Testament story, Adam and Eve having violated Jehovah's instructions are driven out of the Garden of Eden. A curse is placed on Adam.

> "By the sweat of thy brow shalt thou eat bread
> Cursed shall be the ground because of thee.
> By painful toil shalt thou eat from it all the days of thy life" (28).

To the woman, Jehovah said,

"I will make thy pain great in thy pregnancy
With pain shalt thou bring forth children,
Yet toward thy husband shall be thy desire,
And he shall rule over thee" (29).

In both the Greek myth and the Hebrew story woman is a later creation and the cause of man's loss of ease on earth—loss of the Golden Age
when men lived like gods without sorrow of heart, remote and free from
toil and grief, when the fruitful earth *unforced* bare them fruit abun-
dantly and without stint (30).

There is in both these versions of the creation of woman and the fall of
man, of the loss of a mythical life of ease and abundance, and the consequent "curse" of toil and strife placed on man, the strong suggestion
that in essence they tell the tale of the change in man's pattern of living
from that of the nomadic food gatherer and hunter to that of the relatively settled farmer and animal breeder.

It is this which most likely propitiated the shift from matriarchy to
patriarchy. For with the development of agriculture and animal husbandry the human family acquired the character of a social and economic
organism. Heretofore it was essentially biologic in nature. It was not
love, at least not in the sense we understand it, but necessity and the
benefits of mutual services that founded the patristic-economic family.
It served also as the vis-a-tergo of masculine culture.

It is of interest that the Hesiodic poems fall into two categories—those
devoted to farming and husbandry (*Works and Days*) and those that deal
with the origins of the gods (*Theogeny*). *Works and Days* is devoted to
"the life of the farmer, his toil and routines, his slaves, and hired hands,
and oxen" (31). The treatment however, is not entirely descriptive; it is
not merely a handbook on farming. It is also and more distinctively
exhortative and morally demanding. It extols work, work with thought
and in season. "Both gods and men," Hesiod writes, "are angry with a
man who lives idle, for in nature he is like the stingless drones who waste
the labour of the bees, eating without working; but let it be your care to
order your work properly, that in the right season your barns may be full
of victual" (32). Three factors are here united—man, work and order.
Work and order are the anlage of masculine culture.

All living creatures "labor" for their sustenance. In the deeper sense
of the term work, with its innate and unique sense of artful, that is, intended productivity, it can be said that mankind alone works. Both men

and women labored when their nourishment was obtained by gathering and hunting. But as soon as man turned to the hunting of large animals, he became a worker and not merely a laborer, and this was true also of the woman as soon as she began to cultivate a garden. To hunt large animals men must plan the hunt and coordinate their efforts under the ablest among them. Washburn and DeVore observe in *Social Life of Early Man* that

> The male's role as an economic provider had certainly appeared by the Middle Pleistocene (125,000 to 15,000) when men were killing large animals. Hunting large animals was probably based on cooperation, and the band must have shared in the eating. . . . Hunting large animals made children and females economically dependent (33).

"In the evolution of society, the most important rules are those that guarantee economic survival to the dependent young." The emphasis rests on "the evolution of *society*" and on *"economic* survival."

> Human females and their young are efficient gatherers, so the crucial customs are those that guarantee the services of a hunter to a woman and her children. That the resulting family bonds are much more than sexual is shown by the fact that custom in contemporary hunter-gather groups provides that new families may be formed only around males who have proved themselves as economic providers. The maturing human male is dependent upon the adult males not only for food but for years of instruction in the techniques of hunting (34).

The years of instruction to which the young had to submit increased in number and the body of required learning was extended immensely when male farming supplemented in an overshadowing measure food gathering and women's gardening and when the domestication of animals leading to animal husbandry reduced man's dependence on hunting for the main source of his meats.

Agriculture and animal husbandry jointly served as the basic foundation of civilization. Man settled down, first in villages and then also in cities. Now man's genius could operate under favorable conditions to invent the plow, the loom, the wheel and metal working. It is with the introduction of the plow that agriculture became an important male industry. Handling the plow required more strength than the average woman could muster, and particularly so when oxen were used to draw the plow.

The basic inventions of plow, loom, wheel and metalworking lifted man economically above the level of subsistence living, facilitated and encouraged division of labor, specialization, barter and exchange. Commerce necessitated the keeping of accounts and records. Counting, measuring, writing, and ultimately the alphabet—signs that stood for single sounds—were developed. Man began in earnest to order his encounters with experience. Science, religion and law were the products of his efforts. And all the evidence available, prehistoric as well as historic, credits the major attainments in civilization and culture—technology, science, religion, law, literature, music esthetics and philosophy—to the efforts of males.

In his thoughtful and stimulating book *The Human Animal*, Weston LaBarre observes, "Primitive men know rightly that women can make children with their bodies. But it takes men to make men, that is, members of the tribe," the human tribe!

> Moral bonds and cultural structures—styles of thinking—are an area of men's present and future evolution that are not yet and probably never will be made bodily organs and somatized. It may be true that some of the arts—probably pottery, gardening, and weaving—are the inventions of women. But principle or generalization is a male artifact: the *logos*, that is, the endless preocupation of male metaphysics. What connects father and son, male and male, is the mystery of *logos* and logos alone: logos as the literal "word" which conveys linguistic meaning and understanding; logos as laws, agreements, rules, and regularities of behavior; logos as the implicit means and substance of common understanding and communication, and of cultural joining in the same styles of thinking; and logos as shared pattern, within which father can identify with son and permit his infancy, within which son can identify with father and become a man, and within which a male can perceive and forgive the equal manhood of his fellow-man. This does not mean, of course, that women are biologically unable to become great philosophers, creators of literature, or indeed scientists all of whom are concerned with generalization but it does mean, as is historically manifest, that men are more characteristically and inescapably motivated to formulate principles and generalizations. For, biologically, woman are closer to realistic particulars (35).

But whatever the biologic differentiations of men and women are, or may be, it is historically certain that civilization as we have experienced and known it had its origin in and emerged with the patriarchal family, wherein fatherhood acquired a power status and a dominant role.

The patriarchal family successfully met the requirements of evolving society. It formulated and enforced the rules which assured economic survival to the dependent young. The accent here is on economic and not merely physical survival. Economic survival implies training in skills, in discipline and in ever expanding social interrelations. These constitute the core elements of our historic ethos. The patriarchal family prospered and with it mankind, so that with time, homo sapiens, once a rare mammalian, has become relatively numerous—and indeed threatens to overrun the earth. It would be a fatuous redundancy to catalog the great accomplishments of historic civilization; they are common knowledge. But it may not be amiss to note that poetry and literature, law and religion, philosophy and science, the arts, and be it noted in particular, romantic love, are male products emergent from and subservient to the patriarchal family—wherein fatherhood reached its apogee.

We have been long in tracing the rise of fatherhood; the event itself was long in time. And now we need to turn to the decline of fatherhood. This portion of our review is briefer.

Even as the rise of the patriarchal family is to be attributed to the operations of economic-technological determinants, so too can its decline be accounted for. The development of machine technology breached and disrupted the economic integrity of the historical family. It removed the man from field, workshop and home, and harnessed him to the factory machine. It took over the vital domestic operations of the woman so that she no longer spun, wove, sewed, baked, preserved, nor otherwise served man and child in the multitude of ways that made her so precious and essential to their life and well-being. It disorganized the intrafamilial relations and dependencies of husband and wife, parents and children. Fatherhood was depotentiated severely.

The socially disruptive effects of machine technology as concretized in the Industrial Revolution have been described by numerous writers. One of the best among them, Karl Polanyi, wrote in his *Origins of Our Time* (36): "At the heart of the Industrial Revolution of the 18th century there was an almost miraculous improvement in the tools of production, which was accompanied by a catastrophic dislocation of the lives of the common people" (37). "The fabric of society was being disrupted; desolate villages and the ruins of human dwellings testified to the fierceness with which the revolution raged, endangering the defenses of the country, wasting its towns, decimating its population, turning its overburdened soil into dust, harassing its people and turning them from decent husbandmen into a mob of beggars and thieves" (38). This was a society that "had indeed forgotten the shape of man" (39).

Very much of the disruptive effects of machine technology and of the Industrial Revolution is charged to the landed gentry and to the industrial entrepreneurs. "The lords and nobles," Polanyi wrote, "were upsetting the social order, breaking down the ancient law and custom, sometimes by means of violence, often by pressure and intimidation" (40). The blame is properly placed but it only can be a partial blame, for the disruptive effects were inherent in the technological revolution in which *rentier* and *entrepreneur* were major *dramatis personae*. They intensified but did not engender the disruptive effects of the revolution. The more recent experiences of Sweden and of communist Russia, two widely divergent states, confirm this.

Polanyi does not attribute the calamitous effects of the Industrial Revolution only or chiefly to the exploitation of the masses. "The masses it is true were being sweated and starved by the callous exploiters of their helplessness" (41). But, Polanyi astutely observes,

> Actually . . . a social calamity is primarily a cultural, not an economic phenomenon. . . . Not economic exploitation, as often assumed, but the disintegration of the cultural environment of the victim is the cause of the degradation. The economic process may, naturally, supply the vehicle of the destruction . . . but the immediate cause of his undoing is not for that reason economic; it lies in the lethal injury to the institutions in which his social existence is embodied (42).

How sound and correct this affirmation is can be seen in the fact that though living conditions for most individuals in the economically developed countries have improved immensely, the deterioration of the patristic family and of the cultural environment has continued unabated. For in effect the deteriorative process is irreversible. The patriarchal family functionally suited and served a given economic-technological period, one of long duration which, however, in the Western world, is now approaching its end.

There is a tragic consequent to this *fin de l'ancien régime,* for we as yet have nothing to take its place. The disintegration of the patristic family has involved as consequent and concomitant a weakening of the institutions which buttressed its ethos. Religion and law, morals and discipline, are openly flaunted and aggressively challenged. The humble virtues, bearing in mind that the root term of virtue is *vir,* meaning man, those of work, order, discipline, the fulfillment of pledge and promise, of judicious husbandry, neither niggardly and mean nor profligate and wasteful, these have become trivial in the mood of our times.

We are, in short, in a state of social and cultural crisis, an *historical crisis!* "An historical crisis," Ortega wrote in his *Man and Crisis,*

is a world change which differs from the normal change as follows:
The normal change is that the profile of the world which is valid for
one generation is succeeded by another and slightly different profile
Yesterday's system of convictions gives way to today's smoothly, without a break. This assumes that the skeleton framework of the world
remains in force throughout that change, whereas only slightly modified. An historical crisis occurs when the world change which is
produced consists in this: The world, the system of convictions belonging to a previous generation, gives way to a vital state in which
man remains without these convictions, and therefore without a
world. Man returns to a state of not knowing what to do, for the
reason that he returns to a state of actually not knowing what to
think about the world. Therefore, the change swells to a crisis and
takes on the character of a catastrophe. The world change consists of
the fact that the world in which man was living has collapsed and,
for the moment of that alone. It is a change which begins by being
negative and critical. One does not know what new thing to think;
one only knows, or thinks he knows, that the traditional norms and
ideas are false and inadmissible. One feels a profound disdain for
everything, or almost everything, which was believed yesterday; but
the truth is that there are no new positive beliefs with which to replace the traditional ones. Since that system of convictions, that
world, was the map which permitted man to move within his environment with a certain security, and since he now lacks such a map, be
again feels himself lost, at loose ends, without orientation. He moves
from here to there without order or arrangement; he tries this side
and then the other, but without complete conviction, he pretends to
himself that he is convinced of this or that (43).

Crisis man is left "without a world, handed over to the chaos of pure
circumstances in a lamentable state of disorientation" (44).

This is the picture seen in global dimensions and it has its image equivalent in the microcosm, the family, now also in a condition of historical
crisis. The depotentiation of the father has breached and disrupted the
means and processes of ethos transmission. Communication between the
generations has broken down so that even if valid and acceptable information were available, it could not under the prevailing conditions be passed
on. The little black box isn't working now!

It is this, more than the failure of traditional ethos to retain pertinence in our rapidly changing world, that is at the core of the present
day historical crisis. The traditional ethos during its long development
had undergone numerous and radical changes. In none of them, however, was the institution of fatherhood involved or challenged. The
individual father might be rejected or discredited, but not the office

and the role of Father. Indeed, in the past the rebel himself was more than likely to justify his rebellion by claiming that the father was *not a good* father and that he aspired to be a better one.

What happens when the process of ethos transmission breaks down? It has at times in the past broken down, regionally and for comparatively brief periods, because of wars, revolutions, or because of so-called natural disasters. What we observe in such circumstances is that the affected group tends to become lawless. Once more to quote Ortega,

> During periods of crisis, positions which are false or feigned are very common. Entire generations falsify themselves to themselves; that is to say, they wrap themselves up in artistic styles, in doctrines, in political movements which are insincere and which fill the lack of genuine convictions (45). On feeling himself lost, man may respond with skeptical frigidity, with anguish, or with desperations; and he will do many things, which though apparently heroic, do not in fact proceed from any real heroism, but are deeds done in desperation. Or he will have a sense of fury, of madness, an appetite for vengeance, because of the emptiness of his life; these will drive him to enjoy brutality, cynically, whatever comes his way—flesh, luxury, power. Life takes on a bitter flavor (46).

This is a fair and fitting description of the mood that affects an appreciable portion of the people in the Western world—one that will engulf the rest before very long.

People become lawless. That, of course, is not the same as becoming criminal, though some of the lawlessness is likely to fringe on the criminal. It is the young who are most likely to prove the most lawless. After all, they are on the *receiving* end of the communication exchange and currently little or nothing comes over to them, save only perhaps what is to them incomprehensible noise. It is of interest that for the lawless young we have a particular term—delinquency—the core meaning of which is not willfulness but failure, neglect, possibly due to ignorance or to lack of conviction.

It was, I believe, Sheldon Glueck in his pioneering work titled "Unraveling Juvenile Delinquency" who first clearly emphasized the negative influence of the weak or absent father (add to this the domineering, castrating mother) in the engenderment of the delinquent child. But in effect the delinquent is not created—he is engendered. The absent father does not "create" the delinquent, he merely fails (most commonly now he is disenabled) effectively to indoctrinate his children. The result is a protean psychopathology—that of paternal deprivation.

PATERNAL DEPRIVATION

The pathogenicity of maternal deprivation and its effects in terms of developmental retardation and distortions are well known. Since the pioneering work of Spitz and Bowlby, many have investigated the nature of the "the mother-to-infant and child relation" and have described the many ways in which this relation can be disturbed and the numerous and varying untoward consequences of these disturbances.

Incidentally, it is of interest that in these studies attention has been centered on the infant and the child. Seemingly the pathodynamic process has been studied as if it were unilinear and unidirectional. What happens to the child deprived of its mother was the initial and primary concern. What happens to the *mother deprived of the child* has not been explored and investigated. The reasons for this are fairly obvious. The pathologies manifest in the "mother-deprived" child are initial and startlingly evident, hence easy to perceive and to study. Those of the mother are recondite and linked with numerous antecedent experiences and reactions. The child is the passive unit in the mother-child duo, the mother the active and decisive one.

Maternal deprivation may, of course, be the resultant of overriding circumstances and forces, including death, sickness, poverty, other misfortunes, and also, we need add, of bizarre socio-economic theories and philosophies which advocate the herding of children in creches and asylums and of their mother in "fields, shops and factories."

This notation on the one-sidedness of the studies in maternal deprivation is not intended as a carping criticism, but rather to underscore the need to take in earnest the common affirmation that mother and child form a symbiotic combine. In this combine, what happens to the one affects and is reflected in the other. In this purview, maternal deprivation is to be viewed as an interaction, pathogenic, at its minimum in the relation of two. But mother and child form not only a symbiotic combine but also an ecological twain. They provide for each other some of the elements of a setting favoring their respective growth and development. I say "some of the elements," for in effect among human beings mother and child do not form a complete unit and do not normally exist apart. They are usually segments of a family which includes a father, set in a social matrix. The immediate ecological setting of the family is a product of *the* family, while the successive ecological perimeters are determined by the existent basic societal factors and conditions.

As previously noted, the effects of maternal deprivation have been amply recognized and understood, while those of paternal deprivation have as yet been but little appreciated. In a pointed formulation it can be said that the problems relating to paternal deprivation involve both cultural anthropology and psychiatry. Maternal deprivation, in its more grievous forms, is reflected in developmental retardations in the somatic, perceptual and affective spheres. Paternal deprivation is witnessed in the pathologic categories of "primalism," asocial behavior, social disorientation and amorality. The effects, that is, the pathologies, of paternal deprivation differ in degree and kind, in males and females.

All this, I am sure, has a familiar ring. It is reminiscent of Freud's superego and of the role of the Father in its engenderment. "The superego," wrote Freud, "arises as we know from an identification with the father regarded as a model." Freud was rather expansive in tracing the derivation of the superego. He credited it not only to the Father but to both parents. "The parents' influence," he wrote in his *Outline of Psychoanalysis* (Chapter 1), "naturally includes not merely the personalities of the parents themselves but also the racial, national, and family traditions handed on through them, as well as the demands of the immediate social milieu which they represent." Freud further compounds his scheme by postulating the superego as "the heir to the Oedipus complex and that the superego only arises after that complex has been disposed of" (47). The superego then, according to Freud, is derived from many sources, from parents, the milieu, race, nation, tradition, etc. It embraces customs, habits, manners, beliefs, tastes and other characterological elements, as well as conscience, ethics and moral imperatives. Freud also derives the dynamic potentials of the superego from the transmitted and/or resolved Oedipus complex. This superego is the introjected, respected and feared Father.

Diffuse and questionable as this Freudian schema on the derivation of the superego may be, it still contains some precious elements, the most valuable among them the implicit affirmation of the existence of a superego and of its inhibiting and guiding governance of the primal drives—those of the id.

The dynamic relation of the superego to the Oedipal complex is a moot issue, and as initially formulated by Freud, is naive. The "dreaded father" is Freud's universalization of a unique experience, and the "castration fear" is a something not too often encountered in contemporary society. Nowadays mothers are less frightened by the enticing sexuality of their sons, and fathers bask in the affection of their daughters. This is not to reject or to deny the authenticity of the

Oedipal complex, but rather to reduce it to its realistic dimensions. The unresolved Oedipal complex is a frequently encountered pathodynamic state. Associated with it are retardation in maturation, an inadequate ego and not infrequently a cruel, exacting and perverted superego. But for all that, the superego does not "only arise after the Oedipal complex has been disposed of" (Freud). It has its origins long before that in the early and initial awarenesses of the child of the presence of the father and of the father's unique position and behavior in the family constellation, most notably in his relations to the mother. In a normal family, the developing child experiences the mother as a source of nourishment, of warmth, of comfort and affection, and the father as one who makes things happen, who is strong, motoric and directive. The superego begins, to phrase it in the vernacular of ethology, with and as an early imprinting experience. It is for this reason that the early, consistent and effective presence of the father within the family complex, of his effective male relation to the mother and of his function as arbiter in issues of ethics, morals and social mores are of such vital importance to the healthy psychologic growth and maturation of the child. Paternal deprivation is in these respects a grievous experience and the source of a many-form pathology.

Here I must make clear what is all too commonly misunderstood, namely, that the development of a superego is the distinctive attainment of "an apparatus" and is quite independent of the particular commitments by which its existence and operations become manifest. The superego's commitments can and do change with time and with experience. Indeed, the commitments of adult understanding may be the very opposite to those held in youth. *The superego apparatus is made manifest in the individual's capacity to be committed, irrespective of what the particular nature and quality of the commitments may be.** The significant role of the father is to foster the development in the child of a superego apparatus. If the commitments of the father's own superego, which the child is so very likely to introject, are sound, reasonable, socially desirable, and effective, so much the better. But ethical and moral commitments, as was said, may be cancelled out and changed. The superego apparatus, however, if not adequately developed during the early years of the individual, may never be attained in later life. Paternal deprivation, quite like maternal deprivation, is more disrup-

---

*This is not to be confused with Heinz Hartmann's ego apparatus. The latter refers to "such apparatus which sooner or later come to be specifically used by the ego (e.g., the motor apparatus in action)" (48).

tive in the early years of the individual. The consequences may prove uncompensable and unremediable.*

Clearly then, it is better for the child to have an exacting, demanding and firm-to-the-point-of-cruelty father, than to have none at all. It is agreed that the reasonable, exemplary father is by far the best.

It was stated before that the superego begins in an imprinting experience. Substantively, or experientially, this means that in the normal family the child perceives, as soon as he is capable of perceiving it, the presence of a distinctive personage, different from all others about him in tone, posture, mien and most notably in his relations and behavior to the mother. Now imprinting, as has been shown in numerous animal experiments and human studies, in order to serve effectively in the normal development of the organism, must be experienced at the time specifically "programmed" in the organism's innate developmental pattern. The term "imprinting," deriving from the vernacular of the ethologists, was unknown to Freud, yet he had a deep appreciation of the determinate significance of "early experience."

During the last decades a great deal of work has been done on "imprinting" at the so-called critical periods, and it has been clearly demonstrated that "experiences at the critical periods determine," to quote J. P. Scott, "the direction of social, intellectual and emotional develop-

---

* Konrad Lorenz has written pertinently on this subject. Though what is quoted refers specifically to the postpuberty period, it has also a direct bearing upon the earlier period in the individual's life.

"During and shortly after puberty human beings have an indubitable tendency to loosen their allegiance to all traditional rites and social norms of their culture, allowing conceptual thought to cast doubt on their value and to look around for new and perhaps more worthy ideals. *There probably is, at that time of life, a definite sensitive period for a new object-fixation, much as in the case of the object-fixation found in animals and called imprinting.* If, at that crucial time of life, old ideals prove fallacious under critical scrutiny and new ones fail to appear, the result is that complete aimlessness, the utter boredom which characterizes the young delinquent.

"Apparently this process of object-fixation can take its full effect only once in an individual's life. Once the valuation of certain social norms or the allegiance to a certain cause is fully established, it cannot be erased again, at least not to the extent of making room for a new, equally strong one. Also it would seem that once the sensitive period has elapsed, a man's ability to embrace ideals at all is considerably reduced.

"By a process of true Pavlovian conditioning plus a certain amount of irreversible imprinting these rather abstract values have in every human culture been substituted for the primal, concrete object of the communal defense reaction.

"Whether enthusiasm is made to serve these endeavors, or whether Man's most powerfully motivating instinct makes him go to war in some abjectly silly cause, depends almost entirely on the conditioning and/or imprinting he has undergone during certain susceptible periods of his life" (49).

ment" (50). Scott, in an excellent summary-review of the work done in this field, refers to three major kinds of critical-period phenomena that have been discovered. These involved "optimal periods for learning, for infantile stimulation, and for the formulation of basic relationships" (51). The age range of the critical period for the imprinting of "the paternal figure," postulated as the anlage of the child's superego, has not been established. Conjecture based on relevant data gained in other studies would set it from infancy "up to the time when children begin to use and understand language" (52).

Ives Hendrick, skirting the issues of the early genesis of the superego (he credits the well-organized superego to the resolution of the Oedipus complex without tracing the superego back to where and when it was as yet *not* well organized) has nevertheless contributed tellingly to this field of study in a series of papers on the identification of early develop-ment of the ego in infancy. Hendrick defines identification in a fashion congenial to our thought. "Identification," he states, "is a psychological process which originates in the wish to be like another individual in some way, and eventuates in the assimilation of these attributes of the other into stable and quite permanent elements of the total personality." Further, he affirms, "those identifications which contribute to the basic structure of the ego occur very early in life," that is, before the resolu-tion of the Oedipus complex. "They, therefore, are established at a stage of development when the foundations of the personality are not yet stabilized and when the relationship of the infant to others is relatively primitive . . ." (53). What Hendrick posits for the early development of the ego, holds true and valid for the superego, for in essence the budding ego includes the *anlage,* the bud, of the superego, and it derives from the impingement of the father person on the infant.

To summarize in brief: It is argued that the anlage of the superego is an imprinting experience to which the infant is, under normal con-ditions, exposed during the appropriate critical period, i.e., in infancy. The essential imprinting agent is the father. The imprinted effect is the infant's identification with the father, thus laying the basis for the later introjection of certain, mainly ethic, attributes of the father. The car-dinal requisite for the effective realization of the sketched development is the presence of the father, and of his authentic participation in the conjoint activities of the family. Here the term "father" is intended in its pristine sense. Another adult male cannot be fully "equated to father" even when he is in effect serving in "locum patris." The difference may at best be imperceptible; it nevertheless exists, and renders the relation less than ideal. I will not at this point argue the pragmatic considerations that impinge upon the above rather categoric statement, but instead deal with one other core consideration, bearing on the "presence of the father" in the development of an adequate superego.

In traditional Freudian theory, the superego is regarded as the moral antagonist of the id and the strict overseer of the ego. In *Moses and Monotheism*, Freud wrote, "In the course of the individual development, a part of the inhibiting forces in the outer world becomes internalized; a standard is created in the ego which opposes the other faculties by observation, criticism, and prohibition. We call this new standard the superego." Also, "The superego is the successor and representative of the parents (and educators) who superintend the actions of the individual in his first years of life; it perpetuates their functions almost without change" (54). And again, "the superego may bring fresh needs to the fore, but its chief function remains the limitation of satisfactions" (55). The superego is represented as primarily hostile to the id.

Bearing in mind that Freud conceived the superego as the father substitute, it follows then that he likewise conceived the father as an exacting, cruel and prohibiting personage, if not in effect and in reality, at least in the eyes of the child enmeshed in the classical Oedipus complex with its frightening threat of castration.

There is no question of the father's role as a socializing agent, transmitting and imposing upon the child a multiform discipline, the process involving supervision, prohibition and at times punishment. But father also shows affection, encourages, supports, evokes and applauds. This, too, the child "identifies with and introjects." The initial impact may have been a prohibition, but with *the prohibition observed* there came the reward of approval. The child ultimately introjects both the prohibition and the reward of observance. In this combination we find the fountain sources of ego strength and of adequate body image which enable the maturing individual to tolerate and to withstand adversity, frustration and uncertainty. Furthermore, "socialization" is not all a matter of inhibiting and sublimating the id impulses and drives. Socialization embraces ideal, aspiratory elements, and these are fostered not by prohibition but by evocation. The father may in his own being embody "ideals" (in contrast to expected patterns of conduct) which the son can adopt, or the father may project "ideal hopes" for the child which the child accepts. The risk that such projected "hopes" may have a neurotic origin (Freud in effect thought civilization itself was "neurotic") and that they may be unrealistic for the child does not, of course, imply more than that the socializing process may "go wrong," as indeed it frequently does with some individuals. The basic fact is that the superego derives not alone from the introjected prohibition but also from the accompanying rewards and gratifications gained in the observance of the prohibition. There is a faint suggestion of the aforegoing formulation in Freud's concept of sublimation, but sublimation as defined by Freud is a process for the evasion of punishment, of "deflection from the sexual," rather than a source of satisfaction and ego strength.

The appreciation of the superego as a source of ego strength is important, for the individual who has suffered paternal deprivation is generally poor in ego strength and impoverished in ego capital. He is also likely to lack "direction," to be diffuse, uncertain and unstable both in his immediate and in his long-term goals. The paternal-deprived individual thus not only is lacking in his superego (is in effect more or less an affect idiot) but has meager resources for healthy ego satisfactions and reinforcement. In the main, his ego satisfactions derive from the pursuit and gratification of his id drives, and for these reasons he is not uncommonly categorized as an instinct-ridden character.

Writing on the instinct-driven characters, Fenichel observes that their history commonly shows "a frequent change of milieu, a loveless environment, or a very inconsistent environmental influence; the Oedipus Complex and its solution are correspondingly disorganized, weak and inconsistent; some patients simply have never learned to develop object relationships" (56). The role of the father in engendering or contributing to this untoward "anamnestic history" is not explicitly defined by Fenichel, but that it is ponderable and significant is clearly implicit.

By this time it must be clear that the pathologies deriving from paternal deprivation are most prominently witnessed in the realm of the superego. This is a terminal paraphrase of the initial formulation to the effect that the effective presence and operation of the father-person in the family constellation is an essential prerequisite for the child's development of adequate superego apparatus, thus enabling him to be committed to things, persons, principles and values; in other words, to be committed to a definitive ethos.

Here one comes upon the interesting and challenging question: Does not paternal deprivation likewise and similarly affect the development of the ego? The generalized answer must be "Yes," but it needs to be further particularized. Thus, the id we know is given. The ego is materialized in the individual's contacts with *immediate reality*. The superego is in last analysis a product of culture. It is the product of the individual's contact with *"transcending reality"*; with the past and with the future, these mirrored in an exacting ethos. The ego prospers best when it is subject to the judicious governance of both id and superego. Where, because of the weakness of the superego, the id drives predominate, the ego is crippled. Such a person may suffer somatically and physiologically, but the major symptomatology will be manifest in his social, interpersonal, and societal relations.

The individual with a weak superego, the impulse driven character, is not in effect a narcissistic psychopath who, having no superego, can therefore gratify all his demands without consideration for others. He may gain his immediate objectives but invariably he remains unsatisfied, and his dissatisfactions further intensify his pursuit of the id drives.

This order of person is categorized as suffering a character disorder. His problem is primarily that of defective development of the ego complex, principally in the superego component, this deficiency being traceable to paternal deprivation. His difficulties, his pathodynamics, do not conform to the patterns of the classic neuroses in which the integrated personality is suddenly overwhelmed by heretofore well-integrated and controlled impulses. Here there is no borderline between the personality and "symptoms." The "symptoms" *are* the personality. The overall clinical picture of the neuroses, Fenichel noted, has during the past decades undergone a fundamental change. "Instead of clear cut neurotics, more and more persons with less defined disorders are seen, sometimes less troublesome to themselves than for their environment" (57). Such patients, "more troublesome to their environment than to themselves," are in the greater part the "victims" of paternal deprivation.

Paternal deprivation may be suffered in different degrees, and by virtue of a wide variety of circumstances and conditions. War, revolution, political persecutions and other mass upheavals deprive large numbers of children of their parents, and most notably of their fathers.

Paternal deprivation may be total or partial. It may be due to the periodic, physical absence of the father from the home for long or short periods, or it may be due to the ineffectual relation of the father, present, but inadequate in his role playing. It may be due to the aggressive interposition of the mother between the child and the father, rendering his ethos operations ineffectual. In the latter instances, the child is likely to be imprinted by the attitudes and values of the mother, presumptively and by definition not suitable for the development of an effective superego apparatus. Paternal deprivation may, and in our socio-economic system does, in a measure derive from the diminution and obscuration of the role of the father in the family. Not uncommonly the father appears as no more than the present adult mate of the adult female, the mother, to whom the children sense a closer bond, in that they know themselves to be the issue of her body. Whatever may be the effective reason or combination of reasons that result in paternal deprivation, the pathologic effects are to be witnessed in the ego apparatus of the individual and in particular in the superego component. The gravity of the disturbance is generally commensurate with the severity of the deprivation.

The more obvious pathologic categories deriving from a defective superego are well defined, particularly those involving *anti*social behavior—the delinquent, the criminal, the recidivist. What perhaps is less appreciated are the less obvious, less flagrant forms of pathology, which are more asocial than antisocial, and which in terms of the patient are as much self-defeating as imposing on the environment. Here the emphasis should be placed on the fact that the *anti*social personality is to be distinguished from the *a*social one. The former is generally dominated by an underlying hostility to all forms and orders of authority. Such a character is not unaware of his antipathy to authority, to inhibition, to conformity. Not infrequently, he is avowedly antisocial, even when it would be to his advantage to accept authority. In such cases it is not a lack of superego that explains the antisocial behavior, but rather the presence and operation of a powerful but perverse superego apparatus, one fashioned by cruel exactions and experiences.

But the asocial deviant *is* in effect lacking in superego. His asocial behavior is the "normal" issue of his character and personality. He does not plan or intend his behavior; he acts without any marked self-awareness. That others might think his action reprehensible is an item to be noted, but it reflects *their* peculiarity, not his own. When those about him react adversely to his asocial behavior, it may surprise him, but he seldom reacts with any intensity, and is more likely to accept the consequences with the passivity of a somewhat bewildered child.

I have used the pronoun "he" in describing the superego-deficient asocial personality. In this category of character disorders, however, though definitive statistics are unavailable, females appear to be the more numerous. I will not explore the reasons why this may be so. Freud ventured the opinion that women have a different superego formation, and hence "have less sense of justice than men, less tendency to submit to the great necessities of life, and frequently permit themselves to be guided in their decisions by their affections or enmities" (58).

Certain it is that the feminine personality is more intimately proximate to the primal drives, and in their regard will brook less interference by the superego than will the masculine.

I suspect, too, that one of the reasons why the female asocial deviant appears to be more numerous than the male is because contemporary society seems to be more tolerant of the female deviant than of the male.

In a paper titled "Are Psychiatry and Religion Reconcilable?" I have described the asocial male patient.

> A singular feature of these patients was that they were not only destructive of themselves, that is, of their own immediate being and person, but they were even more destructive of those whom they involved in intimate relations, whom they nominally loved; wife, husband, lover, child, brother, sister, friend. . . . They weren't quite like the general run of patients who come to the psychiatrist. What was so basically distinctive of them, and of their pathology, is that they were individuals without an effective super ego. They hadn't ever cultivated or developed a sense of the "ought" or the "must" *in the moral sense.* Yet these were not grossly immoral or even irresponsible people. They wouldn't, say, steal, or lie, or bear false witness. They didn't *violate* mores as the rebel might, they just had no sense for mores. They did outrageous things, things that were as destructive to themselves as to the others involved, their own children for example (as a group they were not prolific); but then they would blink in amazement when subsequent events, the results of their antecedent actions, exploded, so to say, in their faces. Recovering from their amazement they would become indignant, resentful, demanding. How could such things happen to them? How, save that the other person, the boss, one's wife or husband, one's parents, one's children, yes, and even one's therapist, was an idiot, a fool, incompetent, stupid, ignorant, and worse!
>
> Diagnostically, these were cases of personality disorder. But they were not of the so-called psychopathic variety. These were, as I came to understand them, having fathomed the dynamics of their psychopathology, cases of severe deprivation (paternal deprivation). They had not been exposed to the examples or precepts of a relatedness to other beings, at an altruistic, that is, transnarcissistic level. Yet these were not developmentally retarded individuals. They were not "infantile" though they were, in the majority and in the main, self-indulgent. They were not even selfish, though they were self-centered. They had developed into an order of maturity that did not embrace any concern with, or practices bearing on, the meaning of life and its achievements *in a deep relatedness* with others, either with one's immediates, or with mankind at large.
>
> This psychological and personality syndrome or pattern is not a constitutionally determined psychopathy. It is rather experiential in

origin. In physical characteristics there was nothing of significance common to this group of individuals. And even within their common psychopathy they differed radically.

Since I first perceived this order of psychopathy, which I consider to be of a distinctive nature, in other words a definite psychological disorder, I have encountered a goodly number of other, similar cases. These, however, stemmed from quite different social strata. The majority of them have been young women of native American parentage. They differed in many respects from the group I first encountered, but their psychopathy was similar, and the dynamics thereof could likewise be traced to the absence of an effective super ego (59).

Here I will give in brief the case histories of two female patients who to my mind are clear instances of behavior disorders deriving from paternal deprivation. Both patients have much in common.

They are young (broaching thirty), college graduates, handsome and well built. Both are the younger members of old families, noted for leadership in commerce, social service and education. Both patients are talented in music and one shows distinctive competences in mathematics. Both married young, in their early twenties, and had their first children within two years after marriage. Their pregnancies (one has three children and the other two) were uneventful and were enjoyed. The children were normal. Both patients were "more loved than loving." Their respective husbands were much involved in and committed to their mates, more so than the wives to their husbands. In both cases the husbands initially looked up to their mates, prizing their charm, their physical beauty and their social status. Both husbands, be it noted, were "in therapy" when they married, and both married against the advice of their respective therapists. The husbands presented no better nor more decisive father-person images than did the wives' own fathers. The husbands were undoubtedly contributory to the ultimate issues, and failures of, the marriages, but chiefly in that they were unable to inhibit or change the unravelment of the pathological sequences innate in their mates' character defects.

As stated, both patients suffered paternal deprivation, but each in a different wise. Patient A's father was an almost completely closed-in personality, formal to the point of rigidity, burdened with a heavy load of prejudices on morals, economics and races. He was against the government and refused to pay taxes. The government, of course, caught up with him, and the results were almost disastrous. The father was inaccessible both to the patient's mother and the patient. In the younger years of the patient's life, the father divorced and then remarried the mother of the patient. The patient was not much closer to her mother, a rather immature and self-centered person, than she was to her father. Most of her young life was spent in private schools and in the care of maids and governesses.

Patient B's father was the third mate of her mother, and his marriage lasted a mere 4 years. The following and fourth mate of her mother involved the patient in serious sex play. The patient was then 12 years of age, and from the history it would seem that while the sex play was initiated by the stepfather, it was continued for some time with the tacit consent of the patient. The patient's father remarried and lived abroad for long periods, returning to this country only occasionally. In effect then, the patient had very little contact with her father, and her stepfather and her mother's miscellany of lovers contributed little toward the patient's development of a superego. The mother shaped the patient's world, life and value perceptions. The mother lived a Bohemian life, was self-indulgent, narcissistic, parasitic, amoral and arrogant. She was also very beautiful, animated, clever and much adored by a certain order of susceptible men. The patient was completely overshadowed by the mother, was dependent on her and regarded her as an ideal.

We can now revert to the story of the respective marriages of the patients, for here again their similarity is striking. Both patients were willing, if not eager, to marry. Neither one found her sexual experiences in marriage adequately satisfying. Neither had any significant sexual experience before marriage. Each patient soon learned to use sexual accessibility as a weapon against her husband. Each of the patients, but in different ways, resisted the normal demands of a marriage union and sought to go her own way *in* the marriage. They would not compromise nor subjugate their wishes to the overriding needs of the husband and the transcending interests of the union. Patient A left her husband, who was establishing himself in a position of promise at a distant city, and returned to New York where her parents and old friends were living. He, in turn, could not but follow her, giving up his promising position, and suffering in consequence a severe personal and professional crisis that lasted for several years.

Patient B could not refuse any invitation to any party, and when her husband could not accompany her because of work which he had to do, she insisted on going alone and staying out late. Fond of the limelight, she cultivated opportunities to perform in "Bohemian joints" as a chanteuse and guitarist, much to the embarrassment of her husband. Her consistent ambition appeared to be to escape from the exactions of housekeeping and from the commitments of wifehood.

Neither patient had matured sufficiently to effectively and with satisfaction execute the roles of wife and mother.

As noted above, both patients gave birth to their first children within 2 years after marriage. Pregnancy and delivery were uneventful and normal. The children were planned for and welcomed. They were well cared for by their mothers. But even here there was evinced some resentment at the limitations which the children imposed on the mother's freedom of movement. With time, the care of the children was increasingly foisted on husband, hired help and baby sitters.

In both patients there developed a protest against monogamy and an urgent need to sample the affections of other men. Patient B was the more promiscuous and the less discriminating, following in this the patterns of her mother. Patient A was the more discreet, but not very discerning in her choice of sexual partners. Both women were not circumspect in their affairs. Only their optated blindness kept the husbands from seeing what was going on, and only the eventuation of a pregnancy, not to be credited to the husband, forced, in each case, the husband's recognition and acknowledgement of the true state of affairs. It is noteworthy that when questioned and confronted, neither woman attempted to deny the charges of promiscuity and infidelity, nor to set up any defenses. They manifested no strong reactions and no sense of guilt or contrition.

Both patients were in therapy with me for different lengths of time. They sought therapy at the behest of their respective husbands and not because they had any inner urgency. They were pleasing enough as patients, but it was not possible to establish an effective transference. They were present at, but alien to, the therapeutic session and effort. They could intellectually grasp what was uncovered, but they mustered no affective concomitant. They could envision the untoward effects of their behavior and perceive them to be dire, but they remained unmoved, unmotivated, as if it didn't really concern them, their marriage, their children or their husbands.

Therapy was ineffective. The patients progressively withdrew and ultimately dropped out "without a whimper *or* a bang." Nothing prevailed. The marriages were dissolved. My prognosis is that both these women will repeat the patterns of their asocial existence throughout their lives. I do not believe that they can be re-educated. The deprivations they suffered are not compensable and not remediable. With them the critical period for the development of a superego apparatus is long past; they are asocial recidivists in the true sense.

I have described but two patients; my records, as those of every psychiatrist, include numerous such cases. The fact is, as anyone who has practiced psychiatry for more than 25 years can attest out of his own experience, that this order of case is markedly on the increase, among both men and women.

As noted, paternal deprivation is structured into contemporary society. Our modes of living deprecate the role of the father and make it nugatory. The agitation witnessed some years ago about "momism" and the "generation of vipers" was grossly misdirected. It pictured the mother as a conspiratorial character, bent on castrating both father and son. This is sheer nonsense. The mother's role has grown in preeminence and effect because that of the father has diminished in our changing socio-economic system. The functions of ethos indoctrination have been taken over and are badly served by the agencies that have so largely displaced the father, namely, the schools, television, the funny sheets, the glossy magazines, the morbid realism of the ultramodern fiction and advertising. The results are reflected in the growing magnitude of delinquency, both juvenile and adult, and in the far more numerous mass of asocial, ineffectual persons, who because of serious paternal deprivation, are handicapped in the process of self-fulfillment by their inadequate superego.

One concluding comment. This exposition on paternal deprivation is not intended and is not to be construed as an argument for the re-establishment of a patriarchal society. That would be foolish, and besides, utterly impossible. But it does argue that the indoctrinating role of the father is essential for the effective development of the ego complex and most directly in the development of a competent superego apparatus. What should concern us all is how far the indoctrinating, ethos-forming role of the father can be re-established and reconstituted within the limits of contemporary society, and for the rest, how and where we can find and develop the moral equivalent of the Father Person.

REFERENCES

1. BACHOFEN, JOHANN JACOB: *Dasmutterrecht,* Vol. II, Benno Schwabe, 1948, pp. 356, 358, 359.
2. NEUMANN, ERICH: *The Origins and History of Consciousness.* Trans. R. F. C. Hall. New York, Pantheon Books, 1954, p. 48.
3. *Ibid.,* p. 54.
4. *Ibid.,* p. 181.
5. *Ibid.,* p. 92.
6. *Ibid.,* p. 140.
7. *Ibid.,* p. 138-139.
8. *Ibid.,* p. 143.
9. *Ibid.,* p. 147.
10. VAN DER LEEUW: *Religion in Essence and Manifestation,* Chapt. 20, cited by Neumann, p. 148.
11. NEUMANN, *op. cit.* p. 172-173.
12. OATES, WHITNEY, J. AND O'NEILL, EUGENE JR. (EDS.): *The Complete Greek Drama,* Vol. II. Trans. Gilbert Murray. New York, Random House, 1938, p. 252.
13. *Ibid.,* p. 254.
14. *Ibid.,* p. 255.
15. *Ibid.,* p. 270.
16. *Ibid.,* p. 270.
17. JAEGER, WERNER: *Paideia,* Vol. 1. Trans. Gilbert Highet. New York, Oxford University Press, 1944, p. 345.
18. OATES AND O'NEILL, *op. cit.* Vol. I, p. 292.
19. *Ibid.,* p. 294.

20. *Ibid.,* p. 297.
21. *Ibid.,* p. 298.
22. *Ibid.,* p. 299.
23. *Ibid.,* p. 299.
24. *Ibid.,* p. 307.
25. BIDNEY, DAVID: *Theoretical Anthropology,* New York, Columbia University Press, 1953, p. 225.
26. GENESIS 2.22.
27. HESIOD: *Works and Days.* Trans. Hugh G. Evelyn-White, Loeb Classics, New York, G. Putnams Sons (Loeb Classics) 1926, p. 9.
28. GENESIS 2.19.18.
29. *Ibid.,* 2.16.
30. HESIOD, *op. cit.,* p. 11.
31. FINLEY, M. I.: *The Ancient Greeks.* New York, Viking Press, 1967.
32. *Ibid.,,* p. 25.
33. WASHBURN, SHERWOOD L. (ED.): *Social Life of Early Man,* New York, Wenner-Gren Foundation for Anthropological Research, Inc., 1961, pp. 98-99.
34. *Ibid.,* p. 99.
35. LEBARRE, WESTON: *The Human Animal,* Chicago, University of Chicago Press, 1954, p. 212.
36. POLANYI, KARL: *Origins of Our Time,* London, Victor Gollancz, Ltd., 1945.
37. *Ibid.,* p. 44.
38. *Ibid.,* p. 43.
39. *Ibid.,* p. 169.
40. *Ibid.,* p. 43.
41. *Ibid.,* p. 158.
42. *Ibid.,* p. 159.
43. ORTEGA Y GASSET, JOSE: *Man and Crisis.* Trans. Mildred Adams. New York, W. W. Norton, 1958, pp. 85-86.
44. *Ibid.,* p. 88.
45. *Ibid.,* p. 86.
46. *Ibid.,* p. 88.
47. FREUD, SIGMUND: *Outline of Psychoanalysis.* Trans. James Strachey. New York, W. W. Norton & Co., 1949, Chapter 8.
48. HARTMANN, HEINZ: *Essays on Ego Psychology.* New York, International Universities Press, 1964, p. 121.
49. LORENZ, KONRAD: *Ecce Homo!* Encounter, September, 1966.
50. SCOTT, J. P.: Critical periods in behavioral development. *Science* 138:949-958, 1962.
51. *Ibid.,* p. 949.
52. From Scott, referring to work by J. Money, J. G. Hampson and J. L. Hampson, *Arch. Neurol. Psychiat.* 77:333, 1957.
53. HENDRICK, IVES: Early development of the ego: Identification in Infancy. *P.S.A. Quarterly,* 1950, p. 50.
54. FREUD, SIGMUND: *Der Mann Moses und die Monotheistische Religion.* Amsterdam, Verlag Albert De Lange, 1939, p. 206.
55. FREUD, *op. cit.* Chapter 2.
56. FENICHEL, O.: *The Psychiatric Theory of Neuroses.* New York, W. W. Norton, 1945, p. 374.
57. *Ibid.,* p. 464.
58. FREUD, SIGMUND: Some psychological consequences of the anatomic distinctions between the sexes. *Int. J. Psychoanal.* 8:469, 1927.
59. GALDSTON, IAGO: Are psychiatry and religion reconcilable? *Pastoral Psychology,* May 1960.

3

The Psychodynamics of the Triad:
Alcoholism, Gambling, and
Superstition

THERE is more than a suggestion of chicanery in the title of this contribution. For the offer to expound the common denominator of three distinctive categories must in all good sense carry the implication that each of the separate categories is sufficiently well known to permit of comparison and abstraction. This, however, is most definitely not the case with any of the three psychopathies here conjoined—alcoholism, gambling, and superstition. On the contrary, each of them is something of a moot issue, fringed with a fray of divergent and contradictory observations, theories, and arguments. How, then, are these moot issues to be encompassed within a single exposition, and what am I to plead to the indictment that the title is more smart than valid?

Two arguments I would submit: one is pragmatical, deriving from clinical experiences, and the other is theoretical and is drawn from historical experience. Let me deal with the second argument first. It is an historical fact that certain distinctive pathologies which troubled and puzzled physicians over long periods of time—and which they could not comprehend separately—became meaningful and understandable when studied in the perspective of a common etiology. You will surely recall how disparate and confusing were the pathological entities—phthisis, consumption, scrofula, Pott's disease, and lupus—until the time when Virchow propounded and demonstrated the *unity of the tubercule.* Even more remarkable, and more immediate to our own issue, is the "order brought out of chaos" by the comprehension of the common etiology underlying the wide variety of disturbances that include scurvy, pellagra, beriberi, polyneuritis, the Korsakoff syndrome, cirrhotic affections of the liver, night blindness, and a host of other conditions, little understood in the past, but now known to be due to nutritional and metabolic deficiencies.

The moral of this historically validated generalization is that entities that are relatively incomprehensible singly may at times be understood when conjoined. That is the warrant I advance for my attempt to treat the triad—alcoholism, gambling, and superstition. I believe they can be better comprehended in the light of their common psychodynamics than when contemplated singly. Of course, as is nearly always the case, this conviction was not derived from a study of historical precedents and principles, but rather from immediate experience. The historical antecedent only serves to inspire confidence in and to impart validity to the particular experience. It ties it in, so to say, with common knowledge.

The pragmatic experience, which, as you will recall, is my second argument, involved the contemporaneous exposure to three patients—a periodic alcoholic, a prostitute, and a gambler. It was while working with this triad of patients that I was impressed by the common denominators of their disparate psychopathies. A few words first about the patients.

The alcoholic was a man fifty years of age, bearing the name of a distinguished family, the successful head of a large and important industry, married, and the father of several sons. He was a periodic alcoholic, whose drinking bouts were associated with fugues and radical alterations in personality, recessive in character and characterized by behavior completely foreign and repugnant to him in his non-drinking states.

The prostitute—or perhaps I had better refer to her as the ex-prostitute, for she had abandoned that oldest among professions some three or four years before coming for treatment—was a handsome, well-constituted, and physically sound female thirty years of age. She had been born in a capital city of the Midwest, the daughter of Polish-Jewish immigrant parents. Despite her lack of formal education and many years spent as a prostitute, she proved to be an intelligent, informed, and capable person. At the time she came under treatment she was successfully administering a cosmetic business. Her complaint—that is, the symptom that specifically caused her to seek psychiatric help—was a vague dread of some unknown, unspecified disaster that hung over her and impeded, or at least retarded, her "advance in life." She is the "superstition exemplar" of my triad.

The third patient was the gambler. His complaint did not center about his gambling. He rather accepted gambling as a normal and even desirable component of his living pattern—which, I might add, was enormously complicated. His complaint was of a mild and, as it proved, a transient sense of depersonalization. It was associated with and had been precipitated by the development of a psychotic reaction in his older brother. My patient introjected his sick brother.

The patient was forty years of age, a Jew, almost completely illiterate, married, and the father of two children. He was the successful manufacturer of an apparel commodity and employed a goodly number of workers. He had built up his business from "scratch," and had managed it successfully for many years. He was shrewd and intelligent. He gambled consistently, and had gambled ever since he was twelve years of age. He was, as I have already indicated, a man of substantial wealth. He did not gamble to gain money. Nor did he lose much, in the scale of his wealth and income. He gambled, as he phrased it because he *had* to gamble; it temporarily relieved him of some kind of tension, the nature of which he did not understand and could not describe.

There seemed to be but few social or psychological factors common to this motley triad of patients—the well-born, wealthy, socially prominent alcoholic; the robust, keen, self-assured ex-prostitute; and the spare, fine-limbed, sharp-witted gambler, whose odd, perpetual, ingratiating smile mirrored his miserable youth in Poland, where he had been apprenticed to a shoemaker at the age of seven; where in the eruptions of the first World War, dodging the searing menace of German invaders, Polish anti-Semites, Red revolutionists, and white counter-revolutionists, he had wandered with his mother on the byways of the Polish countryside, a mendicant, and a thief by necessity. There seemed to be but few factors common to this triad of patients—at first. But as I came to know more and more of their life histories and could see more clearly and deeply into the dynamics of their psychopathies, I began to perceive in what respects they were kin—what, indeed, was common between them.

This I will propound now, leaving the justification of my proposition to the end. These were three constitutionally able individuals, each successful and effective in an appreciable segment of the totality of their life functions. Yet each of them suffered some crippling personality deficiency that robbed them of the full fruits of their endowments and denied them ultimate effectiveness and happiness. The question I posed amounted to this: Is there a common characteristic in the personality deficiencies suffered by these three, and if so, how is it to be designated, and what may be its derivations or etiologies?

As I brooded upon this issue, it became clear that what was common to these defective personality structures was that they retained within their psychic economy certain atavistic components which impeded their effective operation, something which, like the bronchial clefts, is proper to an early developmental stage, but that should have been outgrown in the process of maturation. In some respects and in some segments of their personalities, these individuals had suffered an arrest in development, and thus presented the equivalents in the psychiatric field of the better understood and more easily appreciated developmental deficiencies to be seen in the somatic field. To be more precise and specific, these patients carried into maturity, and incorporated within their adult personalities, emotional and psychological dynamisms and relational configurations that belong to the pre-adolescent and childhood periods.

During these periods the child is normally and in the true sense of the term at the caprice of fortune. During these years, the laws of cause and effect, of initial act and ultimate consequence, are not only nonoperative with regard to the child, but effectively nonexistent for it. The world of actual reality is a latter-day comprehension, which, indeed, not every one attains. In the child's realm, fancy and fortune (or misfortune) *are* the reality. From the first instant when appeasement is brought to the infant, forcefully dislodged from its earthly Garden of Eden, by some ministering female, and for a good many years to follow, what happens to the child is not related to its own efforts. There is, indeed, no correlation between its inner life and its outer experiences. It does not recognize, it has no knowledge of, causality. This does not, as has been amply demonstrated, hamper the acquisition by the child of simple associational patterns of appreciation and response, not unlike conditioned behavior patterns, nor does it deny the child a rich exercise in autistic thinking.

The thinking patterns of the child are syncretistic, that is "wide and comprehensive, but obscure and inaccurate." The child's logic has been aptly described by Piaget as precausal in quality and nature. The child does not comprehend causality as the adult does. For the child, causality is largely an extension of arbitrary intention, the fulfilment of the desire or the caprice of potent agents, human or otherwise.

The behavior of the alcoholic, the superstitious, and the gambler seems to me to be explicable on the assumption that they have retained within their personality structures, and within their psychic mechanisms, the early pre-causal patterns of comprehending, and dealing with, reality and experience. The gambler behaves as if he were still a child to whom gifts may come by mere solicitation, or by teasing for them, as indeed *is* the case in the child's experience. The superstitious individual still labors under the burden of that capriciousness that characterizes the child's realm in which, by inestimable likelihood, disaster may overwhelm or fortune favor. The alcoholic makes use of still another pre-causality-pattern, that of the denial of the unacceptable reality. Alcohol is merely the most convenient means for achieving that goal. In the magical, pre-causal realm of the child, the real can in the last resort be reformed at will. To the child nothing is impossible, for in its world nothing obeys causal laws.

The child's world, and the child within its world, are normal and proper—to the child. They are, separately and together, particular instances of well-comprehended reality, and must not be misconstrued out of their normal framework. There is no pathology inherent in them. The pathology issues from displacement. To revert to an analogy already employed, bronchial clefts are normal in the embryo, but abnormal in the postnatal constitution. Seen thus, the alcoholic, the superstitious, and the gambler are to be viewed not merely as grown individuals embarrassed by the retention of some childish traits, but rather as sick individuals in whom the retention of pre-adult patterns is a symptom of some serious injury. The crucial matter is not what childish and preadolescent patterns they retain, but rather the dynamics of this retention, the why and how of the arrest in development they suffered. This triad of patients does not operate with childish patterns in the world of the child—but with childish patterns in the realm of the adult. The result is not regression, where consistency is still possible, but distortion and disfigurement.

In this rather brief communication, I cannot dilate upon the dynamics of the arrest in development reflected in this triad. This much, however, I can advance: these patients suffered early and severe deprivations in their affect relations with their parents. They did not experience that rounded cycle of contacts and interpersonal reactions with their parents, most notably with the mother, and also—though this is in the nature of a corollary—with their siblings, that is essential to a healthy development through infancy, childhood, adolescence, and youth. Hence they behave as if harking back to that early period at which they suffered the arresting deprivation. There they appear to be compulsively fixated, and unable to advance.

Let me sketch briefly the early life histories of my three patients. The gambler was born in a little village in Poland, and throughout his youth he was surrounded by poverty and squalor. His father was separated from his mother and lived in a distant village. It was the father's second marriage, and my patient had half-brothers and half-sisters twenty and more years older than himself. He was apprenticed to a shoemaker at the age of seven. And from that age until he married, he had no "home." I mentioned his trying adventures during the years of the first World War and the revolution that followed.

The ex-prostitute lost her mother at the age of five, probably as the result of an infection supervening on an abortion. The father remarried and attempted to reëstablish a home for his children. He did not succeed in accomplishing this, however, and the children were sent to an orphan asylum. This patient had a great hatred for her father, whom she blamed for the death of her mother, and she similarly rejected and blamed her oldest brother.

The alcoholic patient was the son of a self-indulgent, narcissistic mother and a domineering, sadistic father. The earliest memories he had were those of crying bitterly every time his mother left him. Both my patient and his older brother were ceremoniously circumcised—as a punishment for masturbating. Grown of age, having fought in the first World War, having married, and being the father of a young son, my patient happened once to fall ill. Whereupon his father ascribed his illness to sexual overindulgence and offered to finance a vacation trip, provided he would leave his wife at home. Fortunately the father died soon thereafter, or the family might have gone to pot completely.

The three psychopathies herein conjoined have been studied to different extents. Most study has been devoted to alcoholism, least to superstition. It seems proper, then, for me further to expound my thesis, centering my exposition about gambling. Quantitatively, not much has been written on the psychology of gambling, but what is available is of a high order. Edmund Bergler has made both extensive and deep analytic studies of the gambler—whom he quite properly dubs "a misunderstood neurotic." In a penetrating and on the whole acceptable analysis of the psychology of gambling, Greenson observes: "One would expect to find in the history of neurotic gamblers severe deprivation and/or over-gratification in childhood. This is confirmed by the clinical findings."* This is also in harmony with my own observations.

Those who have studied the gambler are in agreement about the principle of his psychological characteristics. Thus he does not gamble to gain money. Money may be the token of his favor, but not the aim of his gambling. The neurotic gambler seldom if ever quits when he has made a "killing." The neurotic gambler stays until he loses, and he seems to

---

*See "On Gambling," by Ralph R. Greenson. *The American Imago,* Vol. 4, August, 1946. p. 70.

have a compulsion to lose. The neurotic gambler appears to know that he cannot win, but acts as if he might. The neurotic gambler behaves as if he were bent on soliciting and teasing Fortune into smiling benignantly upon him and granting him her favors. Neurotic gambling can thus be understood as a compulsive acting out of a plea to the surrogate figures —the mother most likely, but the father also—for a show of favor, for the affirmative response to the questions, "Do you love me?" "Do you approve of me?" "Do you think I am good, and smart, and strong?" It is as if these questions, proper to the child, had for these children, now grown, never been answered adequately in childhood, and thus they remain fixated and incapable of realizing that there are other means for eliciting an appropriate response—the testing of one's worth, for example, in the lists of adult relations.

The gambler is obsessive in his uncertainty—and compulsive in his need to pose the question: "Is Lady Luck with me?" Since a definitive and ultimately satisfactory—that is, reassuring for all time—answer to his query is impossible, the gambler will not "quit" until he is without the means to continue gambling. This will make understandable the gambler's seeming compulsion to lose, for the more he wins, the more means he has wherewith to gamble, and the more intensive becomes the gambling. Release is to be found only in losing.

Bergler and Greenson describe the gambler as one who has regressed to infantile longings for omnipotence. I am rather persuaded to consider him as one who has not successfully egressed out of the child's world of pre-causality. This is equally true of the superstitious and the alcoholic, and for this reason I look upon the triad of alcoholism, gambling, and superstition as developmental deficiencies, and hence as having a common psychodynamics.

This is an issue of large import, for it has a bearing on etiology, prophylaxis, and therapy. Should we grant that this triad does indeed represent the pathology of retained pre-causal patterns of conceptualizing and dealing with reality, then the proper question would be what caused the atavistic retention. Or, more profitably, since physiology is generally more illuminating than pathology, the question might be asked: How does the normal child supplant its precausal logic with the logic of causality, and how and where may this process go awry? This would be the protocol for future studies. I am inclined to believe that the primal injury would be found to have taken place in the early affect relations between mother and child, the father playing a secondary rôle.

I am aware that in this presentation I have touched on large issues which deserve more spacious treatment than I could possibly give them here. But on this score I made my apologies at the very start. It is not alcoholism, gambling, or superstition *per se t*hat fixed my interest, but rather that which is common to them collectively—their common psychodynamics. And in that it is the idea of a psychopathy due to the retention of early pre-adolescent psychological components—within the adult economy—that is outstanding. I have designated this as in the nature of developmental deficiencies or developmental arrests. This type of psychopathology has to my mind not been given the study and attention it deserves.

Because of Freud's emphasis, and that of psychoanalysis in general, we have been much taken up with those forms of psychopathology which are the result of specific traumatic experiences, in which singularly painful, directly injurious happenings had been encountered, and which resulted in neurotic behavior patterns, in ineffective and crippling personality compromises, in the repression of memory, in the splitting of affect from the event or situation with which it was originally associated. Undeniably, Freud's emphasis on the dynamics of these patterns of psychopathology constitutes one of the truly great achievements in the history of psychiatry. No less brilliant and precious was his development of the particular technique of free association which is so effective in the uncovering and in the subsequent correction of these patterns of psychopathology.

Yet there are other sources of psychological morbidity—as Freud himself affirmed —and one such source I have attempted to delineate in this paper. The triad—alcoholism, gambling, and superstition—represent conditions notoriously resistant to therapy. But then it is much easier to reduce a dislocated hip than to grow an acetabular socket where one has failed to develop.

4

The Gambler and His Love

The psychiatrist, unlike the clinician, does not have either ample means or frequent opportunities for testing out his postulations as to the aetiology, the basic pathology, and the therapeutic handling of a given case. Psychiatry has nothing that equals in specific relatedness the tuberculin, the Schick, or the sugar tolerance test. Psychiatry lacks the equivalents of Koch's postulates, so determinate in establishing the authenticity of the causative agents of the infectious diseases. It is therefore rewarding to come upon an instance wherein the patient's own life experience confirms, at a later time, the validity of the formulations, postulated earlier, to account for the dynamics of his psychopathology.

It is such an experience that I wish to detail here. I initially described the patient in a paper published in *Mental Hygiene,* in October, 1951. The title of that paper was "The Psychodynamics of the Triad, Alcoholism, Gambling, and Superstition." The gambler was one of the "triad."

Few gamblers come for psychiatric treatment with gambling as their chief complaint. My patient complained of his sense of depersonalization, not of his gambling. In treatment he reintegrated his personality without much difficulty. After a year of therapy he returned to his accustomed world and its accustomed ways.

Five years later the patient called for an appointment, complaining of what amounted to an acute anxiety. He was again accepted for therapy, and therein we come to The Gambler and His Love.

The gambler, as I reported previously, was married and had two children. He was fond of his wife, as a son might be of his mother. He provided her with all the comforts she desired, but did not share life with her, socially or sexually. She concurring, he arranged to have her vacationing or visiting away from home for the greater part of the year, in Florida, and/or the Catskills. The children were placed in boarding schools. He had never wanted and never thought of legally separating from or divorcing his wife. He was indeed fond of her—in his own way.

The patient was sexually active, mainly with costly call girls and casual women. His business required him to travel frequently and widely. His excursions were enlivened with many and bizarre sexual adventures. But these were more in the nature of an exercise than of an orgiastic indulgence. In telling of his sexual ventures he always spoke as if he had been "external to the experience."

But once something extraordinary happened to him—a woman fell in love with him, and she refused to be put off, or to accept the role of a casual partner. The woman was married and the mother of two children. Her devotion to the patient knew no bounds. She pursued him constantly and responded to his every beck and call. She asked nothing of him but his love.

At first he was emotionally unresponsive, aloof, and casual. He relished her sexually but wanted no involvement. In time, however, the woman prevailed, at least to the extent of engaging him emotionally more than any other woman had ever done before. He even suspected that he was beginning to love her. But the more his affections became involved, the more his suspicions grew. Did she really love him? Was it for the love of him that she was sacrificing her husband (who was in fact a shady character with a criminal record), and her two children? Or, was she just a "bum," and after something other than his love? She had "carried on" with him for 18 months, and during that time had not asked him for any money. That puzzled him greatly, and fed his suspicions copiously. He queried her on every score, and though she offered him infinite reassurance and a thousand proofs of her love, he remained unconvinced and suspicious. He was, to quote him, "tortured, nervous, tense."

And this is the way he set about to gain relief! He enlisted the cooperation of his most intimate gambling crony, and with him conspired to put the woman, his love, to a test. The patient was to leave the city for a week, and during this time the friend was to try and "make" the woman. As it was agreed, so was it done! And then came the *Nemesis*. The patient returning, his friend reported that though he had tried his very best, employing his every stratagem and resource he could get nowhere with the woman. She was, he assured the patient, steadfast in her loyalty, and committed in her love.

But, as I am sure you can anticipate, this did anything but reassure the patient. It only enlarged the range of his suspicions, for now he not only doubted the love of the woman but also the fidelity and truthfulness of his friend.

It was all too much for him, and he came back for help. Under the circumstances therapy could only be supportive with a minimum of uncovering and insight. Yet in the end he managed to regain his singular balance. This is the pattern he followed. He gave up his "love," and simultaneously regained his friend.

The unconscious homosexual component in this constellation is, of course, self-evident. But more interesting and significant is what happened with his compulsion to gamble. He had abandoned gambling during the 18 months of his involvement; now when "the love" was discarded, he resumed it. He gambled recklessly and lost a good deal of money. His game of preference was gin rummy. To this must be added dice and horseracing. He resumed his sexual contacts with call girls and casuals. He made an abortive attempt to "get closer" with his wife. Nothing came of it. And yet, he found living more tolerable. He had returned to the old and endless pursuit of Lady Luck, who never answers but only smiles the enigmatic smile of the Sphinx.

During therapy he reported an interesting dream. "He was walking somewhere in Chicago. A man and a woman tried to hold him up. They took everything from him. He ran to find the cops. Then ran further and finally gave up."

This slice of life, treated as a psychiatric biopsy, confirms, I believe, this much: that the neurotic gambler always plays to lose, that in his gambling he is obsessively teasing his surrogate figure Lady Luck for a show of favor, yet cannot and will not accept "Yes" for an answer. Such an answer does not square with the deeper facts of his life, nor with the unconscious memories of his irremediable deprivations. And in some ways I am persuaded the gambler is right; for who can make up, and what can cancel out, the egregious loss of the mother's assuring love and the father's supportive sanction? Such a one is doomed to wander through life asking unanswerable questions.

More pointedly, the Gambler and His Love are an unrealistic pair. Only the gambler is real. The gambler has no love. He is incapable of love. Gambling is the gambler's addiction, not his love. For love has the requisite of an antecedent ego maturation—to which the gambler has not attained. He is in these respects severely retarded, a victim of his deprivational experiences.

5

On the Etiology of Depersonalization

DEPERSONALIZATION HAS ENGAGED the interest of a goodly number of psychiatrists and has been the subject of much study.

The condition was first effectively described by Krishaber in 1872, under the designation of *De la Nevropathie Cerebro-cardiaque*. Fifteen years later Dugas named the symptom-complex, depersonalization. The literature on depersonalization is quite extensive, the condition having been the concern of neurologists, psychologists, psychiatrists and psychoanalysts.

Paul Schilder, who was intrigued by the problem of depersonalization, referred to it as a "fascinating type of neurosis" (*Goals and Desires of Man,* p. 188), which, in essence, represents "a disturbance in the body image, the psychogenesis of which is not yet known" (*The Image and Appearance of the Human Body,* p. 138). All authors who have dealt with depersonalization agree that the disturbance in what the Germans term "Ich gefuhl" and what Schilder acutely called the body image, constitutes the predominant feature of the disorder. On the other hand, when these authors turn to the problem of the psychogenesis or the causation of depersonalization, "they speak a veritable babel of tongues." This is especially the case with the psychoanalytic authors. Among the genetic factors to which the psychoanalysts ascribe depersonalization may be listed the following: little or no breast feeding or the impersonal bottle or parent (Searl); some shock or severe physical punishment for defiant naughtiness giving rise to a narcissistic wound together with loss of libidinal attachment (Federn, Nunberg, Sadger, Hendrick)—this may be particularly connected with viewing and exhibiting in the Oedipus situation (Sadger) in defiance of the angry restraining looks which are meant to keep the child quiet (i.e., like a piece of furniture—Searl); viewing turned inward

58

instead of outward (as a result, an increase in the scrutinizing tendency —Schilder, Eidelberg, Bergler)—this self-scrutinizing may represent the activity of the harsh parent (super-ego—Oberndorf); an attempt to escape psychic and physical punishment, psychic castration, guilt and castration (Sadger, Hendrick), by acquiring the immunity of an inanimate object (Searl), compensation for their lifelessness by extreme activity and erotization of thinking (Fenichel and Oberndorf) in identification with the frustrating parent, and Oberndorf thinks that there is a clash of homosexual with heterosexual striving.

The non-psychoanalytic authors, though rather numerous, and though their writings on this subject bulk larger than those of the psychoanalysts, have advanced fewer theories on the causation of depersonalization. It is not necessary to review each of these theories, but it will be profitable to take notice of the major ones. The earliest and possibly the most obvious theory traced the etiology of depersonalization to some organic, traumatic, toxic or other essentially somatic-pathological condition. To the credit of the neurologists be it said that they did not long maintain or defend this theory. For though they saw the symptoms of depersonalization in cases of cerebral injury and disease, they recognized the pure case of depersonalization, which is full blown in the total absence of organic injury or disease. Theory then shifted from gross organic pathology to pathological physiology, particularly to disturbances in sensibilities, that is, in what Sharrington termed the exteroceptive and proprioceptive mechanisms. The hypothesis was that the inner and outer worlds of the depersonalized individual *seemed* strange to him because he beheld them strangely. But this theory was soon disproved. In his sensibilities the depersonalized patient functions quite like the normal person. The quest for physiological abnormality was then advanced centrally toward the cerebrum. But here again the yield was nil. The depersonalized patient proved himself in no way functionally inferior to the normal person in any category reflecting cerebral efficiency. Memory, imagination, understanding, the capacity to reason, to learn—none of these showed deviation from the normal in the depersonalized patient. The last theoretical propositions advanced by the non-psychoanalytical authors hold that the genesis of depersonalization is to be found in intrapsychic disorders, in "psychic synthesis" (Janet), in "Aktionsgefuhle" (E. Storrin), in "Hemmung des gesamten Gefuhlslebens" (Oesterreich). At this time the medical psychologist and the non-psychoanalytic, as well as the psychoanalytic, psychiatrists have come close to one another in their theoretical formulations. I must, however, add that not many of them are aware of this.

To return to the plethora of theories on the causation of depersonalization that abound, particularly among psychoanalytic authors, it may be profitable to inquire just what accounts for it. Mayer-Gross ascribes it to the tendency of authors to pick out some detail, some partial symptom in the whole picture, to place it at the center and then to derive "all the rest" from it (Mayer-Gross *"On Depersonalization,"* p. 115). The reason why this is possible is that "the depersonalization syndrome presents a general change of psychic experience, which can, of course, be found in almost every psychic function." (op. cit. p. 115). This means, in substance, that the symptomatology of depersonalization is protean and the particular complaints of the patient are manifold. It is a fact that every sphere of psychic function—affect, sensation, perception, memory, thinking—may become involved in depersonalization, and the patient not infrequently shifts the emphasis of his complaint from one sphere to the other. Mayer-Gross' dictum is, therefore, quite valid, and it does help to account for the origin of so many divergent theories on the causations of depersonalization. There is, however, more to this problem. There is a "mirror side" which we need to consider. Depersonalization is not only protean in its particular symptomatology, but is a component, *in varying measures,* of every major and minor psychopathy. There is, in other words, a specific nosological entity known as depersonalization, and also a generic disturbance in psychic function carrying the same label, which can be found associated with other specific psychopathies.

An analogy from the clinical realm may help to make the above differentiation easier to appreciate: thus, while an acceleration in the pulse beat is associated with all febrile and many other conditions, it is a primary and specific disturbance in paroxysmal tachycardia.

The relation between depersonalization as a specific psychopathy and depersonalization as a component of other psychopathies is of deep interest in its bearing on the problem of psychogenesis and on the problem of differential diagnosis. This relation will be dealt with later on. At this point it is worth noting that many authors have recognized that the syndromes of depersonalization are to be found as components of other psychopathic states. Schilder, agreeing with Nunberg, wrote "almost every neurosis has in some phase of its development symptoms of depersonalization" (*The Image and Appearance of the Human Body,* p. 138). Karl Haug (*Die Storungen des Personlichkeits bewusstseins*), reports and describes depersonalization symptoms following on skull injuries, gross brain injuries, apoplectic incidents, hemiplegias, encephalitis, epilepsy, central nervous system lues; in other systematic illnesses, in intoxications, in neurasthenia, psychasthenia, in hysteria; in manic depressive psychoes and in schizophrenia. Sophie Morgenstern states that "the syndromes of depersonalization can be observed in melancholia, in hysterical and epileptiform deliria, but, most frequently, in the initial states of schizophrenia" (*Psychoanalytic Conception of Depersonalization,* p. 164). She further states, and I would underscore this statement because it is particularly noteworthy, "Lesser states of depersonalization are to be found even with normal people, either after an emotional shock or after physical exhaustion." Mayer-Gross is inclined to go somewhat to the other extreme. He questions whether depersonalization is ever a specific psychopathy. He regards depersonalization as "a nonspecific syndrome occurring in illness of different kinds during the state of minor intensity, and it may remain as it is if the illness is not intensified" (*On Depersonalization,* p. 117). I am persuaded that Mayer-Gross errs when he considers depersonalization to be only a nonspecific syndrome. It is that, but it is also a specific nosological entity, a definite neurosis.

At this point, we need to define in particular detail precisely what we intend or conceive by depersonalization. Should we attempt such a definition in the words of the patient, we would hardly come to an end, for the respects in which the body image may undergo change are innumerable. The patient may complain that his entire body is dead, or that it is light and airy or grown too heavy. He may confine his complaint to some one portion of his body or to some one organ. He may consider his voice strange and not his own. He may look on his hands and "feel" that they belong to someone else. He may even, as one of my patients complained, "feel that he is going into an animal," perceived on the street—in this case, a dog. The patient seldom holds to his changed body image, but is rather inclined to alter it from time to time. To gain a substantial idea of what depersonalization as a psychiatric entity represents, one must subsume the vast varieties of patient complaints and extract from them their common factors. Doing this, we can observe how very fortunate the name *depersonalization* is, and how well it epitomizes the common factors of the syndrome. Above everything else, these patients complain of a loss, of a change, of a degradation in personality. "Where is the gay, carefree, happy young woman I knew before?" was the continuous almost stereotyped lament of one of my patients, uttered with great despair and accompanied with copious tears. The patient, in addition, describes the *new personality* not only as strange, but, also, as outside himself, that is, outside the framework of his memory of himself, and as a compelling personality obliging him to do things not within his volition. The patient is likely to describe these latter appreciations as automatisms, and himself as an automaton.

These, then, are the principal and most important psychopathological features of depersonalization: the patient is aware of a change and a degradation in his personality, and he is aware that much of his overt and other behavior is without his volition, that he seemingly is being manipulated by alien forces. Such objective changes as the patient may complain of in himself and in the external world are secondary to the primary appreciation of the change in his subjective self; they are projections of the primary appreciation.

By this definition of the primary psychopathological features of depersonalization we are brought up against the basic problem of "personality": if we are to understand fully the nature and quality of the change, we need to know and understand the medium in which the change takes place. If we are to understand "depersonalization," we need to understand "personalization." In these connections, I must emphasize that I am concerned only with "personalization" and not with "personality," for the former term reflects the dynamic process of personality, while the latter term connotes a fixed or determined entity. For my purposes, personalization can be equated to ego formation, and depersonalization to a change and degradation in ego strength and intactness. It is in the dynamics of ego formation and ego function that we will, I believe, find the answer to the psychogenesis of depersonalization.

With these preliminary notations and definitions given, I proceed further to define personalization as both a process and a state resulting from the effective interplay of the instinctive drives and the social exactions. In psychoanalytic terms, ego formation and ego function are the resultants of the interaction of the *id* and the *super ego*. In divergence, at least to some degree, from psychoanalytic conceptions, I want to affirm that in the hypothesis advanced only the id and the super ego are conceived as realities with loci and material representation. They are, in other words, embodiments, and, hence, objective realities. The ego, as I conceive it, is a functional entity without embodiment. It is an experiential reality rather than an objective reality. The ego is related to the id and to the super ego as "the spinning is to the spinning top." Or, to draw an example from physiology, as "circulation is to the circulatory system." In this latter instance, the heart, the blood vessels and the blood are the "realities with loci and material representation," but circulation is a "functional entity." The ego is engendered by the dynamic apposition of the id and the super ego. The ego is not, however, passive. It has a function in relation to the id and the super ego. Its function is to integrate the two, so that, speaking teleologically, both the id and the super ego might best be served and preserved. Thus, to recapitulate briefly, the ego is engendred by the inter-reaction of id and super ego, and its function is to integrate both, in the interest of both, as well as of the individual who embodies them. This is, in essence, the theory of ego formation and of ego function. It is also the theory of the process of personalization. On the basis of this formulation, it follows as a corollary that all psychopathology is a disorder in the integrative function of the ego. It follows, likewise, that the disruptive factors that can affect the integrative function of the ego may stem from the id or the super ego, or from both, and that the resultant psychopathology may, therefore, present a very large number of variables in ego structure and ego function.

Depersonalization is a degradation in the integrative functions of the ego. The state of degradation is perceived and appreciated by the ego—by the personality—and is complainingly reported by the individual. Since it is a degradation in the integrative functions of the ego, depersonalization is present and appreciated in practically every case of psychopathology, the exceptions being those with very sudden onset and fulminating development. Conversely, depersonalization is particularly to be noted in the cases which are slow in onset and slow in development. Yet there is a very definite nosological entity properly called depersonalization; there is a clinical syndrome *sui generis* which is depersonalization, pure and simple.

The differential diagnosis between depersonalization as a definite disease and depersonalization as the component of other psychiatric disorders is not difficult. It is made entirely on the basis of exclusion and on the score of the very definite insight into his condition shown by the depersonalization patient. The true case of depersonalization never loses contact with reality, and no matter how fantastic may be the perceived changes within himself or in the outside world which he reports, these changes always remain incredible to the patient. Sophie Morgenstern gives the criterion for differentiating between schizophrenia and depersonalization as follows: "I consider the touchstone of the diagnosis of depersonalization the retention by the patient of the control of the distinction between reality and his morbid sensations. The depersonalized notes that persons and things *seem* changed to him, while he maintains that in reality nothing has changed, whereas the schizophrenic is really persuaded of the change of the world and accepts even the idea of the destruction of the world as a fact."

I am particularly interested in Sophie Morgenstern's differential diagnosis because she sets depersonalization off against schizophrenia. To my mind, this apposition is not fortuitous. Though Morgenstern does not make the point, I have, on my part, long felt that depersonalization could properly be described as a benign form of schizophrenia. The basic mechanisms and a good deal of the symptomatology of both conditions are similar. In this connection, I am prompted to observe that the erotization of thought which Oberndorf finds so pathognomonic in depersonalization is an even more prominent feature in schizophrenia. Finally, and merely to round out the thought, the principal barrier to the development of schizophrenia in the true case of depersonalization is the presence and operation within the patient of a powerful id. Schilder wrote: "Depersonalization is the neurosis of the good looking and intelligent who want too much admiration" (*Goals and Desires of Man,* p. 197); and, again: "It is astonishing how well, even in severe neuroses, this type of person can get along in his occupation" (p. 197). I can underscore both these observations. My own depersonalization patients have been uncommonly attractive, exceptionally well endowed intellectually and very able. Each one of them, despite his neurosis, did well in work and in meeting the common everyday duties.

I have now gone to some length to define what I intend by personalization, having equated it to ego formation and ego function. The ego in my postulation arises out of the interplay of the id and the super ego; the function of the ego is to integrate the id and the super ego. Failure in the integrative process is at the base of every psychopathology. One pattern of failure is described by the name of depersonalization.

At this point, it is fitting to inquire what can contribute to, and what can engender failure in the integrative process.

This inquiry is posited broadly and not in relation to depersonalization only. The most obvious category of causes is that of organic or physiological changes in the nervous system, resulting from disease, from toxic products and from fatigue. These are too obvious to require detailed presentation. Besides, the psychopathology resulting from these causes is outside our immediate concern. Yet this is perhaps the best place to underscore the thought that psychic integration is achieved through the agency of neural elements and structures and that the total bulk, the quality and the differentiation of these neural elements and structures influence, as much as any other factor, the competence—the finesse, we might say—of the integrative function that may be witnessed in any given individual. Furthermore, though this may seem to take us somewhat far afield, we must, in these connections, conceive of a pathology that is not cellular, nor physiological, but that is only relational, a pathology where the disease manifested is the result of the disproportions that exist in the component parts of the neural structures—where, for example, the amount and quality of neural elements available for psychic integration are inadequate to achieve the normal. This concept of a pathology arising from disproportions in the component elements of the individual need not and should not be confined to the nervous system. It is applicable to all phases of the individual, and is intereffective.

I find this a rather provocative thought, related, of course, to Kretchmer's study of types, and to the studies in constitution of George Draper. Yet it differs from the ideas advanced by both Kretchmer and Draper in that it goes beyond merely associating given disorders with given constitutional types or anthropometric data and postulates that disease *per se* may be the consequence of disproportions in the otherwise normal component parts of the individual. This hypothesis may perhaps enable us better to appreciate why it is that, particularly in the realm of psychiatry, the hazard of pathological developments seems to be heightened at critical periods in the individual's life, at puberty, for example, or in adolescence, following parturition, or at the time of the climacterium. These are instances in the individual's life representing epochal changes in the architechtonic pattern of the individual, and it is at these times that disproportions are revealed.

One final hypothesis in these connections: not only is psychic integration mediated through neural elements and structures, and not only is the quality of the integrative function reflective of the quantity and quality of the neural elements and structures, but there is also an architechtonic scheme in the structure, maturation, and hence, in the function of the neural elements and structures through which the integrative function is mediated. Deficiencies and failures in the integrative process may be manifested early and grossly, or may be revealed at different stages in the unfolding of the architectonic pattern.

All this, as I have said, appears to take us far afield, and yet it is relative to the inquiry we have advanced, namely—"what can contribute and what can engender failure in the integrative process?" To the first category of causes, i.e., somatic disease and physiological disturbances, we can now add a second, namely, deficiencies, relative and absolute, in integrative competence, conceived ultimately as being due to deficiencies in related physical and functional endowments.

Failure in the integrative function may also arise out of the condition where *that* which is to be integrated is too violent, too gross either in its own nature or in its relation to the experience of the individual. Here there is no primary incompetence in the integrative function—"the grist tries the mill." Finally, there may be failure in the integrative function simply because it has not been competently exercised. It was not trained adequately to meet normal eventualities.

The pure cases of depersonalization fall under this last category. These patients are not sufferers of somatic disease nor of physiological disturb-ances; they are not the victims of poor endowments, rather the contrary is the general rule; their disorder is neither precipitated nor maintained by any gross or violent experience. They fail in psychic integration be-cause they have not learned, most often have not been taught, to integrate.

Schilder well said that "Depersonalization is the neurosis of the good looking and intelligent who want too much admiration." However, they want a great deal more than admiration. They desire to obtain "infantile satisfactions" within the framework of adult existence, and when they fail to achieve this, as fail they must sooner or later, their depersonalization begins.

Their failure in integration arises out of the predominance of the id drives within their psychic dynamism, and because of the relative weak-ness of their super ego. Their personalization, so to say, leans in the direc-tion of the primitive and of the individual. In this way they represent the mirror pattern of the schizophrenic whose personalization is in the direction of the super ego and away from the id. Between the two, how-ever, there is, I believe, this radical difference: in the schizophrenic the id weakness is of constitutional origin; in the true case of depersonaliza-tion the super ego weakness is only functional; it is only developmentally retarded. The depersonalization case is very frequently amoral in its be-havior, yet it is quite different in this respect from the case of the psycho-pathic inferior personality. The depersonalization case is generally very unhappy; unhappy, too, in its amoral behavior. The patient, however, fails to connect his unhappiness with his behavior.

One of the patients with whom I could work but a short time well illustrates these personalization defects. Attractive, well built, physically healthy, and gifted in many ways, she still managed to live 33 years with-out achieving an adult insight into the ways and values of life. She wanted many things, good things—such as a good home, antiques, silver-ware, good clothes, a circle of friends, the affection and regard of her community, children and love. Yet she remained unwilling, and I say unwilling rather than unable, to "work" for these good things in the ways common to most. She expected to obtain them in her own way, by a smile, by being "good and deserving" in a childish way. She was inordinately clever, but not wise; and this was characteristic of the whole of her life. When, as a young girl, she attracted but could not retain the attention of the neighborhood boys whom she fancied for her boy friends, as her girl companions did with their boy friends, she simply moved out of the sphere and "took up" with an older and wilder crowd. There she "got what she wanted" and gave little in return. Specifically, she worked in a store which sold a luxury commodity and catered principally to men. Here she was the recipient of much attention, of many invitations to dine, dance, visit the theater and to go on weekends. According to her story, she accepted many of these invitations, but indulged in no more than "heavy necking." Asked how she managed to fend against the more importunate of her companions, she said she "always wore a sanitary napkin" and that "scared 'em off." However, the "trick" didn't work always, for on one occasion, according to the patient's story, she was raped. The rape phase of the story is open to question. However, pregnancy, an induced abortion, and a low-grade, long drawn out pelvic infection did follow in the wake of the episode. Whereupon, in due time, sobered but still clever, she married a stolid, coarse and practical witted man, the very antithesis of her former companions. Within this setting of her marriage, however, she attempted to recreate and to perpetuate the life of luxury she knew before, and she thereby estranged her husband, her relatives and her friends. They thought her pretentious, a fake and a snob. This patient, who under treatment gained appreciable insight and was promptly relieved of her depersonalization symptoms, still believed herself "clever enough not to require more therapy." Her parting words, so to say, were, "Doctor, there is nothing wrong with me that a good man couldn't set right," and by "good man" she did not mean a good psychotherapist. The scheme which she evolved was substantially this: palpably her husband was not the right man; hence, it was up to her to find the right man. If she saved her money, and did not spend it on doctors, she could go for "vacations" to Bermuda, to Florida, to Canada. There she was bound to find the right man. The right man would give her everything.

At this point it will be profitable to consider more closely the major symptomatology of depersonalization, and to trace its psychodynamics within the broad scheme of the etiology of depersonalization already sketched. The depersonalization patient complains of changes in his personality, of changes in his body, of changes in the world about him. He complains most often that he has lost his will, or, more affirmatively, that he is an automaton, moved or affected by forces that are no part of his volition.

Viewed collectively, the depersonalization patient's complaints sum up to the proposition that "things internal as well as things external have changed." This proposition establishes two correlated conditions: first, that there exists for the patient a memory of *"things as they were"*; and, second, the suspicion, if not the full realization, that the changes are not in the things perceived, but only in the perceiver. Janet well cites as a contributing cause of depersonalization *(sentiments d'incomplétude)* "the memory of the manner in which our thoughts functioned time past" (Pierre Janet, *Les Obsessions et la Psychasthénie*, p. 545). According to our hypothesis on the etiology of depersonalization, things in effect *have* changed in the patient. He *has* experienced and *is* suffering from a state of dysintegration, that is, an abasement in the integrative function of his ego. His personality, his ego, *is* different, and his complaint, in that respect, is at least partially correct and valid. He recalls the quality of his previous function and finds the current one different in contrast. But the patient not only complains that he is different, he particuarizes his complaints. First and foremost he complains of the loss of his will, of his state of automatism. This complaint points to a condition of prime significance in our study on the etiology of depersonalization. For in substance here, too, the patient is correct in his complaint. The impulsions he experiences and which seem to him to be outside of his ego are, in effect, those of the unintegrated id and of the unintegrated super ego. In normal functions the ego is not ordinarily conscious of the interplay of the id and the super ego, or, to the mild extent that it may be, the ego *does* experience the sense of inner conflict, and may even experience some mild symptoms akin to those of depersonalization. But these experiences are still within the realm of the normal. In true depersonalization some of the impulsion and, to a lesser degree, the super ego impulsions are, so to say, torn loose, and their impact upon the ego has a violent effect giving rise to the sense of an external compulsion or of automatism. An illustration drawn from clinical experience can serve to illuminate this matter. As long as the contractions of the heart are normal we are insensible to or only mildly aware of them. But when an arrhythmia develops, we become acutely aware of the heart, and we know in a very unpleasant way that it is not beating "according to our volition."

Pursuing this matter further, we find that the complaint of automatism not only has quality but substance, too: the patient *feels* that he is an automaton, and the feeling stems from certain acts which he performs.

It is the nature and quality of these acts that most clearly reflect their id or super ego genesis. One of my patients complained that she felt "she was going into a dog"; another had the compulsion to ask with regard to everything she saw "where will it be a hundred years from now"; a third one complained he had no body. The changes which the patient complains of in his body image and those which he "sees" in the world about him are, in effect, and are to be interpreted as, symbolic of his difficulties in psychic integration. It is futile and misleading to look for the origin of these "changes" in some alteration in the perceptual mechanisms of the body. These "changes" are akin to those experienced in dreams and are to be similarly understood. At this point, I want to turn to the matter of self-observation which Schilder, at least in his earlier works, considered to be important in the etiology of depersonalization. The existence of a tendency to self-observation in depersonalization patients is undeniable, but that it is a primary cause of depersonalization I rather doubt. In its pathological degree it is the consequence, or an associate effect of, rather than a cause of, depersonalization. The sense of psychic dysintegration, like the extrasystole and the cardiac arrhythmia, compels self-observation. It is more than likely that once this process of self-observation is initiated it becomes self-perpetuating in a vicious cycle of "looking because of seeing." This, in turn, must contribute further to the dysintegration of the ego.

I want now to give a résumé of the material presented.

It will be appreciated, I am sure, that much of the aforegoing presentation is founded upon the antecedent works of others who labored to illuminate the genesis of this disorder. Wherever it was pertinent I cited "the man and his work." But, in some instances, it was not feasible to give derivations. Nor was it always quite proper to do so, for the application of some thoughts was at such variance with their original intent that their author could hardly be expected to recognize them, and doing so would be likely to disown them.

It will be profitable, however, to trace some of the antecedent thoughts and theories that find representation, partial or otherwise, in my presentation. At the very core of the problem of depersonalization is, as we said, personalization, which we, in turn, equated to ego formation and function. Freud describes ego function as a militation between the id and the super ego. Freud conceived the ego to be a differentiated portion of the id. The theory of ego function which I have advanced substantially agrees with that of Freud, save that instead of picturing the ego as a sort of innocent "middle man" caught between the two conflicting personalities,

I see the ego as a dynamism that both results from and favors the effective interplay of the id and the super ego. *Ego function is integration: ego strength is derived from effective integration.* Where there is dysintegration, there is ego weakening, or ego weakness.

The integrative function of the ego has been appreciated and described by many students of the psyche but not in quite the way I have elaborated it here, that is, in terms of the id and the super ego. Pierre Janet, for example, considers the diminution of "mental synthesis" as the primary cause of depersonalization, and from this postulate he derives the multiple associated feelings of unreality and automatism. This is reflected in the following citation, drawn from his *Les Obsessions et la Psychasthénie* (Interpretation of symptoms, p. 545-6):

"There are," Janet wrote, "three important phenomena which play a role in the creation of the sentiments of incompleteness. These are: first, the diminution in the mental synthesis and, in consequence, the diminution in the systematization and in the unification of the elements conjoined in the field of consciousness; second, a reduction in mental complexity of the numbers of elements, sensations, images, movements, emotions which ordinarily fill consciousness and which give us the sentiment of reality and of the present; third, the memory of the manner in which our thoughts functioned in the past, of its unity, its richness, the comparisons between the past state and the present and the inevitable interpretations which derive from these comparisons."

Janet, however, is not very precise as to the causes of the failure of mental synthesis. He postulates as possible causes fatigue and exhaustion, as well as constitutional inadequacy. These postulates, which are basically correct but which do not suffice to account in full for the genesis of depersonalization, have been neatly summed up by Janet in the address which he delivered at the Harvard Tercentenary Celebration entitled *Psychological Strength and Weakness in Mental Disease.*

Ribot expresses similar ideas relative to the origin and function of the ego. "The unity of the *ego*," Ribot wrote, "is not that of a mathematical point, but that of a very complicated mechanism. It is a consensus of vital processes, co-ordinated first by the nervous system—the chief regulator in the bodily economy—and finally by consciousness whose natural form is unity."

The integrative character and integrating function of the ego is very ably formulated by a number of German authors, notably by Ernst Störring, Konstantin Oesterreich and Karl Haug. Each of these has dealt extensively and very ably with the problems of depersonalization, and collectively they reveal keen insight into the dysintegrative feature of depersonalization. Where these authors seem to me to fall short is in understanding what it is that produces the dysintegrative state. Reading their very illuminating studies one is impelled to feel that these men very ingeniously deciphered some difficult code but found the decoded messages composed in a language they did not know. Their case histories literally glisten with revealing incidents, yet the authors are blind to their meaning. They reassure us, for example, that when the patient says he is feelingless, he is incorrect, he *has* feelings. But they stop at that point and do not venture to inquire *why* the patient says he is feelingless, what he *means* to say, what function his palpably erroneous statement serves. They are lacking in the insight which psychoanalytic theory and experience could provide them. But they do have a superior understanding of ego structure and ego function, and they correctly understand what is psycho-physiologically at fault in depersonalization. They do not, as I said before, *seem* to grasp the specific pathodynamics of the conditions.

The psychoanalytic authors, in contrast, seem to me to have paid far too much attention to the secondary phenomena and to the episodic aspects of their depersonalization cases. They appear to me thus to have failed to conceive and to deal adequately with the basic psychopathology and with the psychodynamics of depersonalization. In this connection I want to venture a criticism, which I believe can justly be directed at a goodly number of present-day psychiatrists. Too many of them base too much of their theory and practice on what I would call "episodic preconceptions." They seek for unique episodes, for specific traumatic experiences, to account for the neurotic conditions and behavior of their patients, expecting to find in these episodes the specific etiology of the patient's complaint. Of course, there are such cases; and they are very gratifying cases, because it is in such that the psychiatrist works miracles. But the majority of psychoneurotic patients are not of this order. They are individuals whose psychological disability has been cumulative, and whose psychopathy can be conceived and understood only in terms of their total developmental experience. Therapy with such patients must be directed not to the uncovering of the specific traumatic incident, the memory and meaning of which is presumably lost in the primal darkness of the unconscious, but rather and most often toward their further education, their re-education, or both, in personalization, in effective psychointegration.

The depersonalization case is eminently representative of the major portion of the psychoneurotic patients, and the study of its psychodynamics is broadly revealing and instructive. It affords insight into basic and elemental psychopathological processes. It is, no doubt, for this reason that the condition has engaged the deep interest of so many competent men, among them our own Schilder.

BIBLIOGRAPHY*

FEDERN, P.: Some variations in ego-feeling. *Internat. J. Psychoanal.*, 7: 434, 1926.

———: Narcissism in the structure of the ego. *Internat J. Psychoanal.*, 9: 401, 1928.

GRIESINGER, W.: *Mental Pathology and Therapeutics.* London: 1867.

GUTHEIL, E.: Depersonalization. *Psychoanalyt. Rev.*, 17: 26, 1930.

HAUG, KARL: *Die Storungen des Personlichkeits Bewusstseins.* Stuttgart: F. Enke, 1936.

HESNARD, A.: *La signification psychoanalytique des sentiments dits "dépersonnalisation."* *Rev. franc. de psychanal.*, 1: 87, 1927.

JANET, P.: *Les Obsessions et la Psychasthénie.* Paris: 1903.

———: *Le Sentiment de Dépersonnalisation.* Paris: 1908.

———: *Psychological Strength and Weakness in Mental Disease.* Cambridge, Mass.: Harvard University Press, 1937.

KIRSHABER, M.: *De la Névropathie Cérébrocardiaque.* Paris: 1873.

LÖWY, H.: Die aktionsgefühle. *Prague. med. Wchnschr.* 1908.

MALAMUD, W.: The sense of reality in mental disease. *Arch. Neurol. & Psychiat.*, 23: 761, 1930.

MAYER-GROSS, W.: On depersonalization. *Brit. J. M. Psychol.*, 15: 103, 1935.

MORGENSTERN, S.: Psychoanalytic conception of depersonalization. *"Journal of Nervous and Mental Disease,"* 73: 164, 1931.

NUNBERG, H.: Ueber depersonalisationszustände im lichte der libidotheorie. *Internat. Ztschr. f. Psychoanal.*, 10: 17, 1924.

OBERNDORF, C. P.: Depersonalization in relation to erotization of thought. *Internal. J. Psychoanal.*, 15: 271, 1934.

———: Feeling of unreality. *Arch. Neurol. & Psychiat.*, 36: 322, 1936.

OESTERREICH, T. K.: *Die Phaenomenologie des Ich in ihren Grundproblemen.* Leipzig: 1910.

PICK, A.: Zur pathologie des ich bewusstseins. *Arch. f. Psychiat.*, 38: 22, 1904.

RIBOT, T.: *Diseases of Memory.* London: 1882.

SCHILDER, P.: Selbstbewusstsein and Persönlichkeitsbewusstsein. *Monographien aus dem Gesemtgebiete der Neurol. u. Psychiat.* Berlin: 1914, vol. 9.

———: *Entwurf zu einer Psychiatrie auf Psychoanalyt.* Leipzig: 1925.

———: *The Image and Appearance of the Human Body.* in Psyche Monographs. No. 4. London: 1935.

———: *Goals and Desires of Man.* New York: Columbia University Press, 1942.

SEARL, M. H.: Note on depersonalization. *Internal J. Psychoanal.*, 13: 345, 1932.

STEKEL: *Die 'Sprache des Traumes.* Ed. 3, Berlin: 1927.

STOERRING, E.: Die depersonalisation. *Ztschr. d. Neurol. u. Psychiat*, 98: 462, 1933.

TAINE, H.: *De l'Intelligence.* Paris: 1870.

WEBER, A.: Ueber nihilistischen whan und depersonalization. *Abh. a. d. Neurol. Psychiat., Psychol.* 1938.

WITTELS, F.: Psychology and treatment of depersonalization. *Psychoanalyt. Rev.*, 27: no. 1, 1940.

---

*This is a selected bibliography, drawn from a much more extensive list of of works which I have found directly pertinent to the points of view treated in this contribution.—I.G.

6

Prophylactic Psychopathology: The Rationality of the Irrational in Psychodynamics

THE APPRECIATION of the essential rationality of the irrational we owe to Sigmund Freud, who propounded and demonstrated it, specifically in his *Psychopathology of Everyday Life,* and more generally and consistently in his elaborations of psychoanalytic theory. It is not my intention therefore to reargue or to elaborate upon such matters as the forgetting of names and words or the making of mistakes.

I intend rather to analyze the significance in psychodynamics of grossly irrational, and crucially determining actions which are highly complicated and which are deliberately, that is not unconsciously, executed by otherwise seemingly intelligent persons. It is my intention to demonstrate that while in the perspective of the collective norm such actions are not only irrational but also patently neurotic, they are in effect, in the internal psychodynamic tension states of the individual, neither irrational nor neurotic, but rather reactive and sanitizing. I hope also to throw light on certain problems involved in the therapeutic reconciliation of the patient with his own past irrationalities, for, in my experience, unless a reconciliation is effected, the patient is not fully cured, and is likely to suffer a rankling, self-recriminating, self-disparaging, compulsively fixated preoccupation with his so-called "stupidities."

To illustrate and to support my thesis I will cite, rather briefly, three cases. These I might add, have successfully completed therapy, and are now living full and effective lives. In describing the persons involved I have for understandable reasons altered certain superficial particulars, but I have in no respect tampered with the psychiatric data. Each case involves a woman. The first to be described was in her middle forties; the second was in her middle twenties; the third had just turned twenty. Each of the patients was exceptionally well gifted, physically, in intelligence and otherwise. They were also well educated.

The oldest of the three was the wife of a banker, and the mother of two children, both in their teens. To all appearance she had led a satisfactory married life, and had drawn some pleasure in sharing her husband's business affairs and activities, in caring for their two children, and in being active in a modest social circle. Shortly before she came under therapy, while her husband was abroad, this patient *ran away* with her masseur. She left her children behind (they were away in camp), withdrew a substantial sum of money from the bank, took her husband's car, and with her masseur set out for parts unknown. She left a letter for her husband in which she upbraided him for many and sundry faults, sins, and crimes. She did not tell him that she was running away with someone, nor what she thought or wished to do about their marriage and their children. She just ran away!

To fully appreciate the utter irrationality of this action so freighted with grievous consequences, one needs to bear in mind that the patient was a soft-spoken, gentle, and well educated person. The masseur was a man, some twenty years older than she, married, poorly educated, and as it turned out, a rather pathological personality not above taking both her money and her car, and threatening to make a scandal, when he was later asked to return the spoils. She had known him only a few months before taking off with him. His ambition was to go West, and to open a saloon. She was to provide the funds and to help him run it.

Neither of the "elopees" thought to change the license plates of the car, and so the police were easily able to follow their transcontinental trek. On my counsel no police action, other than keeping check of their whereabouts, was taken. When they reached their journey's end the husband went forth to fetch his wife and had no difficulties in bringing back with him a contrite, bewildered, and much depressed person—up to then, so gentle, pliant, and obedient a mate. I might add that the husband, though not at all contrite, was yet as much bewildered, and depressed, as his wife.

Contemplating this experience as an episodic unit one must ask, just what is its dynamic significance in the life of the patient; what function did it serve in her psychic economy? However, before attempting to find the answer I want to make certain that we understand the question precisely. Here we want and need to know not primarily *why she ran away*, but rather *what the running away did for her*. For an action is not alone the resultant of definable antecedent psychic determinants, and itself a powerful and fateful determinant of subsequent psychic states and of behavior; but over and above all this, it is of profound import to the psychic economy of the patient. Its very irrationality, and the deliberateness of its execution more than suggest that it has an uncommon function, that it is the witness of some crucial intra-psychic adaptation, readjustment, or compensation. It serves to reestablish psychic homeostasis. It is my impression that while we pay close attention to, and minutely analyze the derivations of such irrational behaviors, we commonly overlook the inherent (as against the derivative) significance, that is the psychodynamic function of the actions. This fault, I believe, arises in the unwarranted assumption that if we know *why* the person did a something, we know all we need to know about the act. Of course such is not the case at all, first because conceivably the antecedent determinants could find expression and issue in a variety of different actions, and second because the actually effected action cannot but have dynamic significance and meaning independent of its antecedent determinants.

I have already committed myself on this score, affirming it as my conviction that the irrational act of the type under consideration has the effect of sanitizing, that is of rendering the person *sane* or whole. It serves to equilibrate the psychological dynamics of the person involved. Before advancing the argument further, I am impelled to once again underscore that the crucial factor in our inquiry is not *why* a given action took place, but rather what the dynamic significance of that action is in the psychological configuration of the *Actor*.

Let me illustrate the issue by citing a case given by Freud. This case, I must observe, is remote from those we are considering, since it involves the so-called accidental loss of a prized object, and not the deliberate execution of a complicated, grossly irrational and fateful action. But it will serve to accentuate the difference between the *why* of an action, and the *import* of this action to the actor. The case is as follows.

A man lost a highly prized mechanical pencil which he had had for two years. Analysis elicited the following facts: "The day before, he had received a very disagreeable letter from his brother-in-law. . . . The effect connected with this letter was so powerful that the next day he promptly sacrificed the pencil which was a present from his brother-in-law in order not to be burdened with his favors." (pp. 239, 240, Psychopathology of Everyday Life, N.Y., Macmillan, 1919). Here we are told "why" he lost the prized pencil, that is, because he had received a disagreeable letter. But, we do not know just what import the action of losing the pencil had to the offended man. The guess that it was in order not to be burdened with his brother-in-law's favors is hardly impressive. One might speculate why the man didn't break the pencil, or misplace it. But in the end, the really crucial question is: What did the man gain or accomplish by losing the pencil? This inquiry is quite different from the one that asks—*why* did the man lose the pencil?

At this point I want to briedfly describe the other two cases. The older of the two, in her middle twenties, married, the mother of a young child, when abroad with her husband and child, once gave a rendezvous to three men, her husband, her lover, and an older man who was seeking her favors, at one designated place, and for the identical time. The three arrived at the specified place, *at* the same time. As a consequence she was full of confusion and bewilderment, not knowing what prompted her to do something so utterly "stupid." This was not the only instance of irrational behavior in her rather complicated and trying life. But it was patently singularly irrational. Yet this young woman was inherently neither stupid nor irrational. On the contrary, the fact that she survived all the ordeals and vicissitudes of her young life attests to her inborn good sense, her fine intuition, and her keen intelligence. But all this made more prominently stark the irrationality of that "multiple rendezvous."

The third patient was a young woman just turned twenty. She was a beautiful, statuesque person, gifted in languages and music, and with fine aesthetic sensibilities. She was an earnest youngster, eager to marry, and to have a home and children. Yet, while still in college, this young woman managed to invite and to accomplish being raped. Then she seduced a man some ten years her senior, first to have sexual relations with her, and then to become engaged to her. Subsequently she abandoned the engagement and went abroad, ostensibly to continue her studies. This, as a matter of fact, she did in a measure. But more prominent in her experiences abroad was first, a number of casual affairs, and then a liaison with an older, well educated but deeply neurotic man. The failure of this liaison and certain resultant complications brought her under therapy.

I am aware that this last case is seemingly quite different from the two preceding cases cited. The actions here reported are not as patently nor as grossly irrational. They resemble more closely the type of behavior which we designate as simply neurotic. Despite this I deem this case to be on a par with the others, not simply neurotic, but characterized by irrational behavior which yet has a rationality in the psychodynamics of the patient.

Here we come up against a troubling question. In the broad sense of that term all neurotic behavior is irrational, while at the same time it is also meaningful. What then distinguishes the cases I have cited from the general run of neurotic cases and what renders the rationality of *their* irrational actions particularly distinct and significant? Are they not all alike, simply particular instances of psychopathology? To this the parabolic answer is that surely they are all instances of psychopathology, but that as particular instances they are sufficiently distinctive to constitute a unique order of pathology. In order to argue the issue further I want to call upon the experience and evidence of *clinical pathology.* Here too, ever since the time of Virchow, it has been understood that all pathological phenomena are meaningful, and biologically rational. But over and above this valid generalization, it has been demonstrated that some pathology is *anaphylactic* in ultimate effect, while some is *prophylactic;* in other words some reactions serve to advance the disease, while others favor the sufferer's recovery. Perhaps one of the most interesting and most impressive illustrations of these two orders of pathological reactions, i.e. anaphylactic and prophylactic, is witnessed in the so-called Koch phenomenon in tuberculosis. Koch observed that when a guinea pig is inoculated subcutaneously with a minimal dose of tubercle bacilli, it develops in time a chronic tuberculous ulcer at the site of the inoculation. If it is then inoculated subcutaneously with tuberculosis a second time at a different site, there will again develop a tuberculous ulcer at the second site, but this ulcer instead of remaining chronic, will in time slough off, and the tissue involved will heal over. The allergic changes following on the original infection result in what amounts to prophylactic pathology in relation to the second inoculation. It favors the animal's recovery at the site of the second "injury." That is all to the good when the tissue involved is the skin. But if instead of the skin the lungs become involved in a secondary infection, then what was a prophylactic reaction in the skin becomes an anaphylactic reaction in the lungs, for the sloughing off of the involved tissue results in lung caseation and cavity formation, both of which drag the patient down. Parenthetically I might add that the rationale of the use of B.C.G. vaccine lies in the belief that its use will yield prophylactic results and block the anaphylactic sequences of ordinary tuberculosis infection.

I am sure you will gather from this that I consider the three cases I cited as instances of "prophylactic pathology." The rationality of the irrational in the psychodynamics of these cases is to be witnessed in the fact that their irrational actions served to help them regain a measure of inner ego balance. In the longer run it favored not their disease but rather their recovery and maturation.

Before detailing the dynamics of the rationality in the irrational, I am prompted to offer a second and simpler illustration of what I have termed prophylactic pathology. The normal peristalsis of the gastro-intestinal tract, at least in the lower two-thirds of the esophagus, is in the direction from the mouth to the anus. Reversal of peristolic movement is therefore always indicative of pathology. Vomiting, by that token, is pathological. But as can be easily appreciated, though essentially pathological, it can also be prophylactic, as when by emesis the body ejects noxious matter. In such an instance the action is still pathological in character but sanitizing in effect.

That, basically, was the essential quality and effect of the irrational actions of the cases cited; though they were pathological in character their effects were sanitizing. The patients gained a something which favored their well-being.

Now let us see how this actually worked out in the cases cited. Of necessity I'll have to be rather saltatory and brief in my accounts, but the gross pattern will, I believe, be clear enough. Thus, as I am sure you anticipated, the first patient was, despite all appearances, far from happy in her marriage. The actuality was that she had been the long suffering mate of a self-centered, demanding and domineering man, who had "seduced" her when she was rather young, and who married her only after she had threatened to commit suicide. Though she was by far the better educated of the two, he was the older and the more worldly. She looked up to him when she first met him, and for many years thereafter. Time and experience taught her so assess him more realistically, but she was unable to readjust her relations with her husband so as to bring them in line with reality. He persisted in considering and in treating her as he did when she was a youngster of eighteen, ignorant of and inexperienced in life. Why at eighteen she was both ignorant and inexperienced is "the tale of her antecedent years" and its exposition would serve to illuminate the *why* of her marriage, and the reasons for her irrational elopement. But since my concern is primarily to make clear the meaning of the action itself rather than of its determinants, I must ask you to "pick up" the story of the case at the time of the elopement. Confronted with the frustrating circumstances of her life she seemingly had but few ways out. She might, but palpably did not want to continue to submit and to suffer the degrading position in which she was placed. She could not directly confront her husband and amiably or reasonably work out with him a realignment of their respective positions. He would not be responsive to such an approach and could not for lack of insight appreciate any need for a reassessment of their relations. He was happy in his position and could see no warrant for change. Any hint of dissatisfaction on her part he could credit to her "queerness," and to her unreasonableness. Thus entrapped in what amounted to totally frustrating circumstances, she took what to her seemed to be the only way out: the elopement. I need not underscore the fact that at the time of her elopement she had only the acute awareness of her long endured frustrations, and no insight at all as to the significance of her actions. Her behavior was that of a woman who "could stand it no longer," and not that of a clever, intriguing, conspirator who aimed to attain her goals by devious routes and manipulations. That in the end her actions did lead to a workable and tolerable adjustment in her relations with her husband was not the immediate resultant of her deliberate intentions but rather the effects of what I have termed the prophylactic pathology which she "suffered." Some credit must also be assigned to her therapy, but it is conceivable that she would not have come for therapy did not the "cataclysmic impact" of her elopement jolt her husband into the realization that he really "didn't understand."

The wife's elopement did in actuality have a cataclysmic effect upon the husband. He discovered that not only did he need his wife for such common uses, domestic and business, as he was wont to have, but that indeed he loved her. His dismay at her departure overshadowed his feeling of outrage. He was more eager to have her back than to be avenged on her or her paramour. In effect then she did achieve what to her was vitally necessary, that is, not only the evidence of being wanted, and of being loved by her husband, but also the show and the recognition of her native power and her prestige position in the complex of her family. Heretofore she was as nothing, and by this grossly hazardous and highly irrational action she did achieve some ultimate rationality in her life.

I am naturally aware of the many other ramifications of this case and some of these must come to your mind. I cannot, however, and do not want to deal with them now. I need only cite so much of the case as is requisite to the illumination of the rationality of the irrational in psychodynamics. Before leaving this case I do, however, want to underscore several small but significant items which highlight the indwelling intelligence of the irrational behavior. Thus it is patent that this woman eloped with a man who could hardly have ever proved satisfactory as a life's companion. He was too old, too much below her in education and in social position. There is in this more than a suggestion that had she been in earnest (on the unconscious level) she would have elected a more likely and more acceptable partner. As it was, her elopement could not *stick*. That she did not change car plates is to my mind an added witness that she unconsciously wanted the elopement to be an "escapade" rather than an "escape." That she elected to run away with a masseur, who in the gradiant of her husband's social scale would rank "beneath his dignity" also has its significance, among other things suggesting the order of intimate concern, preoccupation and satisfaction which she craved but did not obtain from her husband. Nor was it entirely accidental that the elopement occurred shortly before the husband returned from Europe and while the children were away at camp. Indeed on close inspection the elopment has the craft marks of a clever, very clever dramaturge who plotted on the theme that "all is well that ends well."

Because of the relatively ample treatment of the first case I can be more compact in dealing with the other two. The second case as will be recalled was that of "the triple, simultaneous rendezvous." The essential facts in this case are as follows. The patient was the daughter of a world famous artist. She was born abroad, and came to America during her early teens. Her parents were divorced when she was very young. Her mother remarried shortly after the divorce. But the patient spent most of her childhood and youth in boarding schools. She did live in her mother's home for awhile, but that had tragic consequences, for the mother by this time had become a chronic alcoholic, and upon the child fell largely the burden of caring for her mother during her alcoholic stupors, and during the painful periods of contrition that followed on sobriety. The patient saw but little of her father. She was a good student, indeed somewhat precocious. She went to college in the Midwest, and while she relished academic and campus life, she suffered deeply from loneliness and the feeling that she was, as she phrased it, a "universal orphan." Her mother's unexpected death interrupted her college life, and brought her back to New York. Here she made the acquaintance of a sympathetic but neurotic and inadequate young man. He fell in love with her and persuaded her to marry him. He won her consent, substantially because he offered her a home. But it was his mother's rather than a separate home. His mother was amicably separated from her husband, and lived with her grown-up son, she providing all the wherewithal, and he "pursuing the arts." My patient's marriage meant the acquisition of a child's home and the equivalent of a mother, rather than the fulsome adventures and experiences of wifehood and domesticity. Yet what she gained in marriage, even at this level, was so much greater than what she had had before, that she was for a while quite happy and content. Parenthetically it may be added that at that time she probably would not and could not have undertaken a marriage that would have exacted the taking on of greater responsibilities and the fulfilment of greater obligations. At any rate, for some time both she and her husband, and also her mother-in-law were happy living together. "It was quite like a doll's house." But then, my patient found herself pregnant, and the "doll's house" was thrown into a turmoil. Practically everyone, even including her father, urged her to have the pregnancy aborted. But she stood out against all such counsel and carried her child to term. This involved much heroic effort on her part, for no one in her immediate circle was able to give her much attention or support.

The birth of her son had a profound effect upon her husband. He was incapable of the role of parent, and he resented not only the intrusion of the stranger, but also the loss of his playmate, his wife. He made an abortive and unconscious attempt at suicide, inhaling a vaporized insecticide, and thereafter complained of a variety of nervous disturbances.

The mother, thinking a stay abroad would help, and probably also to be relieved of the troublesome mess, sent the young family to Europe. She paid for their trip and gave them a monthly allowance. The money was sent to the husband, and my patient, without any resources of her own, was dependent upon him for everything.

The sexual life of the couple was fairly satisfactory during the early marriage period. But when the wife became pregnant, and increasingly thereafter, the husband found fault with her in various ways. Concomitantly the frequency and satisfaction of their sexual relations declined. After the birth of the child and the phantom suicide attempt, the husband entirely ceased to cohabit with his wife. He repeatedly disparaged her, describing her as ugly and sexually repugnant. At this point, the patient developed an intimate relation with a friend of her husband, the so-called lover of the triad. But this man too was rather weak and inadequate. The husband knew of his wife's relations with this friend and tolerated them without protest. The friend on the other hand accepted conditions as they were, and made no attempt to change them. My patient's intimacies with the friend of her husband gave her little ego satisfaction. At this point irrationality broke through and she made a rendezvous with her husband, her lover, and an older man who had been pursuing her for some time. The result, of course, was tragi-comical. The three met, regarded each other and her with some astonishment, spoke of inconsequentials, and left, each to go his own way. She remained behind to ponder on her "folly." And as she pondered it she forged the resolution to resolve her nightmarish existence. She decided to return home, without her husband. She appealed to her father and he gave her the money for her return. Shortly thereafter she came for therapy.

Seeking for the rationality in her irrational actions one can perceive that "the triple rendezvous" had for its ultimate purpose, and indeed had the effect, of bolstering and replenishing her all-too-severely battered and depleted ego. In a subtle way she cancelled out, she counterbalanced each of the trio with one or both of the others; the husband with the lover; the weakling lover with the older man, and the older man with both. This collective trio of suppliants, past, present, and future, somehow gave her a sense of being desirable, for two sought the very favors which her husband disparaged. Furthermore in contriving it so that none gained her favor, though they came in hope, she had the satisfaction of being in the dominant position. I speak here as if the rendezvous had been plotted and the results anticipated. That was true only on the unconscious level. On the conscious level she knew only that she was impelled to bring the three men together at one time in one place. And when they came she was flustered, confused and angry with herself for being so "stupid." Yet, as indicated, following on this irrationality she took effective steps to set her life aright. One interesting point is to be noted here, that concerning the older man. Just why was she impelled to exhibit him to the other two? Why was she not content to merely reject his advances? The dynamics for her behavior became clear during her therapy. The older man won her sympathies by first playing the role of the experienced counselor. He thus served her as a father substitute. When he declared himself to be in love with her, and attempted sexual intimacies, she felt betrayed and traduced, and reacted accordingly.

The third case I will describe even more briefly. The patient was the only girl in a family of three children. Her mother was an illegitimate child, and the first of her own children, a boy, was conceived out of wedlock and foisted as his own on the man she married, my patient's father. The mother revealed this deceit some ten years after her marriage. The father had been married once before, and had been abandoned by his first wife. The marriage of which my patient was issue was never good. The partners quarelled, and were in constant conflict. My patient was literally caught between them. The father was fond of his daughter and when she grew into young womanhood became even more devoted to her. This antagonized the mother and caused her to pour all her wrath upon the child's head. She charged her with "playing up to father," of taking his side against her, and in general of failing to do her part as a dutiful daughter. She edged her out of the house, exiling her to a boarding school. All this of course only served to embitter and thus to worsen relations between husband and wife. A paranoid-like reaction chain was thus engendered. The more the father defended the daughter the more certain the mother was that her daughter conspired against her. In this paranoid-like cycle, the mother further and more intensively abused the daughter, charging her now, among other things, with gross immorality, with incest, and with other forms of sexual promiscuity. As can be readily appreciated, though the father favored the daughter, and defended her against the mother, he was not effective as a parent and was no counter-foil to the mother's abuse. He could only protest, he could not undo or even compensate for the mother's hurt. In these circumstances, which were further complicated by the patient's failure when at college to "make a sorority," and by her awareness of her social gaucheness and her lack of experience, she broke through *irrationally*. She contrived to get herself raped, and became thus at one and the same time the center of a minor "cause célèbre," and an "experienced woman." Father came out to see that the right thing was done. She transferred to another and for her a more acceptable college. Mother for the time was frightened, and hence less abusive.

The next move was to seduce a male co-student, some years her senior, to have sexual relations with her and to become engaged to her. He, however, proved rather weak and uninteresting, and so she dropped the engagement, then persuaded her father to send her abroad, ostensibly to continue her studies. I have already detailed her experiences in Europe, these including several promiscuous affairs, and a more earnest and endur-ing love relation with an older, highly educated and badly neurotic man. The failure of this love affair was the decisive experience that brought her under therapy.

In analyzing the dynamics of this patient's irrationality it is patent that she was caught between a "castrating" mother and an "incestuous" father. She resolved both conflict and tension situations by cancelling out one against the other—the incest tension *and the* castration menace, first in the rape episode, then in the seduction of the co-student. Her flight to Europe and the subsequent adventures, winding up in her more mature love affair with the older man, were in effect an extension of her equilibra-tion process. When on her return from Europe, disillusioned in her last love relationship, she came for therapy she was ready to "integrate" both of her parents and to function effectively within the framework of her reality as an adult woman.

I trust that in delineating the essentials in these cases I have at least made clear the meaning of what I intend by the rationality of the irrational in psychodynamics. Now I am impelled to develop in greater detail the basic physiological function of this involved process which I have also designated as prophylactic pathology. First, however, I would recall to your minds, a saying common among the older analysts and psychotherapists, to wit, "the neurosis is always right." I must confess, when I first heard it from my old mentor, Brill, I didn't quite understand it. How could the neurosis be right since it was precisely the neurosis of which the patient needed to be relieved? But I discovered in time that the phrase was intended in a particular sense, to wit, that the neurosis must be permitted to work itself through in its own unique way. In that respect we are required to be not only permissive but also patient and *very* understanding. Concretely what happens is that despite our own best efforts and also those of our patients, they, the patients, at times persist in pursuing a line of action or a pattern of existence which is not only neurotic in character but even destructive in effect, all this as I have said despite full insight both into the derivation and the quality of the action. This pattern of behavior, *during therapy,* is in some ways even more baffling than such instances of "behavior irrationality" antecedent to therapy as I have exemplified in the three cases cited. In both instances, however, and under both circumstances, outside and in therapy, the psychophysiological process is identical. Stated at its simplest: it is prerequisite to a change in polarity that a full potential of the opposite polarity be first established. This is a principle which the wisdom of the populace has embodied in such wise saws as "It's darkest ere dawn," and "It always gets worse before it gets better." It is the principle which Norbert Wiener has so brilliantly expounded in his *Cybernetics.* Here we see a concrete instance of his negative feed-back pattern. Indeed we can clearly conceptualize the very radical difference between what I have designated as prophylactic pathology, and the psychopathology of say the compulsive, obsessive or paranoid case, which is anaphylactic in character, by thinking of the first as operating in an effective feedback circuit, and the second in a defective circuit. Wiener describes both types of circuits; the first being of the negative order and the second of the positive. The positive feed-back pattern results not in "homeostasis" but in accelerated oscillation or, as Wiener phrases it, "in noise rather than communication."

The aforegoing, to my mind, validates and illuminates the empirically derived principle reflected in the dictum "the neurosis is always right."

And now one thing remains to be said, that concerning the treatment of the type of patient described in this contribution. It is not enough for the therapist to understand the dynamics of the patient's behavior, and to utilize this understanding in effective therapy. It is imperative that the patients themselves should comprehend the rationale of their irrational actions, and that they should be emotionally reconciled to them. Failing to do this they will carry with them a rankling, self-recriminating, self-disparaging, compulsively fixated preoccupation with their so-called "stupidities." The preoccupation may be encapsulated, but will be a complex, in the true sense of that term, and will drain the patient's libido. To reconcile the patient with his irrational behavior it is first necessary to lay bare to him the deeper dynamics of his behavior. This involves more expositional and didactic effort and a different role from that which the therapist is accustomed to put forth and to play. It also involves a change in "stance," the patient being taken, so to say, behind the scenes, to witness the play of the psychotherapist's own judgment and knowledge.

This implies some indoctrination in fundamental psychodynamics and some specific anatomizing of the patient's psychopathology. Ordinarily such indoctrination is undesirable, but in the instances defined here it is imperatively necessary. For the patient cannot integrate his irrationality on the basis of the "transference indulgence" afforded him by his therapist. The conflict which he faces is the derivative of a transgression, not against others, whom the therapist may represent and "take over," but against his own multi-part ego. He must work through his conflict deeply and thoroughly, or he'll have no peace.

I leave this subject with the conviction that there is vastly more in it than I have been able to elaborate. Much remains to be explored and expounded on the difference in the patho-dynamics of the so-termed prophylactic and anaphylactic psychopathologies.

7

Psychiatry and the Maverick

SPEAKING IN THE NAME OF Socrates, Plato in the Phaedrus states, "There are two kinds of madness, one resulting from human ailments, the other from a divine disturbance of our conventions of conduct" (1). Of the divine kind, Plato distinguishes four types, each ascribed to one of the gods. Thus the inspiration of the prophet is credited to Apollo, that of the mystic to Dionysus, that of the poet to the Muses, and the fourth, the madness of the lover, to Aphrodite and Eros.

In a previous exchange between Socrates and Phaedrus, Plato had affirmed that madness is not invariably an evil. "In reality," he stated, "the greatest blessings come by way of madness—that is heaven sent" (2). And Plato further observes, "Madness was accounted no shame nor disgrace by the men of old, who gave things their names; otherwise they would not have connected that greatest of arts, whereby the future is discerned, with this very word, 'madness' and named it accordingly" (3).

And by way of summing up that portion of the dialogue, Socrates concludes, "So let us have no fears simply on that score; let us not be disturbed by an argument that seeks to scare us into preferring the friendship of the sane to that of the passionate" (4).

The concept of divine madness was common to Greek thought. Professor E. R. Dodds, in his scholarly work *The Greeks and the Irrational* (5), points out that it was Democritus who first talked about poetic ecstasy, maintaining that the finest poems were those composed with inspiration and by the holy breath. Democritus denied that anyone could be a great poet *sine furore* (6). If any man come to the gates of poetry,"

Throughout this paper the terms maverick, gifted person and genius are used interchangeably. This usage is explained at the end.

86

Socrates affirmed, "without the madness of the Muses, persuaded that skill alone will make him a good poet, then shall he and his works of sanity, with him be brought to naught . . ." (7).

In this connection it is of interest to recall the cryptic story of an encounter between Democritus and Hippocrates, the latter having been summoned to Abdera to treat Democritus, considered by his co-citizens to have turned mad. In the story it is related that Hippocrates came away from this encounter persuaded not only that Democritus was not mad, but that, on the contrary, he had plumbed the depths of human wisdom. Mad were those who counted Democritus mad (8).*

Hippocrates, as is well appreciated, excluded the gods from the pathodynamics of human disease. The gods had no share in the engenderment of the so-termed Sacred Disease, nor in any other human disorder (9). Hippocrates, in other words, was no Platonist, and in general he eschewed the philosophers and their speculations.

Hippocrates traced all thinking and feeling, both in health and in disease, to the one *organ*—the brain. "Men ought to know," wrote Hippocrates, in the off-quoted passage from the *Sacred Disease*, "that from the brain, and from the brain only, arise our pleasures, joys, laughter and jests, as well as our sorrows, pains, griefs and tears. . . . It is the same thing which makes us mad or delirious, inspires us with dread and fear, whether by night or by day, brings sleeplessness, inopportune mistakes, aimless anxieties, absentmindedness, and acts that are contrary to habit. These things that we suffer all come from the brain when it is not healthy. . . ." The corruption of the brain Hippocrates charged to phlegm and to bile (10).

Plato's division of madness into the constitutional and the divine was not favored by the generations of Greek and Roman philosophers and physicians who came after him.

Nor did the pupil and later critic of Plato, the most learned of men— Aristotle—accept the Platonic category of divine madness. Where Plato perceived the influence of Apollonian inspiration—the order of madness that is heaven sent—Aristotle, quite as Hippocrates, saw only the effects of black bile. In the book *Problemata* Aristotle asks, and answers, the rhetorical question, "How does it happen that all those who have achieved pre-eminence in philosophy, politics, literature or art clearly are of a black

---

*This story, of course, is no more than an artful conceit, one that was elaborated at a later date in the fictitious and forged correspondence alleged to have passed between Hippocrates and Democritus.

bile temperament and some among them sicken because of their black bile—even as among the Heroes it befell Heracles?" (11).

In effect the concept of divine madness was not propagated beyond the time of Plato. Those among the ancients who treated of madness, of the disorder of the mind—Galen, Soranus, Aretaeus of Capadochia, Caelius Aurelinus, Celsus—considered the disorder to be caused by physical agents and conditions. There was, for those who treated of the matter, but one order of madness, that resulting from human ailments. There was no credence in any other order— and none in divine madness.

Neither Plato nor Aristotle had any followers competent to propagate and to elaborate their master's teachings. More significantly, it was not long after the founding of Aristotle's Lyceum in 335 B.C. that Greek civilization entered upon a slow progressive decline.

In the third century B.C., Greek civilization, in the words of Professor Dodds, was entering not as it would seem on the Age of Reason, but rather on a period of slow intellectual decline which was to last, with some deceptive rallies and some brilliant rearguard actions, down to the capture of Byzantinum by the Turks. In all the sixteen centuries of existence still awaiting it, the Hellenic world produced no poet as good as Theocritus, no scientist as good as Eratosthenes, no mathematician as good as Archimedes, and the one great name in philosophy and the philosophic viewpoint he engendered, transcendental Platonism, was believed to be extinct (12).

But as history was to demonstrate later, transcendental Platonism was not extinct but only dormant. When classical culture was reborn in the Renaissance, Plato also returned to life. Transcendental Platonism was transmuted and absorbed into Christianity. Plato's divine madness was rechristened the poet's inspiration and, for the believing, in St. Augustine's phrase, "divine illumination."

Having discussed at some length the origin and destiny of the Platonic category of divine madness, and because we are shortly to deal with its modern equivalents, it is here pertinent to establish, as clearly as we can, what Plato intended and what we understand by divine madness. One thing is certain; divine madness embraced nothing of the widely held belief that all types of mental disease are caused by supernatural interference—the belief that so tragically prevailed during the late medieval period. On the score of madness "resulting from *human ailments*," Plato was as well informed, if not as experienced, as Hippocrates. This is impressively reflected in the book titled *Laws* (XI-934). Therein Plato wrote, "Now there are many lunatics and their lunacy takes many different forms.

In the case just mentioned it springs from disease, but there is another source of lunatics who owe their madness to an unhappy native tendency to angry passion, further strengthened by ill training, a kind of men whom any trifling dissention will provoke to clamorous and scurrilous reviling of each other, conduct always and totally out of place in a well ordered society" (13).

Plato's divine madness had only this in common with madness per se, that it, too, effected a disturbance of the "conventions of conduct." But it differed from madness per se essentially in this—that it took nothing away from man. It was, on the contrary, a gift, Apollo's gift to the elect. It was the gift of Apolline mediumship "which aims at knowledge, whether of the future or of the hidden present" (14). Divine madness was thus the gift and the destiny of the gifted man, the Eternal Maverick.

Here it may profit us to conjecture why Plato was so deeply concerned with divine, with Apolline madness, why he termed it a madness, and was so keen to distinguish it from the other madnesses. Most likely, this preoccupation derives from the experience of his own life, for Plato himself was, after Prometheus and before Christ, one of the greatest among the historic mavericks. "Plato's contemplative life," writes Werner Jaeger (15) "was not a gentle retirement, but was imposed by the tragic opposition of destiny to a natural ruler born out of his time." Not all mavericks take refuge in a contemplative life, but they are all, in varying measures, "out of time." They cannot be otherwise, and from this derives their divine madness.

In his Apology, Socrates pleaded that he could not but attend to the voice of his inner god, his daimonion (16). That *was* his madness, and it cost him his life. Plato recognized the compelling force of divine madness. Plato never urged that Socrates should have behaved in any other way. He never says that the jury (who condemned Socrates) could have been wiser or better. It was, Plato affirms, inevitable for both sides to be what they were, and fate took its unalterable course (17). This Platonic position attests to Plato's penetrating understanding of destiny's unalterable course. For given the jury, the normal, and *the maverick*, the upper variant, condemnation was inevitable. In the deepest sense of destiny, the two are interlocked. Without the normal there can be no maverick, and there is divine madness only because the others are so very sane. Yet Plato was not totally fatalistic about fate. Had he thought it completely unalterable he would not have conceived nor composed his great Republic.

There is a timeless issue in the tragedy of Socrates and it is revealed most clearly in Plato's struggle to fathom it. This issue remains unsolved to this very day, and to this very day the pursuit of its solution revolves about the Platonic ideas of *Paideia* and *Arete*, terms which are only meanly translated as education and excellence. Paideia, according to Plato, could be practiced but arete could only be cultivated, provided, of course, the potential of arete was initially given. Now, the gift of arete is the singular mark of the maverick. It is this which distinguishes him from all the rest. Socrates consistently sought out the exceptional young men, fit for the highest intellectual and moral culture, for these and their like possess quick intelligence, good memory, and eagerness to learn. Yet for all their gifts, unless they are properly educated, such men cannot attain all they want to and at the same time make others happy. This caveat should be noted clearly for herein lies the core problem of the maverick —of the upper variant; how to attain what he would in arete and at the same time make others happy; in existential terms, how to be and yet escape the hemlock cup.

Socrates had great faith in education, meaning paideia. Until he was confronted with the charges of corrupting the youth of Athens, he had no doubt but that the people, the demos, would favor the order of education he avowed and practiced. Not even when he was warned that disaster might strike him, as in the words spoken by Callicles, the Athenian man of the world, the realist in the *Georgias* (18), Socrates remained uninvolved, seemingly disbelieving the warnings. He said he did not fear "for no one who is not utterly irrational and cowardly is afraid of the mere fact of dying; it is evildoing he fears" (19).

Plato himself, be it noted, was not so sanguine either about education or the demos. When Socrates was executed, Plato, together with the other disciples of Socrates, fled to Megara.

Plato's *Republic*, considered with *Laws* as the greatest of his works, is structured as a utopia, that is, a hope beyond the range of realization. At the end of Book IX of the *Republic*, when the perfect state has finally been constructed, Adimantis (who with Glaucon, both brothers of Plato, sustained the dialogue with Socrates) says, "I think it (the envisioned Republic) can be found nowhere on earth." "Perhaps," answers Socrates, "there is a pattern of it hidden up in heaven for him who wishes to contemplate it. But it makes no difference whether it exists now or will ever come into being" (20).

Plato's immediate and intimate sense of discouragement, amounting almost to despair, yet a despair fringed with some remote hopes, can be gathered from his known letters, notably the one numbered seven. This letter is addressed to the friends and companions of Dion of Syracuse.

In this letter Plato comments on the execution of Socrates—"the justest man of his time" (21), on the treacheries of the tyrant of Syracuse, Dionysus the younger, and on the assassination of Plato's intimate friend Dion. "The human race," Plato wrote, "will not see better days until either the stock of those who rightly and genuinely follow philosophy acquire political authority, or else the class who have political control be led by some dispensation of the providence to become real philosophers" (22).

Plato himself took no part in the government of Athens and, anticipating the query why he had never addressed the Assembly, he wrote that "Plato was born late in his country's history, and the people, when he came to them, were already rather well on in years and had acquired from his predecessors the habit of doing many things at variance with his advice." He would have been delighted to advise the people, he avowed, "if he had not supposed he would be risking his life in vain without accomplishing anything." "No serious man," Plato continued, "will ever think of writing about serious realities for the general public so as to make them a prey to envy and perplexity" (23).

I have dwelt this long on Plato and on his concept of divine madness because Plato was the first among the philosophers to define the singularity, the uniqueness, of the "gifted man," and to describe his plight and destiny among the demos, the commonality, the normals.

Concern with the "gifted man," with his divine madness, died out, as we saw, with Plato and was not revived for near to two thousand years. Why was this so? One thing comes to mind at once. To recognize the variant, one must first have a lively awareness of the normal, and for *that* one must have a sense of individuality. A sense of individuality first emerged in Homeric Greece and it attained a high degree of sharpness and refinement in the third century B.C. "In the glorious spring of the free Hellenic spirit, in those centuries full of promise that followed the age of Homer, between the dissolution of the early orders of society and the consolidation of the Attic civilization of the fifth century B.C., there came the first succession of independent personalities of European stamp . . . shadowy figures for us, but nevertheless unmistakable" (24). The flowering of Attic culture in the century and a half from the Persian wars to Aristotle and Alexander deeply affected personality formation and character (25). There was a great redirection of intellectual interest, brought about by the changes of social life in democracy, with its urgent practical problems and with the upheavals it suffered, especially after the Peloponnesian war (26). "A new stage was reached in the conception of individuality: individual action was no longer the expression of the communal consensus, but was based on reflection—yielding the individual a firm basis and a fixed standard for his conduct in life" (27). "The individual began consciously to *use* the tradition instead of being used by it" (28).

All this cleared the stage for the variant to play his fateful role and to gain recognition as the perennial tragic character in the social drama. "In this epoch," writes Georg Misch, "choices between widely varying alternative ways of living opened out before men as never before, and the State left ample room for free activity, until, from the third century of the Christian era, the despotic rulers and the Church authoritatively stereotyped the culture that had accumulated" (29).

We have noted that the decline of Greek culture began in the third century B.C. The reasons for that decline are numerous and mooted, but the evidence of that decline has been astutely described in the phrases "loss of nerve" and "retreat from rationalism." "For a century or more," writes Dodds, "the individual had been face to face with his own intellect and freedom, and now he turned tail and bolted from the horrid prospect" (30). Individualism was engulfed by the resurgent conglomerate mass, and it disappeared. It did not emerge again until the Renaissance. During the long interval there were men of divine illumination, but not of Apolline inspiration. Madness was of one order; the others were not mad, but possessed. Men could believe in demonology; they could not conceive of divine madness.

After Hippocrates the four most significant physicians in antiquity were Soranus of Ephesus (first century A.D.), Aretaeus (second century), Caelius Aurelianus (fifth century), and Galen (130-200). Each of these wrote on mental disorders, but none accepted the category of divine madness. "If maniacs do compose poetry or orate on astronomy and philosophy," wrote Aretaeus, "they do so not because of divine inspiration but because of their previous education" (31).

Soranus, as transmitted to us by Caelius Aurelianus, in his work titled *On Acute Diseases and On Chronic Diseases,* in the section *Madness or Insanity,* first refers to Plato's two orders of madness, then cites the opinions of the Stoics and of the School of Empedocles, the latter holding "that one form of madness consists of a purification of the soul, and the other in an impairment of the reason resulting from a bodily disease or indisposition." Soranus dismisses all but that madness resulting from bodily disease or indisposition and bluntly affirms, "It is the latter form of madness that we shall now consider." He concludes his exposition with the affirmation: "Thus those who imagine that the disease (madness) is chiefly an affection of the soul and secondarily of the body are mistaken. For no philosopher has ever set forth a successful treatment for this disease" (32).

Galen, whose influence on medicine lasted from the second century A.D. up to the eighteenth century, was partisan to Plato's theories on the soul, defending them against Aristotle, but he rejected Plato's two categories of madness (33). "The soul," wrote Galen, "is the slave of the body and is consequently dominated by the body" (34). Psychic functions, Galen affirmed, are centered in the brain and all orders of madness have their origin and causes within the body (35).

It would not here profit us, nor is it possible under the circumstances, to survey the theoretic postulations on the causes of mental illness advanced by physicians from the time of Galen's death until the modern age. For our concern is not with psychiatric theories as such, but primarily with the concept of divine madness and of this there was no thought at all for more than 1200 years. The divine illumination of the Church fathers and the inspirations of the saints bear no relation to Apollonian madness. Nor, most important to note, does the mass of disorders that come under the rubric of demonology. None of these was divine madness. It was not until the Renaissance that the concept of divine madness revived, in part no doubt as a consequence of the rediscovery of Plato and also because of the reemergence of individuality in the Renaissance man. But now the philosophic concern with divine madness was transmuted into a concern with the source and nature of genius. Poet, painter, author, the artist in whatever medium, was deemed an inspired person—gifted if not by God, then by the latter day equivalents of the Muses.

According to Scaliger (1561), "the *dichter* creates in a godly wise." Tasso (1587) wrote: *"Non merita nome di Creatore, se non iddio ed il Poeta."*—"None merits the name Creator save God and the poet." Philip Sidney, in his Apologie for Poetry (1591), compares the author with the Divine Creator.

That the issue of divine madness was thus transmuted can be readily understood, for the Renaissance was singularly the Age of Genius, the heyday of the gifted; yet it soon became evident, even as it had been in ancient Greece, that there was a price to pay for giftedness, in suffering, ostracism and even death.

During the sixteenth, seventeenth and eighteenth centuries the concept of genius was elaborated by numerous thinkers and came to embrace a number of specific qualities such as ingenuity, originality, outstanding creativity. It also in time became tinged with the suspicion of madness, or at least with marked mental and emotional divergences. Vasari, in his biography of Raphael, speaks of the madness, of a something wild, disordered and fantastic, to be encountered among painters. Other writers, Ficino, Aretino, Scaliger, Erasmus, treating of other creative individuals and of genius in general, expressed similar opinons (36).

In time two opposing schools of thought came into being, the one maintaining that the genius was an exceptional, gifted person, inspired, and a law unto himself; the other holding that genius was madness and that the genius, the so-termed gifted person, was such only *because* he was mad. How earnestly each school of thought held to its opinions, how intense was their conflict, how extensive and copious were their respective literatures is now difficult to imagine. Lange-Eichbaum's work, *Genie-Irsinn und Ruhm,* proffers a monumental history and a compendium of these divergent schools of thought and the literature they produced. Lange-Eichbaum, be it noted, belongs to the genius-madness school. He denies that the genius is a *gifted* individual. The genius, he maintains, harbors no gifts, is neither genetically nor biologically endowed. He affirms this in an emphatic statement: *"Genie stellt uberhaupt nichts Angeboren-Biologischer vor"* (37). Lange-Eichbaum classifies genius as a something *Bionegative,** that is, a something sickly or sick, *"Krankliche oder Kranke."*

The outstanding protagonist of the genius-madness theory was Cesare Lombroso (1836-1909). His initial and highly provocative work on this theme was published in 1863 under the title *Genio e Follia.* His last work on this subject was published in 1907 and was titled *Genio e Degenerazione III.* Lombroso in effect considered genius the product of a degenerative process, primarily psychological in character and mainly epileptic in nature. Lombroso's theories stirred up a great deal of controversy and psychiatrists, among others, took sides for or against them. It is of interest that Griesinger (1817-1868) and Forel, two of the outstanding psychiatrists of the period, were favorable to Lombroso's theories, while Kraepelin, Havelock Ellis and Bleuler rejected them.

The Lombroso controversy, for all its intensity, led nowhere. It did, however, have one salutary effect; it stimulated the study and publication

---

*Bionegative: ein Begriff, der hier zum erstenmal gepragt wirder umfass alles, was ungunstig abnorm ist hinsichtlich der Lebensfunktionen und (oder) der Nachkommenschaft. Also Missbildungen, Entwicklungshemmungen, ungunstige Variationen (samt ihrer Vererbbarkeit) und schliesslich, als die extremste Unterabtellung, alles ausgesprochen Krankliche oder Kranke.

of what came to be known as pathographies, that is, psychoclinical studies of noteworthy persons, their lives and attainments. This "literature," as we recently witnessed, can stir up deep and intense emotions, as did Freud's study with Bullitt on the life of Woodrow Wilson.

It is of interest to inquire why the Lombroso controversy died out. In part no doubt because Lombroso's theories were extreme and untenable. Genius *could be mad*. Numerous pathographies reveal this clearly. But the critical intelligence would not be persuaded that the genius was such *because* he was mad, nor that genius was in itself a madness. However, it is not likely that the controversy was dissipated by a simple exercise in logic. It took something more decisive—a novel and promising approach to the problem of genius to dissipate Lombroso's arguments. This was provided by Sir Francis Galton's study of *Genius and Heredity* published six years after Lombroso's *Genius and Madness* appeared. It had been maintained that genius was not genetically transmitted, but Galton demonstrated that it was indeed in a large measure hereditary. By careful biographic studies Galton showed that there is a tendency for genius to run in families; that eminent men tend to have eminent offspring. It should, however, be noted that Galton used the term genius in a more catholic, in a broader sense, than did Lombroso. He embraced in the term all uncommonly gifted individuals, from the barely outstanding to those of the highest and rarest order.

But at the time Galton wrote his historically significant book, he had no way to measure giftedness nor did he have any criteria by which to demonstrate objectively that the genius was indeed a genius. Galton depended on the historical datum of the individual's reputation among his contemporaries.

Galton, who was a half cousin to Darwin, was himself a good deal of a genius, and he tackled the problem of "gauge and proof" of ability with distinctive ingenuity. He sought to quantify mathematically the evidence of ability. After fourteen years of work on this problem, he published in 1883 the results of his studies in a book titled *Inquiries into Human Ability and Its Development*. This work marked the beginning of scientific individual psychology and of mental testing. "Galton," writes Boring, "believed that quantitative measure is the mark of a fullgrown science and he adopted Quetelet's use of the normal law in order to convert the frequency of occurrence of genius into measures of its degree: that is to say, he set up a scale of lettered grades of genius from "A," just above average, up to "G," and to "X," which represented all grades above "G" (38). He found that "G" level was attained by only one man in 79,000 and that of "X" one in a million. Galton linked all degrees of ability in one continuum and created the means for their measurement.

The history of the development, elaboration, and refinement of psychological tests is immensely interesting, but it has only a secondary bearing on our subject; we may not pursue it further. This much, however, should be noted. The mental tests provided the base for a clear concept, at least in one dimension, of genius, the gifted person, the maverick.

As previously avowed, I have used the terms genius, gifted person, and maverick as if they were interchangeable, and referred to one specific order of person. In a significant sense they *are* interchangeable, and they *do* describe a unique order of person. Yet some refinement and definition is at this point desirable. Every gifted person has an element of genius about him. The capital "G" person is the highly gifted person whose giftedness, on Galton's scale, ranges between "G" and "X." The others rank lower, but irrespective of rank they are all gifted. They are likewise variants from the normal, in an upward direction. They are all in that sense "mavericks." In applying the term "maverick" to this unique order of persons, my intention is not to signal their statistical position, but rather to focus attention on the singular psychological characteristics which carry with them distinctive and sometimes grievous psychiatric liabilities. These are the individuals who are liable, in Plato's terms, to "divine madness," a type of madness which, as my long excursus into history has shown, has been little understood and which even now is but inadequately appreciated in psychiatry.

The term "maverick" is of recent origin; it gained currency in 1872. It designates an unbranded creature, one that is outside of the herd. The gifted person is by virtue of his giftedness liable to exclusion from the herd, and he himself finds it natively difficult to integrate with the herd. The herd, the human commonality, finds it difficult to comprehend the maverick, feels him to be alien, and by his difference challenging and menacing. The commonality reacts to the maverick in a variety of ways. It derides him, rejects him, abuses him, and in the ultimate may destroy him, either slowly or in a burst of passion. In a great measure the behavior of the commonality toward the maverick depends upon the ways in which the maverick relates to his own giftedness in the presence of the herd. Both Socrates and Plato were mavericks, but only Socrates was put to death.

Giftedness is a heavy burden to bear and can crush the individual even where the commonality is indifferent and uninvolved. In social existence, the gifted individual needs to learn how to coexist with his own giftedness, how to reconcile his own version of *being* with that in evidence all about him. The task is exacting and hence little wonder that so many among the gifted withdraw from social coexistence to live in their private realms. It is this negative resolution of their difficulties that gave rise and appears to validate the genius-madness formula.

The gifted individual is "afflicted-blest" with divine madness, for in varying ways in different degrees, he perceives, comprehends, and relates to his environment and to the flow of experience in ways different from those of the normals in whose midst he is placed. His differences are not merely quantitative, but even more emphatically substantive. He perceives not so much more of what is the shared vision, but a something different. He is like the fabled child who saw the king not raggedly dressed but stark naked, while all the others saw him dressed in finery.

This madness of the maverick *is divine,* and it is incurable. The maverick can learn to live with his madness and indeed to profit in it for himself and for the larger group. But he cannot abdicate his madness save by self destruction.

Since the maverick cannot but be a maverick, what are the possible consequences of his interactions, as a maverick, with the overwhelming larger mass of normals? It is to be assumed, as is most commonly the case, that the herd is not favorable to him, is on the contrary hostile, and hence will make sport of him, abuse him, reject him, and otherwise injure him. The maverick's reaction, especially during his formative years, is likely to be one of three possible choices: He may withdraw from the group and become an isolate. He may "fight" the group in an endless, indeed lifelong battle (as did Schopenhauer and Nietzsche), becoming in the process increasingly hostile, cynical and misanthropic. Or he may gain a measure of acceptance among the crowd by playing the clown, a resolution masterfully executed by Bernard Shaw.

The maverick during his initial efforts to articulate with the mass may serially try each of these patterns before settling on one. I suspect that many among those who cannot but withdraw and become isolates take refuge in schizophrenia. To paraphrase this in a more telling version, I am persuaded that among the schizophrenics there are numerous mavericks whose giftedness, and the world about them, proved more than they could fuse into a life worth its burdens.

But the crucial question must be asked—is all this inevitable? Are there no other ways? Is it not possible for the maverick to have a rewarding existence among the herd, even though he does not bear its brand mark? This you will recall was the question Plato asked, and seemingly answered in the negative. Given Socrates and the jury (the demos), he said condemnation is inevitable. It is fate! But as we need recall, Plato did not blot out all hope. There still was paideia and arete. We who have the advantage over Plato in that we can scan a longer stretch of history, know that not everywhere nor at all times was the maverick uniformly rejected and persecuted. There were times of relative tolerance for the maverick, as in fifth century Athens and during the early Renaissance, when, indeed, the maverick was prized as pioneer, explorer and innovator, the avant garde of human culture. But history also shows that such periods of tolerance are rare and of short duration. Apart from this there is the germinal problem of the gifted man living effectively with his own giftedness in the world which even when it is tolerant, nay, more, is receptive, still stands out in stark contrast to the perceptive and inner life of the maverick. This contrast to which the maverick is subject and constant witness is in itself a great challenge.

Madness is the special preserve of the psychiatrist. Does then the divine madness of the maverick fall within the psychiatrist's field of concern, or is it to be left to the sociologists, the esthetes, the educators? The question is vain, for on closer examination it is clearly evident that the choice is not as open as all that. In the end, and frequently before that, many among the mavericks *volens nolens* come face to face with psychiatry and the psychiatrist. Some come as bewildered patients at odds with the world, others are embroiled in serious controversies, in futile and misdirected revolts, and still others are in conflict with the law. An increasing number, I find, are parents, themselves mavericks, who are bewildered by the giftedness of their children and do not know how to deal with them.

But then what results when maverick and psychiatrist confront each other? The results, I am afraid, are not always good and, indeed, sometimes are very bad. For the psychiatrist, trained to deal with abnormality, is chiefly concerned with the lower segment in the distribution-curve of normality, that is, with the lower variant. Classically and traditionally, the psychiatrist's efforts are directed to the bringing, or lifting of the variant, back to the normal. Furthermore, the psychiatrist shares and suffers with the rest of the normal world the tyranny of Reality. The psychiatrist is neither trained to nor is he prone to ask "What reality? which reality? whose reality?" There is a risk in asking such questions, for the inquiry may lay the questioner open to the suspicion that he is himself a bit mad. Witness the fate of such as Trigant Burrow and the younger Wilhelm Reich, who did ask such questions! But such questions *are being asked* by philosophers and by the literati. However, philosophers and men of letters do not treat patients. They can only mirror the problem, they cannot resolve it. Neither can the psychiatrist, entirely and all by himself. Still the problem falls squarely and inescapably to his lot, for as noted before, in the last analysis the psychiatrist is called on and is required to deal with the painful and wretched consequences of its nonresolution—as friend and advisor to the courts of law, as keeper to the incarcerated in the mental hospitals, and more frequently as guide and sustainer to those wrecked in their efforts to be themselves and yet to live with the others.

We need to be forthright in this matter; nothing in the present-day training or education of the psychiatrist, psychoanalyst, or other, prepares or qualifies the psychiatrist to deal with the primary, basic "abnormality" of the maverick—his giftedness—his divine madness. At best the psychiatrist can deal only with the consequent or secondary problems, and even there not much better than symptomatically. At best the psychiatrist may prove *himself* tolerant and permissive in the posture which, if verbalized, would sound thus—"Well, of course, if you choose to be that way, it's *your* affair and it's all right with me." Still there is an unspoken "but" in this posture which the patient is not likely to miss. It runs thus—"But, of course, if you had any sense you'd give up your nonsense and become a real fellow. The reality, you know, requires, etc., etc."

Mavericks understandably are not fond of psychiatrists. They shy away from them. When they are artists, they are fearful, unreasonably and erroneously so, that therapy would interfere with and perhaps even deprive them of their artistry. The maverick may be ill and unhappy, but with a healthy instinct he does not want to be made normal. His authentic psychiatric need is to be explained to himself, to comprehend himself, and in that knowledge to learn how to achieve arete in himself and yet give pleasure to the others. It can be done. But the maverick cannot be helped to understand himself in the parlance and dynamics of the oedipus complex, castration anxiety, orality, or id drives. Nor can his problem as a maverick be illuminated in terms of organ inferiority or the sublimation of unfulfilled infantile wishes. His basic difficulty derives from his being a maverick, and this conditions and generally aggravates all the problems which he encounters in the adventures of growth and development. But it is his condition of *being a maverick* and the consequence thereof that require initial illumination and insight. Without that, treatment of the rest is most difficult, if not impossible. In the paraphrase of a story told of Freud, the patient needs to be helped to understand that he doesn't *suffer* from a superiority complex—he is superior—and that this is no mean "disability." Understanding this, the maverick can also learn to understand and to tolerate the differences between himself and the rest, to understand and make allowances for the suspicions, antagonisms and jealousies he is likely to engender in the less gifted. He may even learn how to anticipate them and thus avoid or evade them. In such understanding he may gain tolerance, patience and humility, thereby increasing his arete—and also bringing pleasure to others. In learning this for and about himself, he may also apply this knowledge in the paideia of his children, for mavericks are prone to produce mavericks.

How is the psychiatrist to achieve all this with his maverick patients? First and foremost, by becoming aware of, and thus learning to recognize, this order of patient, not as yet listed in the standard classification, and then by understanding in depth the dynamics of the maverick's intra- and interpersonal difficulties. The rest in understanding and therapeutic procedure should not be difficult to gain and master.

I want to end my exposition with an *apologia*—apologia meaning not excuse but explanation. I have given no case material either in the development of my theme or in illustration and support of the theories advanced. That was not for my lack of such materials, but because I could not include it, the space for this presentation being limited. I chose rather to present an historic survey, and that for the reason that "the proper care and treatment of the maverick" is not only a challenge to psychiatry, but is in effect of vital importance to mankind, to the maintenance and advance of civilization and culture. History shows that society has been cruelly intolerant of its upper variants. It may be kind and rewarding to its persons of talent, but not to the upper variants who challenge society's cherished values and accustomed ways. The annals of history are replete with the records of gifted men and women whom society would not gladly harbor, but instead rejected, persecuted, and destroyed. Was not Aristedes, surnamed the just, banished from Athens precisely because he was just? In exiling the law giver Hermodorous, the friend of Heraclitus, the Ephesians decreed this, "Let no one be best among us, or if one must be best, let him be elsewhere and with other people." In our times we are aware of the receptions given to Darwin and to Freud. These prevailed against great odds. But who is to tell what numbers of such like did not prevail, but succumbed? Society could never afford to be so profligate with its gifted members and can afford it even less so now.

And who shall bring this to the awareness and before the conscience of mankind if not the psychiatrist? In the courts of man's judgement the maverick needs a pleader and defender. Let it be the psychiatrist.

REFERENCES

1. PHAEDRUS: 265. From the translation of R. Hackforth *In* Hamilton, Edith and Cairns, Huntington, (Eds.). *The Collected Dialogues of Plato,* Bollingen Series, LXXI, New York, Pantheon Books, 1961.
2. *Ibid.*
3. *Ibid.*
4. *Ibid.,* 245-b.
5. DODDS, E. R.: *The Greeks and the Irrational.* Berkeley and Los Angeles, University of California Press, 1964, p. 64-101.
6. *Ibid.,* p. 82.
7. PHAEDRUS: 245-a.
8. For an interesting rendition of this fictional meeting of Hippocrates and Democritus, *See* Boisessette Gaston: *Life and Teaching of Hippocrates.*
9. The author of the Hippocratic Prognostikon, however, seems to believe that certain diseases have "something divine about them."
10. HIPPOCRATES: *The Sacred Disease* XVII-XVIII. Loeb Classics, translated by W. H. S. Jones, New York, Putnam's Sons, 1923, p. 175.
11. Cited in Leibrand-Wettley: *Der Wahnsinn.* Munchen, Karl Alter Freiburg, 1961, p. 81. Cicero in Tusculanum describes as melancholics Heracles, Lysander, Aias, Bellerophon, Empedocles, Plato, Socrates, and others, notably among writers.
12. DODDS, *op. cit.,* p. 244 (phraseology slightly modified).
13. PLATO, *op. cit.*
14. DODDS, *op. cit.,* p. 69.
15. JAEGER, WERNER: *Paideia.* Translated by Gilbert Highet, New York, Oxford University Press, 1945, Vol. 2, p. 83.
16. PLATO: *Apology,* 40-a.
17. JAEGER, *op. cit.,* p. 73.
18. PLATO: *Georgias,* 486 b.c.d.
19. PLATO: *Georgias,* 522 d.e.
20. PLATO: *Republic,* Book IX, 592 a.b.
21. PLATO: *Letter VII,* 324 e.
22. PLATO: *Letter VII,* 326 e.
23. PLATO: *Letter V,* 322 b. and Letter VII, 344 c.
24. MISCH, GEORG: *A History of Autobiography in Antiquity.* Cambridge, Harvard University Press, 1951, Vol. 1, p. 67.
25. *Ibid.,* p. 95.
26. *Ibid.,* p. 100.
27. *Ibid.,* p. 100.
28. DODDS, *op. cit.,* p. 237.
29. MISCH, *op. cit.,* p. 183.
30. DODDS, *op. cit.,* p. 246.
31. SEMELAIGNA A.: *Etudes Historiques sur l'aliénation mentale dans l'antiquité.* Paris, 1869—cited by Zilboorg and Henry: *A History of Medical Psychology.* New York, W. W. Norton and Co., 1941, p. 75.
32. DRABKIN, I. E.: *Caelius Aurelianus on Acute Disease and Chronic Diseases.* Chicago, University of Chicago Press, 190, p. 535-541.
33. DE DOGM-Hipp. et Platon III, 7, Book V, p. 337. *In* DARENBERG, CHARLES: *La Médecine Histoire et Doctrines.* 2nd Ed., Paris, Didier et Cie, 1865, p. 81.

34. ZILBOORG: p. 91, A. Semeligne, *op. cit.*, p. 189-190.
35. *See* SPRENGEL, KURT: on *Galen, Versuch einer pragmatischen Geschichte der Arzneykunde,* halle, 1823.
36. LANGE-EICHBAUM, WILHELM: *Genie-Irsinn und Ruhm.* Munchen, Ernst Reinhardt, 1928, p. 30.
37. *Ibid.,* p. 433.
38. BORING, EDWIN G.: *A History of Experimental Psychology.* New York, The Century Co., 1929.

8

Dream Morphology: Its Diagnostic and Prognostic Significance

IN THE COURSE OF MY EXPERIENCE with dream analysis and dream interpretation it became clear to me that the structure or pattern of the
dream—that which I choose to call dreamaturgy or dream morphology—
has diagnostic and prognostic significance, independent of and sup-
plementary to both the manifest and the latent dream content. By dream
pattern I intend specifically the structure of the dream, the scheme of the
story told, and the *manner* in which it is told; its background, its actors,
their doings and sayings, the dream's continuity or discontinuity, its co-
hesiveness or lack of congruity—all of this, I repeat in emphasis, apart
from and independent of the symbol significance of the dream content.
The dream thus viewed is perceived as a *Gestalt*. It proffers, among other
things, an indication of the way in which the dreamer *fashions* his dreams,
for each patient follows his own pattern of dreaming. His dreamaturgy,
like his handwriting, is unmistakably and consistently his own. Yet within
each individual's pattern there is scope for many variations, and the
changes perceived reflect the patient's progressions and regressions during
therapy. By the token of the witnessed changes in the dream pattern it is
possible to gauge what progress the patient is making and to deduce
certain prognostic indices.

In attempting to establish the basic dream patterns, I arrived at 4
morphological categories. These are as follows: first, the dream that has
the pattern of a consistent story; second, the dream that has the pattern
of a *montage*. This order of dream is composed of disjointed, episodic
elements, which, however, are projected upon a common and consistent
background. This category also includes the "multiple dream," that is the
dream that comprises several dreams dreamt serially in one night. The

third category embraces the dream that meanders. This type of dream changes its vernacular, shifts its terrain, and is distinguished by its disjointedness and inconsistency. The fourth category embraces what may be best described as the amorphous dream. In this order of dream we perceive only vague and poorly delineated characters who execute few definite actions, and who in the main register only diffuse emotional overtones and nuances.

The following are representative examples of the four dream categories. I give the dreams as they were reported. Here is a dream of the first category.

> A few girl friends were spending the night at my house. My father was in the hospital and my mother was away for the night also (don't know where). Had an appointment with you and it was arranged that you come to the house. There were two other friends and myself and we got into bed. Myself and Joan in one bed, and Mary and someone else in the other twin bed. You arrived and we started talking right in the room. After a few moments I got up and said to you that I thought it would be best if we went into another room. It was slightly embarrassing. You agreed. After our session you were getting ready to leave, and I suggested you spend the night since my folks were not home. Their room was available. You accepted and lo and behold mother came home later that night unexpectedly. Some surprise and confusion existed for a short while and I think you shifted to the couch in the living room.

The story told in this dream is consistent and well formulated. Contrast this dream with one of the fourth category, that which I have labeled amorphous.

> Something about H: He said he had two things which hurt him. It and something else. I said why don't you put penicillin powder on it, it sounds like a boil. We went on a long trip through Italy. Anita also went in another car. Ethel or someone like her brought dresses —many, a certain type of them, she said, one couldn't wear. A. and I went to P. to tell him we wouldn't come for Thanksgiving. E. the maid then came and said if we went downstairs there was a big party going. We went, masses of people, sat on different sides of the auditorium. Theatricals some famous men, Sorpo or Soyol. A. was somewhere also. A. and I left after a while.

This dream, in contrast to the first, is formless. It has no obvious "plot" and "tells no tale." It is in fact basically amorphous.

An example of the second category, that of the montage, is the following dream:

Something to do with the M's. A. is working there Saturday only and I visit him there and help out too. Not sure. We are planning to get married. Last day for working there and I do something wrong or something happens. Anyway I am to be beheaded. I have the rest of the morning until 2:00 o'clock while Mrs. M. goes somewhere. At first don't really take it seriously. Gradually realize that I am really going to be beheaded. When Mrs. M. comes back she is a little sorry but it is too late to change things. Start trying to think of ways to get out of it. The execution is going to take place on a special boat on the river. Somehow gets to be a whole group of girls which is going to be beheaded and Mrs. M. fades from the picture. Something about girls simply not being able to handle something on board ship correctly and therefore having to die. Nobody is being very whole-hearted about executions but has to go ahead. Postponed for a few hours because Lourdes did not come in time. We are taking showers and getting ready for the executions. Two men are watching me and admiring my body. Across the hall in another shower stall is a man without genitals but otherwise masculine figure. Then I am consulting with. A. as to what would happen if I would not go. See the ship coming in. Everybody is there as we go aboard ship. Everybody is dressed up in elegant gowns and the whole thing begins to have the coloring of the guillotine days. I am still terribly ambivalent whether to try an escape or not. There is some concept that we will revive but rather lifeless or somehow changed. Finally I decide to escape but feel somewhat ashamed about it and also afraid. Even if I get away with it—will live with the burden of fear. In the meantime the first girl is being made to hold her neck over pot of boiling water to "steam it up" in preparation for the knife, and I begin to realize full impact of what is happening. Some fellow outside the door stands guard but he is cooperating with my running away. Calls boy friend who is out hunting and tells him to go back to the ship with the bloody knife to cover up my running away.

This pattern is, I feel, well named a montage. Distinctive and seemingly disjointed parts of the dream are superimposed upon a uniform background and are thus linked together. One can discern an intended pattern, though its discernment calls for close scrutiny. The principal motif here is a *beheading* and the locus is a "special boat on the river." All the rest is ancillary to the tale told.

Less well organized, but still not without pattern is the dream of the third category: the meandering dream that changes its vernacular, shifts its terrain, and is indeed distinguished by its disjointedness and inconsistency. The following is an example of this order of dream:

Somehow I was a young fellow in school but something which I do not recall was wrong with this and for the rest of the dream I was a girl. I came to visit me in the college room or my office. The girl I was talking to had on a red dress and was sitting on the window. She began hanging out of the window more and more and I begged her to stop because I was getting worried that she would fall out of the window. She laughed and said she would not get hurt and showed this by suddenly swinging her whole body out of the window, hanging on only by her hand. Then suddenly she let go and I was terrified and sure she had fallen but she came up again a moment later, laughing. I was astonished and asked her how she had done it. She said that when she was a child she was sick and had to exercise her muscles so that now she has very strong muscles.

Then I went to X., a small town some distance from the college. I don't remember what I did there but was waiting for the bus back, standing in a doorway, talking to some fellows. At least one of them was Negro. Then someone came down from upstairs and made some comment that frightened me a little. Another fellow, who had joined us later, went outside and I asked him to stay with me until the bus came. He seemed pleased that I asked him, put his arm around me and smiled. I had been afraid to ask him because I did not want him to think I was prejudiced against Negroes.

Then somehow I went into the building. Lot of girls from the college there. There was a swimming pool in the center and stairs going up one side to a platform which overlooked the pool. Started to walk up the stairs. There were girls all along the stairway, and there was quite a commotion. Then I noticed that all along the stairway and in the pool was a big collection of slimy animals and entrails and fish. I made a lot of jokes along the way and got all the way to the top. It was then that I realized the water was also full of these things and that I could not expect to swim.

Girls starting to make coffee *upstairs* by adding water to a thick, syrupy mixture like condensed milk. I told *her* that the bus was due in 3 minutes and that in fact it had arrived. I ran down but it had left. However, I saw it turn into the terminal and I ran there and caught it just in time. I thought *two* of the girls had not made it, but when we arrived they got out too and I could not understand how they got there so fast. They had some adventure, asking someone to drive them or something and that is how they got there.

This dream as can be observed is loosely constructed. It begins in "the college room or office," then shifts to the town X. The dreamer then enters a *building,* and there comes upon a *swimming pool.* Coffee is served —upstairs; the bus is due in 3 minutes. The dreamer first "misses the bus," then catches it at the terminal, and finally winds up by wondering how the other girls got there "so fast."

In the four dream categories given, we observe a progression from the most consistently patterned and well-integrated dream to the one that is in effect patternless. I submit that the quality of the pattern of the dream is in numerous ways meaningful and significant. Thus I am convinced that the well-integrated dream, the one that tells a clear tale, bears witness to the fact that the dreamer has an inner appreciation of the nature of his difficulties, albeit on the unconscious level. As a corollary of this it follows that the less well-organized the dream, the greater the difficulties the patient is experiencing in perceiving, in appreciating, and in formulating his psychological problems. Since *insight* is both a prerequisite to and essential *in* effective therapy, the pattern of the patient's dream can serve to instruct us on the depth and extent of insight that the patient possesses. By observing the changes perceivable in the dream pattern of a given patient's dream we can construe the extent, rapidity, and direction of his progress. By the same indices we can also observe the patient's resistances, their intensity, endurance, and alterations. In general it will be found that as the patient gains insight his dream pattern will move away from the amorphous and toward the first category—that of the consistent story.

I am sure I need hardly underscore the fact that these generalizations, though valid, present far too simple a picture of the subject matter. They cannot and must not be applied to specific instances and to particular experiences without added elaboration. Thus dreams do not usually embrace the entire complex of the patient's difficulties. Preoccupation may therefore shift from one set of difficulties to another; indeed, as is common in experience, the resolution of one difficulty may serve to bring relief only to unmask or to uncover other, and at times even greater, difficulties. In the light of this it is to be expected that the dream pattern will change accordingly. New and emergent conflict elements will tend "to confound rather than to clarify the plot," to obfuscate rather than to render consistent the dream. But this too can be grist to the therapist's mill, for if a shift is observed from the consistent to the less consistent dream pattern, the therapist may be alerted to the upsurging of new materials. Here it may not be amiss once again to underscore just what is intended by consistency within the dream pattern. The reference is to the morphology, to the structure pattern, of the dream. No consistency in the sense of the reality logic prevailing in the real and awake world is intended or involved. In the meaning given, all that takes place in *Alice in Wonderland* is bound together in a consistent pattern. Were *Alice in Wonderland* a dream, as in a sense it was and is, it would be classified as of the first category.

I mentioned the uniqueness of each patient's dream pattern. This too is noteworthy, and can prove illuminating. Thus certain patients consistently dream (and/or report) compact dreams, worked out in the manner of a syllogistic exercise. Others are rather prolix. Even when the essential pattern is consistent, their dreams are expansively conceived and executed with a largess of circumstance and action. Such are in the main the dream patterns of patients who prefer the indirect and tangential approach, even as the compact dream is common to the "direct and logical" personalities, those with limited or restricted affect exchange.

In the main it will be found that the dream pattern is a function of the personality of the patient. Indeed it could hardly be otherwise. Since therapy not infrequently modifies personality pattern, it is to be expected that the dream pattern will undergo corresponding change; and it does!

In describing the four categories of dream patterns I emphasized what I call their gross morphology. It was not then desirable nor is it now possible to detail the finer morphologic elements perceivable within each category. The tale told by the dream may not only be more or less consistent, but it can also be told with special attention to the logicalness of incidents, with a marked awareness of moods, with fine details as to colors, odors, and tastes, and with other marked and noteworthy characteristics, as noteworthy in their absence as in their presence. These finer morphologic dream factors also are a function of the personality pattern of the patient.

In preparation for this rather brief communication (brief in the sight of the magnitude of the subject) I naturally canvassed the literature to see what, if anything, of a similar nature had been observed and reported by others. I did not survey *all* the dream literature, and hence it is possible that I missed some pertinent material. But granting this possibility, I still found little touching on the subject of dream morphology, and nothing comparable to the thesis I here present. It is noteworthy, however, that A. E. Maeder, of Zurich, in 1913 termed the dream "an autosymbolic phenomenon" and described two *kinds* of dreams. In the first "the action is lively or direct, energetic." "This quality," Maeder wrote, "may be made use of in prognosis, be it in the sense of an intensely progressive achievement or of an active resistance." The second kind of dream Maeder described as marked by indifference, indecision, vagueness, awkwardness, doubt, stagnation, or fixation. These too, according to Maeder, have "a certain prognostic meaning for the contemporary phase."* Maeder described a third order of dream—one that is teleological and anticipatory in character. It is unfortunate that Maeder did not

---

*The Dream Problem, p. 29. Nervous and Mental Disease Monograph Series No. 22.

pursue this subject further, for dream morphology is for certain a most pregnant and promising study.

It was Freud who affirmed that the dream is the royal road to the unconscious and so indeed it is. Unfortunately, Freud himself, and especially his followers, have perhaps unwittingly, there being so much to do and to study, created the impression that the unconscious is the Dantesque region of the personality, where the repressed and the primitive abide in stygian darkness. Here and there, among Freud's writings one catches a glimpse suggesting that after all, he "knew better." But to Freud, the dream was, in the main, an adventure whereby repressed impulsion, uprising from the unconscious, evaded, deceived, and otherwise eluded the censor, and emerged as wish fulfillments.

The dream mechanism is, however, capable of greater achievements, and the unconscious is vastly more than the region to which the unacceptable and the inexpressible are banished. The unconscious embraces a vast portion of the total mechanism of the personality—and it has an integrative and an adaptive competence that is often anticipatory to, and at times transcending, that of the conscious and rational faculty. In the unconscious lies the deeper wisdom of both the body and the person. It is from this most significant resource and power of the unconscious that dream morphology derives its validity and importance. For the dream is an intelligence of the unconscious and the grammar, syntax, and pattern of its communication, whether it babbles and falters, or speaks knowingly, are no less pertinent than the elements it seeks to utter and portray.

The dream is indeed an autosymbolic phenomenon. It is the most immediate and the most intimate of the person's psychological operations. In this purview the dream might be credited with greater revelatory significance than any of the now utilized projective techniques.

9

Dynamics of the Cure in Psychiatry

AT THE very basis of the science of the healing art lies the problem of how the physician effects a cure. Since the most ancient of times the very best among physicians have been impelled to venture some judgment on this score.

The Greeks, the Romans, and their heritors held that it was only nature that heals. The physician merely treats—*Natura sanat: medicus curat*. This dictum was tersely paraphrased by Ambroise Paré—"Je le pansay, Dieu le guarit" ("I bandaged him, but God cured him"). This affirmation of the physician's limited function is likewise reflected in the terms "therapist" and "therapeutics"; these words are derived from the Greek term θεραπων, which means "servant." The physician's modest pretensions, wherein the greater credit for the cure is given to nature or, in later times, to God, may indeed have stemmed from his inherent humility. Some skeptics, however, have suggested that they served him rather as a shield against blame. For if the issue of a case rests with nature, or with God, then, should the treatment fail or the patient die, the physician can disclaim responsibility. Palpably, it must have been God's wish or nature's intention, and not the physician's fault.

But whatever might have motivated the physician's modest pretensions, fulfilling his obligations as a scientist he at all times held to some theory on the causation of disease and had some concept of the dynamics of the cure.

The two were ever intertwined, and medical history clearly shows that the concepts of the dynamics of the cure were consistently related to the prevailing theories on the causation of disease, so that in any given period the prevailing theory on the dynamics of the cure mirrored the prevailing

110

theory on etiology. Treatment and etiology can be taken as the two interrelated components which together summate the prevailing science of medicine.

How the dynamics of the cure related to the theory of the cause of disease is reflected in the following historical data.

When the physician conceived of disease as resulting from an imbalance in the humors of the body, that is, from a dyscrasia, he sought to effect a cure by reestablishing harmony in the humors. This he undertook to achieve by means of diets, purges, emetics, sweats, and the like. When the physician ascribed disease to evil spirits, he practiced exorcism. When the physician became an iatrochemist, he administered crude chemical elements, aiming at the reestablishment of the chemical harmony of the body, which he assumed had been disturbed in the disease process.

In the 18th century, when the etiology of disease was conceptualized in terms of "sthenic" and "asthenic" states, the two cardinal remedies were antispasmodics and stimulants—opium and alcohol (1).

When, in the 19th century, histology came to the fore, and Virchow developed the science of cellular pathology, the theory of humoral pathology was rejected, and with it also much of the therapeutic practice based thereon.

Later still, when cellular pathology was, in turn, overshadowed by the great achievements of Pasteur and Koch, the etiology of disease was conceptualized almost entirely in terms of micro-organisms, and therapy, in terms of vaccines, antitoxins, and immune sera.

Psychiatry, which for many centuries was an integrated part of the science and the practice of medicine, shared in the prevailing theories, both as to etiology and as to dynamics of the cure. This is neatly reflected in certain terms still common in psychiatric vernacular—terms which by the evidence of their derivation illuminate also the "systems" of medical thought wherein they were coined. Thus, melancholia, phrenitis, mania, hysteria, and splenitis not only designate certain morbid conditions but point also to certain specifc theories on the causation of psychiatric and other disorders. But psychiatry, as a distinctive medical specialty, did not come into being until comparatively recent times. It is not therefore germane to our purpose to dwell on the dynamics of the psychiatric cure as conceived of in ancient times. We need, rather, to confine our studies to the past 150 years. Yet I must make it clear that by this circumscription I do not intend to disparage the antecedent generations of medical men or to deny that among them there were many excellent psychiatrists and psychotherapists. I am not one of those who holds that psychiatry is the creation of modern science. On the contrary, I am quite certain that historically the "psychotherapist" antedated the "clinician." It is not psychiatry as such but only the specialty of psychiatry that is of modern origin. Hence if one desires to study the singular dynamics of the psychiatric cure, one is obliged to limit oneself to the time during which the etiology of mental and emotional disorders, and the rationale of their treatment, became and remained the predominant concern of a group of men who ventured definitive theories thereon. There is some arbitrariness in this time limitation, but it derives not from me but from the historic reality.

Medical history, I have said, teaches us that "the dynamics of the cure is mirrored in the prevailing theory on etiology." Reviewing the past 150 years, we find that the theories on the etiology of psychiatric illnesses, which held and still hold sway, can be listed under eight descriptive headings: (1) the daemoniacal-moral, (2) the hereditary-constitutional, (3) the toxic-traumatic, (4) the asthenic-disintegrative, (5) the repressive-analytical, (6) the ergological, (7) the socio-environmental, and (8) the ecological.

I have listed these theories in their approximate historical sequence, the oldest first and the newest last but it must be recognized that the neatness, both of their designation and of their order, is, in a measure, an artifact of systematization.

There may be some difficulty in recognizing the first division, that is, the daemoniacal and moral, as among the prevailing theories on the etiology of psychiatric disorders. This is, in part, due to the fact that some medical historians have overemphasized Christian demonology and witch hunting. The daemoniacal-moral theory is to be understood in terms not of the Christian devil, but of the daemon of Socrates, and as it is today propounded by Carl Jung and by Maeder. I shall treat this much misunderstood and much underrated etiological theory later.

In contemplating the remaining seven etiological theories, one cannot but recognize that the scope for therapeutic effort which they singly allow differs very greatly. Thus, the psychotherapist can palpably do but little to countereffect malignant constitutional and hereditary factors, and that little is not psychotherapeutic in character. As much must be said of the psychotherapist's function in relation to the toxic-traumatic factors. At best, his task is to diagnose differentially the psychopathology due to toxic and traumatic causes and that due to other causes. Detoxication and the repair, where possible, of trauma do not generally lie within the psychotherapist's competence and obligations.

The therapy practiced by those who subscribed to the asthenic-disintegrative theory is largely in the nature of seclusion, rest, reeducation, and the softening and lightening of the trials and burdens of life. Here, though the psychotherapist's role is somewhat more active, it is still a minor one in the total operation.

Summating, then, the three categories, the hereditary-constitutional, the toxic-traumatic, and the asthenic-disintegrative, we see that in effect they afford relatively little scope for immediate psychotherapy. Within their logical framework, the dynamics of the cure operate far less in and through the person and skills of the psychotherapist than in and through the physical and environmental agents which he may employ, or which, as is more commonly the case, are employed by others under his remote supervision and according to his instructions.

At this point I want to comment on certain seeming incongruities in my recitation. I have listed eight etiological theories in the presumed order of their historical sequence. But they do not form a "chain" of theories. The later one does not necessarily link to, or displace, the earlier one. It may modify the significance of antecedent theories and constrict their applicability. But in actuality the eight listed etiological theories are currently coexistent and to some extent complementary. They form the synthetical body of etiological lore. Historically, however, these theories were each advanced, if not as the solely valid, certainly as the dominant and the superior theory on the etiology of psychiatric disorders.

I underscore this because this historical actuality enables us to divide the history of modern psychiatry into two distinct periods: the period antecedent to and the period following on the introduction of psychoanalysis by Freud. The first period, extending from the late 18th until the beginning of the 20th century, can be designated as the organic, physiological, and descriptive era. The period following is best labeled as the era of dynamic psychiatry.

Before turning to the time since Freud, it will profit us to observe more closely the stage setting of his advent. Between 1800 and 1900 the structure and the operations of the nervous system were intensively studied. Interest in the immediate problem of the etiology of mental illness and in the dynamics of the psychiatric cure waned. It was expected that such problems would be dissipated by the very revelations certain to issue from the anatomicophysiological studies then so feverishly cultivated. Many, and among them Theodore Meynert, Freud's teacher, denied that psychiatry, as distinct from neurophysiology, could ever become a legitimate specialty. Mental and emotional disorders, they held, were the result of physiological and organic disturbances in the nervous system and hence belonged in the field of neurology.

There was still another reason that psychiatry was in a state of "suspended animation" during the second half of the 19th century—it was, in effect, fixated by a great expectation. The period was surcharged with great hopes. Many earnest scientists entertained the most extravagant ideas on what medicine was likely to discover "on the morrow." Psychiatry, too, was awaiting the dawn of a new era. It was anticipating some great issue—something like the discovery of the "germ of insanity" or a specific serum or antitoxin against the neuroses and the psychoses.

Toward the very end of the 19th century a "something" did come forth. But it did not conform to what had been anticipated, and it was not welcome. That something was Freud's psychoanalysis. Freud's theories cut across the assurances, and disturbed the complacencies, of his contemporary world. Psychoanalytic theory was most disturbing precisely because it was not mechanistically oriented. Freud did not challenge the validity of what was known of neural structure and neurophysiology. He had been a neurologist before he turned to psychiatry. Freud, however, denied that the totality of human behavior could be accounted for on the basis of neuroanatomy and neurophysiology. Furthermore, he challenged the usefulness and denied the ultimate effectiveness of the then common modalities of psychotherapy—of hypnotism, suggestion, persuasion, reeducation, and electro-stimulation.

Freud advanced an entirely new theory on the etiology of the psychoneurosis, that of repression. And for the treatment of the pathology resulting from repression, he developed a fundamentally new and novel technique, that of free association. Both these theories were in time greatly elaborated by Freud himself and by his disciples. They, however, remain the foundation basis of psychoanalysis. "It is possible," wrote Freud (2), "to take repression as a center and to bring all elements of psychoanalytic theory into relation with it." Zilboorg (3), also affirms: "Unless the method of free association is carried through, the process of a new affective reintegration of the personality as a whole cannot achieve its therapeutic or scientific goal."

Because psychoanalytic theory has permeated so much of current psychiatric thought and practice, it is desirable to examine closely the theory of psychoanalytic etiology and the dynamics of psychoanalytic cure. To particularize the processes of repression, one may note that Freud postulated the existence of the id, which embraces the primal urges: the superego, which is the socially oriented, inhibiting, conscience-including component of the psychic organism, and the ego, which is, in effect, that part of the psyche immediately in contact with reality, and which impinges upon, and is impinged upon derivately by, both the id and the superego.

This tripartite division of the psychic mechanism was not original with Freud. It is an ancient trinity found almost universally in philosophy, psychology, and religion. What is original with Freud is his theory on the conflict between the id impulsion and the superego, resulting in the repression of unacceptable impulsions.

Two factors in this formulation must be noted carefully, namely, that the repression is an unconscious act—it does not reach awareness—and that the repressed impulsion is not annihilated but may become operative and influence emotion, mentation, and behavior in vicarious, and not understandable, ways. The emergence and operation of the repressed are reflected in the psychopathology of everyday life, in dreams, and in the neuroses.

Because unconscious material, according to Freud, cannot be reached by any deliberate effort in recall but will well up in uncensored thought, free association, again according to Freud, is the essential and all-powerful therapeutic instrumentality of psychoanalytic psychotherapy.

To round out this exposition of the dynamics of the psychoanalytic cure, it is necessary to note that unconscious repressed material when brought into awareness is, according to psychoanalytic theory, deprived of its psychopathogenic energy and the integrated and integrative powers of the ego are thereby increased and improved. Lest I be later challenged on the last point, let me add now that I am cognizant of the fact that mere recall of repressed material is acknowledged by some analysts to be insufficient for "a cure." But this acknowledgment is a late acquired insight and, as a matter of fact, constitutes not an amplification of the original theory, but, rather, a challenge which is in effect tantamount to a contradiction of it. I shall deal with this issue later.

Freud's theory of repression and his theory of recall by free association are both brilliantly conceived. Furthermore, experience shows that the formulations of psychoanalytic theory are valid in many instances. Certainly, as already observed, the theory of repression is supported in much of the psychopathology of everyday life, in the dream process, as revealed through dream analysis, in a good deal of hysteria, and in the obsessive and compulsive neuroses. But, when all this is granted, pertinent and troubling questions remain to be resolved. Accepting, as one must, the reality of repression, one is yet obliged to differentiate between repression as a psychic mechanism and repression as a psychopathogenic process.

That repression is as frequently and as dominantly psychopathogenic as Freud maintains is open to question. The analysts themselves recognize this, professing that "during the last twenty years or so it has become obvious that the mere uncovering of the unconscious is not enough. Not even full recollection of the forgotten events of one's life and the liberation from their repressed state of the various unconscious representations as well as affects, is enough" (3).

Repression may be, and in some instances is, the most prominent and the most powerful psychopathogenic factor. Repression is to some degree present in and contributory to every case of neurosis. But there are other psychological factors which to the unprejudiced student appear to be as powerfully pathogenic as, and more widely operative than, repression. Among these, deprivation is the most significant. By deprivation I intend the lack of some experience, or function, essential to healthy normal maturation. The orphan, the child of a broken family, the unloved child, the overindulged and pampered child, the child of immature and inadequate parents, the child born into times and circumstances of social turmoil and instability—such children are likely to suffer deprivations in physical, social, and psychic experience, deprivations which in the extreme will cripple them irreparably, and which in the more modest degrees may result in asocial, inadequate, and neurotic function and behavior. In such instances the dynamics of the cure cannot lie in "free association," but must depend, rather, on substitutive and corrective experience, and in this the psychotherapist can play an important and determining role. Since a great number of crippling deprivations derive from untoward interpersonal relations which the patient experienced, mainly during childhood—relations to parents, sibling, other family members, nurses, and teachers—the countertransference of the therapist, to use this rather apt analytic term, provides an opportunity and a means for healing. "The therapist," as Franz Alexander has phrased it in another connection (4), "must assume an attitude towards the patient which in the light of the patient's history appears appropriate to undo the pathogenic influences." I would add, "not only to undo but also to amend," for the cure is not always and ever a matter of "taking away." Oftener it is a task of "adding a something that was missed."

Only a few among the so-called orthodox analysts have recognized the pathogenic import of deprivation. That concept, however, was implicit in the ergological theories of Meyerian psychiatry.

To pursue further the dynamics of the cure in psychoanalysis, we need to examine more closely the τέχνη of free association. Zilboorg, in his paper (3), freely grants that the true psychology of psychoanalysis remains unknown and will remain so until the processes involved in free associations are fully understood. These processes, he affirms, are little known. Despite that, he describes free associations "as requiring a deliberate weakening, or attenuation, of that conscious part of the ego which deals with the outside world in order to permit the unconscious trends to slide, as it were, into the preconscious and from there to come to the surface and slip into the conscious" (5). This is neatly phrased, but it does not meet the challenge of the crucial question: In free association, what is the Censor that censors the Censor? The obvious fact is that free associations are never free. Free associations are subjet to the same laws of psychological determination as those that govern all thinking.

It is patent that the therapeutic function of free association is greatly overassessed and much misconceived in psychoanalysis. For one thing, all recall, whether "directed or free," is unconscious, and such benefits as are derived from what is termed free association stem largely from the permissive atmosphere which embraces both the patient and the therapist, rather than from any presumed attenuation or deliberate weakening of any portion of the ego or the superego.

We can concur with Zilboorg's statement that "psychoanalysts know little of the process and the laws of free association." However, this is not tantamount to saying that little *is* known about free association. The ignorance appears, rather, to be confined to the psychoanalysts. Experimental psychologists, for example, know a great deal about free association. They have long been concerned with the dynamics of free association, and historically, be it noted, there was a school of analytical psychology (6) before there was one of analytical psychiatry. Furthermore, one of the original and principal propositions in analytical psychology is embodied in psychoanalytic theory. That is the postulate that all "mental life is directed, purposive, motivated, and cannot be explained as being governed by the chance clashing of elements derived haphazardly from without" (7). Freud, similarly, advanced the postulate that both thought and action are determined by wish and motive. Heinz Hartmann would have us believe that Freud anticipated these findings of the analytical psychologists (8), but R. Adamson wrote in 1884 that "thinking is motivated," and F. A. Bradley stated in 1887 that "thinking is controlled by the object of thought" (9).

The "operation of thought," which embraces free association, has been studied since the time of Aristotle, and most intensively during the past 100 years. The idea that all thinking is motivated, directed, and monitored, that it is therefore not free, is almost universally accepted by all schools of psychology. The sole exceptions are the Pavlovians and the behaviorists, who espouse a modern version of the ancient associational theory. But here we need to emphasize that all thinking, not merely that reflected in so-called free association, is motivated and directed. The distorting emphasis on "free association" found in psychoanalytic doxy would make it appear that only in the "material" produced by free association can one find clues to the patient's conflicts and repressions. This is most certainly not the case. Freud himself, it will be recalled, observed that in the case of Mrs. Emmy he was struck by the lack in her formal recitation of any references to her sexual life and experiences:

> I was also struck by the fact that of all the intimate information imparted by the patient, the sexual element . . . was entirely lacking. . . . What she allowed me to hear was probably an *editio in usum Delphini* of her life's history (10).

Freud did not need to elicit her "free associations" to ascertain the existence of this blind spot. It proved as obtrusive in her deliberate story as it would have been patent in her dreams.

It is not my intention to deny that "free association" is likely to be more productive of significant anamnestic and "forgotten" material than is orderly deliberate recitation. I would, however, deny that "free association" is a unique process of mentation, involving, as it is postulated, an attentuation, and deliberate weakening of any part of the conscious ego. What is termed free association is in essence no more than the basic processes of thinking and recall, exercised in an extraordinarily permissive atmosphere. The psychotherapeutic situation and relationship facilitate what the world at large denies—a broad, inclusive, leisurely, judgment-withholding, sympathetic scrutiny of past experiences, present problems, possible alternatives, and much more beside.

Rado has also come to appreciate the cardinal significance of the permissive factor in the therapeutic relationship. Discussing Breuer's patient and the release she experienced when she vented her anger, Rado (11) observes:

> Another crucial point is that the patient *felt free* to recall the incident responsible for her rage. Had she feared that Breuer might criticize her, she would have remained silent or vented her anger on Breuer.

I have belabored the subject of free association because, although it is badly understood, it has become a shibboleth in psychoanalysis. As such, it not only impedes progress in psychoanalysis but also is responsible for much drag and lag in therapy, the waste of much good money, and the loss of precious time. There is something of magical expectancy in the orthodox evaluation of free association— the expectation that if the patient recumbent will but free-associate long enough all things, including the good life, will ultimately come to him. This, like all magical expectation, constitutes nonsense.

On the other hand, for the achievement of good therapeutic results, it is essential that the psychiatrist, and even more so the patient, should acquire a thoroughgoing, all-embracing knowledge and understanding of the patient's experiences, reactions, rationalizations, and attitudes. For this the patient must have the opportunity for and the circumstances conducive to full and uninhibited recall and recitation. The permissive relationship of the therapist is here the essential prerequisite. But this relationship does not necessarily involve the patient in interminable, meandering verbigerations, nor does it preclude the offering of directions and suggestions by the therapist. On the contrary, if the therapist will draw his clues from the "motivations" patent in the overt behavior and in the formal recitations of the patient, he will find in them profitable guidance to the anamnestic terrains to be explored. He and the patient will thus the sooner acquire a clear understanding of the significant components of the patient's total experience. Therapeutic expeditiousness and therapeutic effectiveness will thus be favored.

All this obviously presupposes much more active participation in the "therapeutic process" than is countenanced in orthodox psychoanalysis. On this score it were easy to opine—"so much the worse for orthodoxy." But that would do no justice to the historical validity entombed in the objection. Then, besides the orthodox analysts, we need to bear in mind some among the clinical psychologists, and some among the social workers, to whom the concept of nondirective therapy is so very precious, and to whom the opposite carries so much of anathema.

As far as Freud and his early associates are concerned, we need to recall that they were inordinately sensitive to "therapeutic activity," for to them it meant a kind of "moralistic busybodyness," with which they were all too painfully well acquainted. Griesinger had no sympathy with "the moralising ideas that were held by bigots regarding the treatment of insanity" (12). Yet under the heading of the more direct moral action for the purpose of restoring mental health, he advised that morbid ideas which repress and conceal the former (healthy) individuality must "be uprooted and destroyed, while the old ego must as far as possible be recalled and strengthened" (13).

This is a far cry from the therapeutic activity which seeks to guide the patient in the exploration of certain segments of his history wherein he might find insight into the derivations of his past and current difficulties. As far as nondirective therapy is concerned, it can be summated as a grotesque on psychoanalytic passivity. Its devotees aim to out-Caesar Caesar.

Nondirective therapy is, in effect, inconceivable. This so-called therapy is not really a therapy but only a game in which one of the players picks up and repeats the last few words spoken by the other as an inducement to continue the game.

All therapy must be, as all life is, goal-directed. The catch, of course, lies in whose goal is to be pursued and by what bearings the course is to be plotted. The current situation of the patient; his difficulties; the patterns of his past performances, successes, and failures; his own hopes and ambitions, all must serve as the coordinates by which the goals of therapy are to be charted. The therapist must scrupulously refrain from intruding upon the patient his own preconceptions and his unrelated therapeutic ambitions. Therapy must draw its ultimate goals from the realities and potentialities of the patient, and from none other. But without goals, without the sense and perspective of direction, therapy can only be a phantom march, a mere marking of time.

Schilder aptly phrased this issue (14):

> It is the important task of the physician to develop the patient's personality according to the capacities, endowments, and characteristics of the patient. He (the physician) will be better able to do so if he has the conviction that the other human being is an entity of its own and is valuable in so far as it is a definite person.

Rado treats this matter even more pointedly (15).

> The aim of psychoanalytic therapy is to increase the patient's capacity for enjoyment and active achievement in life by lifting him to a higher level of psychodynamic organization. . . . An adequate plan for modifying the patient's life performance must first consider the relation of available means to desired ends. It must include an itemized list of problems; an itemized list of tools; a set of instructions as to how to put the latter to work.

All this presupposes, nay, indeed, stipulates, not merely an uncovering of the past, essential but much overrated, but also an assessment of the current situation, the available resources, and the possible goals.

Here I needs must begin the summation of my exposition. The dynamics of the cure in psychotherapy, seen historically, reflects the emergence of diverse theories on the etiology of psychiatric illnesses. The older pre-Freudian theories are easy to comprehend. They are founded on limited, but valid, morbific causes. The amplitude and scope for specific psychotherapy which they inspired and allowed were likewise limited, and the dynamics of such therapy was simple and patent. With the advent of psychoanalysis the picture changed radically. Derived from an ingenious and intricate system of psychodynamics, the etiological theory of repression was advanced to account for much of general psychopathology, particularly of the psychoneuroses.

De-repression by the technique of free association was accordingly developed by Freud, and the dynamics of the psychoanalytic cure was spelled out in terms of "making conscious the unconscious, removing the repressions, and filling in the gaps of memory. . . . We do nothing more for our patients but enable this one mental change to take place in them; the extent to which it is achieved is the extent of the benefit we do them" (16).

The etiological theory of repression and the dynamics of the psychoanalytic cure by free association I have subjected to critical analysis and evaluation.

The etiological theory of repression, while valid to some degree in much of psychopathology, and entirely adequate to account for certain given disorders, is nonetheless propounded in orthodox psychoanalysis with such catholic embrace as to prove ultimately erroneous in substance and corrupting in effect. It is erroneous when it ascribes to repression what is due to other causes, and it is corrupting because it impedes the appreciation of those other causes. I then analyzed the alleged uniqueness of free association, pointing out that it is essentially an exercise of the normal process of thinking and recall. What *is* unique to free association is the permissive atmosphere of the therapeutic relationship. This enables and encourages the patient "to be more candid with the physician than he ever dared to be with himself" (11).

We thus come to the conclusion that the dynamics of the effective psychiatric cure embraces much more than de-repression by means of free association, even as most of psychopathology is traceable to much more than repression.

The dynamics of the psychiatric cure cannot, and must not, be cramped within a neat formula. It cannot be summated by a pat phrase. In reviewing the ascendency and decline, during the past 100 years, of the various theories on the etiology of psychiatric disorders, one cannot but be impressed with the fact that they were most in error where they sought singularly to account for all psychopathology, disallowing the validity and the pathogenic operations of other factors, propounded in other theories. It is at this point that I am impelled to bring up again the daemoniacal theory of etiology. This theory, as I observed, is sadly misunderstood, since it is confused with "witch hunting" and the "Christian Devil." In actuality, it impinges on the id of psychoanalysis and on the *élan vital* of Bergson. It was best propounded by the Greek philosopher Heraclitus, who wrote that, "Ethos is man's daemon." Unfortunately, this, even in translation, we now find difficult to comprehend, unless, of course, we try very hard, for, said Heraclitus, in the daemon there is a logos which connects knowledge of Being with insight into human values and conduct and makes the former include the latter (17). There are a good daemon and an evil one, or, more precisely, the good daemon, as well as the logos, can be corrupted. But in the light of the good daemon, such a one as inspired Socrates, logos can comprehend the law divine, "the law by which all human laws are nourished" (18). In recent decades we have experienced in the cruel totalitarianisms, both large and small, the sovereignty of evil daemons. In the contemporary vernacular, there can be no doubt that evil, corroding and corrupting "climates of opinion," can, and do at times, prevail, that they are noxious both to individuals and to the community, and that such evil climates of opinion may become manifest in psychopathology. Yet the fact must not be overlooked that essentially the primal daemon is good, and that it can give new life to conscious knowledge. Of this daemon it may be said what Mephistopheles said of himself—that it is "Part of the Power not understood, which always wills the Bad—and always works the Good" (19). But this subject is far too complicated and involved to be treated at the end of a rather lengthy presentation. Let me, therefore, but round off this item by pointing to the radical change in social, cultural, moral, and esthetic values which our own times have experienced and which I, for one, find sharply reflected in the difficulties of our contemporaries seeking psychiatric help.

Let me add that the psychotherapist who is not cognizant of the existence and of the operations of the daemon, or, knowing it, fears the daemon and thus cannot bridle *that* power which, willing the bad, always works the good—such a psychotherapist is indeed badly handicapped. He will never understand what is meant by prophylactic psychopathology. He will never really plumb the depths of the human psyche.

But, to return to the dynamics of the cure in psychiatry, I have said that no neat formula or pat phrase can summate it. Yet it is possible to name and to describe the principal components and the main operational sequences that are involved in the achievement of the psychiatric cure.

I shall begin with the patient. He is the primary factor in the dynamics of the psychiatric cure. His innate competences, his willingness to cooperate in the therapeutic process, the intrapsychic pressure which motivates and impels his quest for help, all these not only profoundly affect the ultimate issue but also influence and regulate the therapeutic process.

Freud, with his felicitous ingenuity in coining phrases, described the relationship of the patient to his therapist in terms of the transference neurosis. In essence, this means that the patient's attitude and behavior toward the therapist are of the same order as those which basically produced the untoward effects which brought him under therapy. How the therapist deals with the transference neurosis is crucial to the issue. Basically, he must be permissive. Unfortunately, some therapists consider this to be the alpha and omega of therapy. It *is* the alpha; it is not the omega! The patient is manipulatable. His competences, his willingness to cooperate, the intrapsychic pressure which he experiences, these are not absolutely given and inalterable. They are dynamic potentials which can be degraded or intensified; they are energy quanta which are convertible. The skillful and purposive manipulation of the patient's potentials is in effect the very essence of the art of the psychotherapeutic process. It is here that an appreciation of the daemon is a prerequisite, for without this appreciation the therapist is fearful and lost. He is compelled to yield the therapeutic initiative to the patient and he himself to withdraw into the refuge of passivity.

This brings us to the second principal component of the therapeutic dynamics in psychiatry—the therapist. He not only must be informed in the data of psychiatry and skilled in the techniques of psychotherapy, but must, in addition, be "wise in the ways and meaning of life." It was Freud, I believe, who said that no therapist can bring the patient farther than he himself has gone. To be wise in the ways and meaning of life, the psychotherapist needs must know a great deal more than psychiatry. He needs must be a humanist both in learning and in being. In this an appreciation of the history of the profession and of his own specialty is most beneficial. The historical perspective induces humility, inspires hope, broadens one's vision, and teaches one to be earnest in enterprise, but not humorless in the face of reality.

Given the principal components, we can now turn to the operational sequence in which the dynamics of the cure in psychiatry becomes manifest.

Initially the patient comes to the psychiatrist with a complaint. The complaint is the patient's version of what "troubles him," or of "what *is* the trouble." Almost always the version is wrong; that is, it does not conform to the objective reality. Despite that, it is imperative that the patient be encouraged and helped to formulate and to express his complaint. This is the first step in the anamnestic process. When the complaint has been well formulated, the second phase is entered upon—that of recitation and recall. In effect, this is a parade of the patient's history, given freely, amply, and in a measure repetitively. The patient's history may, will, and should deal with recent and contemporary experience, no less than with the past. The recitation and recall must be projected against the patient's complaint, to assess what, if any, relationship there may be between the one and the other. In this operation the therapist functions like an intelligent echo, giving back to the patient his very own words, but suggesting new contexts and new meanings. This process in time yields the third operation, namely, the reassessment and reorganization of the anamnestic material. A word must be said in amplification of this. In psychoanalysis, major emphasis has been placed on recall of forgotten and repressed material. Recall is both real and valuable but plays a less important role in the dynamics of the cure than the reorganization, i.e., the reassessment of remembered experience. The child, the young person, the immature and inexperienced young adult, remember well enough, but they all too often draw distorted and erroneous conclusions from their experiences. Such distortions and errors must be corrected. In this process the transference effects of the therapeutic relation, as well as the extra-anamnestic effects, are of crucial import. What I intend by this can be summarized briefly. The patient can best reassess and reorganize his experiences with and under the guidance of the therapist. The terms "interpretation" and "insight" are applied to this process, but these are somewhat neutral designations. They do not reflect the powerful operations of that force which derives from "what the therapist stands for." Furthermore, and that is what I intend by extra-anamnestic effects, the patient cannot gain recovery and derive effective therapy solely from the contemplation—no matter how deep and detailed—of his past experience; for those ends he requires certain new experiences, which in a measure are derived from the actual person-to-person relationship of patient and therapist.

The final step in the operational sequences of the cure in psychiatry lies in implementing, motivating, and acting on the therapeutic gains. The psychoanalysts speak of this in terms of breaking, or terminating, the transference. This formulation places the emphasis on the patient-therapist relationship, with the initiative in the person of the therapist. It should, rather, be conceived in terms of the relationship of the patient to his immediate world, with the therapist endeavoring not to break the dependence but, rather, to dissipate it by encouraging the patient "to apply his gains in the real world"—to love Rome more, rather than Caesar less. This phase of therapy calls for the exercise of much skill and wisdom on the part of the therapist.

Such are the principal components and operational sequences that enter into the dynamics of the cure in psychiatry. Again, I need not elaborate what must be clear to all, i.e., that the listed steps and items are not, in actual operation, as distinct and sequential as they are given in the recitation.

Two of the eight etiological theories which I list at the beginning of my presentation I have not as yet touched on; these are the socioenvironmental and the ecological. Actually, however, I can do little more than mention them, for they are, so to say, at the peripheral zone of psychiatric research and study. Marxian economists and communist scientists have advanced the theory that much, if not most, of the psychiatric disorders are "economically determined." I can recall when Frankwood Williams, returning from a visit to Russia, enthusiastically reported that with the advent of the proletarian revolution there was a most remarkable drop in the incidence of the psychoses and neuroses. But that, of course, was a delusion. The relation of socioeconomic factors to the etiology, incidence, and issue of psychiatric illness is being studied, particularly in the United States, with fine discrimination and competent skills, by many men.

In these studies, psychiatrists, sociologists, anthropologists, ethnographers, and demographers are combining their skills and competences to assess the psychological effects of the socioeconomic matrix upon the individual and upon the group. We needs must await the issue of their studies. Yet even now we know that the social and economic components of the individual's environment can and do affect his personality, his sensitiveness to and tolerance of stress and frustration. Poverty, instability of the home, a degrading environment, the experience of being one of a minority group which is socially not accepted, or is disparaged, all such experiences are in effect both traumata and deprivations and may contribute to manifest psychopathology. A plethora of the world's goods and overprotection, of course, can also contribute to the engenderment of psychological difficulties. The psychological effects of the social matrix are, however, subtler than these crudely patent instances show. The near future, I suspect, will teach us much on this score.

The ecological theory is, in effect, a much broader development of the thesis propounded in the socioeconomic theory. This concept is the modern counterpart of the Paracelsian micromacrocosmic picture. It has been sketched by James Halliday (20). I myself (21) have attempted to formulate the ecological theory in several contributions on social medicine, and also in a chapter entitled psychosocial medicine. Fundamentally, the ecological theory holds that man is a creature of his own world, and, to put it somewhat cryptically, even as he does unto his world, so is it done unto him.

I wish to end this presentation by emphasizing one important factor. I have attempted to describe, to analyze, and to evaluate the principal theories on the etiology of psychiatric disorders current during the past 100 years and to deal with the dynamics of the psychiatric cure envisaged in each. It is most important to the scientifically guided physician to operate within the framework of a clearly defined theory of etiology and therapy; otherwise, he degenerates into an empiricist. With all that, however, it is important that he bear in mind that it is the man, the therapist, who avails and prevails—with, or against, the theory. In the ultimate, the dynamics of the cure derives more from him than from his theory. My own psychiatric mentor, A. A. Brill, was wont to say: "The most important factor in psychotherapy is the therapist." Experience certainly validates this dictum, which I urge you to bear in mind; otherwise, theory, intended as a supporting scaffold, is likely to become an imprisoning cage.

REFERENCES

1. BROWN, JOHN: *Elementa medicinae*, Edinburg, C. Elliot, 1780.
2. FREUD, S.: *An Autobiographical Study*, Ed. 2., authorized translation, by J. Strachey, London, Hogarth Press, 1952.
3. ZILBOORG, G.: Some sidelights on free associations, *Internat. J. Psycho-Analysis 33*: 488, 1952.
4. ALEXANDER, F.: *Congrés international de psychiatrie*, Vol. 5: Psychothérapie psychanalyse, médecine psychosomatique. Evolution et tendances actuelles de la psychanalyse, Paris, Librairie scientifique Hermann & Cie, 1950.
5. HARTMANN, H.: *Grundlagen der Psychoanalyse*, Leipzing, Georg Thieme, 1927.
6. STOUT, G. F.: *Analytic Psychology*, London, S. Sonneschein & Co., 1902.

7. HUMPHREY, G.: *Thinking—An Introduction to Its Psychology*, London, Methuen & Co. Ltd., 1951, p. 9.
8. HARTMANN, *op. cit.*, p. 65.
9. Cited by Humphrey, *op. cit.*, p. 26.
10. BREUER, J. and FREUD, S.: Studies in Hysteria, authorized translation by A. A. Brill, in *Nervous and Mental Diseases Monograph* Series No. 61, 1936, p. 74.
11. RADO, S.: Recent advances of psychoanalytic therapy, *A. Res. Nerv. & Ment. Dis., Proc. 31*:42, 1953.
12. GRIESINGER, W.: *Mental Pathology and Therapeutics*, translated from the German (Ed. 2) by C. Lockhart Robertson and J. Rutherford, London, New Sydenham Society, 1867, p. 59.
13. GRIESINGER, *op. cit.* p. 483.
14. SCHILDER, P.: *Psychotherapy*, New York, W. W. Norton & Company, Inc., 1938, p. 166.
15. RADO, *op. cit.*, pp. 50 and 51.
16. FREUD, S.: *Transference; in a General Introduction to Psychoanalysis*, English translation of revised edition by Joan Rivière, New York, Liveright Publishers Corporation, 1935, p. 377.
17. JAEGER, WERNER: *Paedeia*, New York, Oxford University Press, 1943, Vol. 1, p. 180.
18. JAEGER, *op. cit.*, p. 181.
19. GOETHE, J. WOLFGANG: *Faust*, Part I, Scene iii.
20. HALLIDAY, JAMES: *Psychosocial Medicine*, New York, W. W. Norton Company, Inc., 1948.
21. GALDSTON, IAGO: *Psychosocial Medicine in Recent Advances in Psychosomatic* London, Sir Isaac Pitman & Sons, Ltd. 1953; Social medicine and the epidemic constitution, *Bull Hist. Med.* Baltimore, 1951; *Social Implications of Dynamic Psychiatry: Social Medicine—Its Derivations and Objectives*, New York, Commonwealth Fund, 1949.

10

Psychosomatic Medicine — Past, Present, and Future

PSYCHOSOMATIC medicine is well on the way to becoming a singular specialty. It now has its coterie of practitioners, its specialty publications, its journals, its monographs, and its historical treatises. True, it is still lacking an international society and a specialty board. But if things move as rapidly and in the same direction during the next 10 years as they have in the past 25, we may expect in the not-too-distant future, both a worldwide society and a specialty board.

These are eventualities which I, for one, do not envisage with pleasure or satisfaction.

Psychosomatic medicine is singular because, unlike all other specialties, it does not revolve about a technological skill, such, for example, as radiology or surgery; or about a definitive system or organs, as is the case, say, with ophthalmology or gastroenterology; or about an age span, as do pediatrics and gerontology. It is not even a nosological specialty, as are those of syphilology, phthisiology, or the neoplasms. Psychosomatic medicine is a singular specialty in that it essentially espouses a distinctive pathological dynamism. It advances the general principle that emotional tensions, chronic or acute, are often discharged in ways that upset the normal physiological equilibrium of an organ, thus initiating the somatic changes that produce disease. Psychosomatic medicine is chiefly concerned with the relationship of emotional tensions to organic and functional disorders.

A great deal is implicated in this simple statement—vastly more than one is at first likely to appreciate. Indeed, psychosomatic medicine, in its superficial aspects, is all too seductively simple, and hence tends to entice the simple. This is one reason why it is said, and in some instances with

128

warrant, that the psychosomaticists, if I may use that abominable term, among the psychiatrists are suspected of being clinicians, and among the clinicians, of being psychiatrists.

I shall have a good deal to say about the numerous implications of psychosomatic medicine. At this point, however, I want to discuss the recency of psychosomatic medicine. On several occasions, and most recently in my paper on "The Roots of Psychosomatic Medicine" (1), I have argued that psychosomatic medicine is "a strictly modern term," and that "there is nothing in the vernacular of antecedent medicine that can be construed as the homologue of psychosomatic."

These affirmations have been challenged by several colleagues. They contend that in the past many medical authors have employed, if not the precise term "psychosomatic," such varied combinations of the terms "psyche" and "soma," "mind" and "body," "mental" and "physical," and in such ways, as to constitute valid equivalents for the term "psychosomatic." Margetts (2) has written an illuminating paper on the history of the use of the term "psychosomatic," which seemingly gives solid support to those of my colleagues who take issue with me on the recency of psychosomatic medicine.

Nevertheless, I must hold to my judgment. It is indeed true that all of our instructed and experienced physicians, from the time of Hippocrates down, have appreciated the reciprocal relations of psyche and soma and have employed some conjunction of these terms to designate that relationship. But psychosomatic medicine, as we know and understand it today, as it has been advanced by Alexander, Grinker, French, Stokes, Wittkower, and Halliday, to name but a few, bears about the same relation to the psychosomatic preoccupations of times past as the atom of the "H-bomb" bears to the atom of Democritus. The fact is that psychosomatic medicine, as we know it today, is not a direct-line derivative of the psyche-soma preoccupations of our medical elders, and it profits us little to lump together all the references to psyche and soma to be found in medical history, and to argue therefrom that ours is an ancient preoccupation.

Present-day psychosomatic medicine *is* historically and actually unique. And it is unique in this: that essentially it constitutes a movement to counterbalance and to correct some of the erroneous and corrupting ideas and viewpoints propagated in organicist medicine. However, it must promptly be added that these errors, these corrupting ideas, have so deeply permeated the data and the mentation processes of present-day medicine that even those who are devoted to the study of psychosomatic medicine do not entirely escape them, and are not completely free of them.

To be specific on these scores, psychosomatic medicine *should* be holistic in its orientation and ecological in its embrace. And yet, it is still largely committed to the primitive concept of specific etiology and to the "time and sequence chain of causality," wherein the linkage is a *cause*, emotional tensions which discharge in ways to upset physiological equilibrium, thus initiating somatic changes, and producing disease.

In my paper "Biodynamic Medicine Versus Psychosomatic Medicine" (3), I exposed in some detail the corruptions which psychosomatic medicine has carried over from organicist medicine. I need not, therefore, reargue the issue here. I want, rather, to elaborate the historical antecedents of present-day psychosomatic medicine and to give support to my contention that psychosomatic medicine came into being as a corrective to the faults of organicist medicine.

It is most interesting and very significant that the earliest exponents of psychosomatic medicine were the psychoanalysts. Freud himself was a pioneer in this field. In his "Studies on Hysteria," published in 1895, he reported on the case of Miss Lucy, the English governess in Vienna, whose symptoms turned out to be dependent on the repression of a forbidden attachment to her employer. It was in the discussion of this case, which Freud had treated in 1892, that he first described how the active process of repressing an incompatible idea results in the substitution of a somatic conversion.

This case history is a pristine instance of a psychosomatic disorder, conforming to the now classical definition—"emotional tension discharged in ways that upset normal physiological equilibrium and initiating somatic changes that produce disease." Freud was too busy developing and promoting psychoanalysis to cultivate also the specialty of psychosomatic medicine. That enlisted the interest of a number of his associates and disciples, notably Deutsch, Ferenczi, Groddeck, and Jelliffe. The last-named was without doubt the most ingenious, erudite, imaginative, and inspired pioneer in psychosomatic medicine. Jelliffe had a most comprehensive grasp of all the implications of psychosomatic medicine in relation both to clinical medicine and to psychiatry. Yet I observe with some disappointment that he has received but scant credit for his original and massive contributions to psychosomatic medicine.

I shall have more to say concerning Jelliffe's pioneering work in psychosomatic medicine. Here, I want to revert to Freud's case—Miss Lucy—and to his theory of the conversion of repressed emotional into somatic disorders. This theory was not only original in the highest sense, but also most revolutionary. It ran afoul of the prevailing schools of thought. It was indeed diametrically opposed and contrary to all the fundamental principles of the biological sciences, then deemed sacred and eternal. What Freud postulated was nothing less startling than that physical changes, that is, demonstrable alterations in the functions and structure of cells, tissues, organs, systems, and of the body entire, could be effected by the psyche. The psyche, be it noted, did not then, and does not now, fit into any of the known categories of "energy and matter."

Here a brief excursion is indicated in order to sharpen our perspectives and to set forth more clearly the originality and profundity of Freud's theory on the conversion of repressed emotions into somatic disorders.

It is an historical fact that many physicians, long before Freud's time, recognized that the psyche in general, and the emotions in particular, affect the operations of the body. The vernacular, in its many and felicitous expressions, such as "eating one's heart out," "can't stomach that fellow," "he gives me a pain in the neck," shows that not alone the learned but the common man as well knew that the soma mirrors the psyche, and vice versa. But the catch had always been in the how of the trick. *How* does the soma affect the psyche, or the psyche the soma? It is simple enough to perceive that they are ligated. The challenge lies in establishing the *nature* and the *dynamics* of that ligature.* Freud's merit and originality lie precisely in this, that he was not content merely to affirm that psyche and soma are ligated, but went further and postulated a theory to describe and to account for the ways by which, and because of which, the psyche affects the soma—and produces disease. That was his theory of repression. This theory he elaborated to embrace the two-way relationship of psyche-soma and soma-psyche. Freud considered the syndrome he labeled anxiety neurosis to be the somatic witness of a "psychic repression," while hysteria he held to be the psychic witness of a "somatic repression" (4). This is Freud's elaboration of this theory:

> In each of them [that is both in anxiety neurosis and in hysteria], there occurs a deflection of excitation to the somatic field instead of psychical assimilation of it: the difference is . . . this, that in anxiety-neurosis the excitation is purely somatic, whereas in hysteria it is purely psychical.

---

*If I mistake not, that is at the root of Hans Selye's researches today, and I know that Harold Wolff and his associates, as well as Grinker, French, Alexander, and their associates, have been and are working intensively in the exploration and on the illumination of just this problem.

It is not relevant to our purpose to establish whether Freud's postulates are correct or not, nor does it matter whether we do or do not accept them as such. It is, however, pertinent that we fully appreciate the fact that in this theory Freud argues that the psyche affects the soma through purely psychological means.

This is a rather bold statement, which I permit myself only in the interest of emphasis and clarity. It suffers the fault of historical foreshortening or condensation and distorts the actuality. What I mean is that at the time Freud first advanced his theory of repression he himself was not too clear, or certain in his mind, that repression *was* purely a psychological operation. He entertained the idea that possibly repression might in effect operate through some toxic chemical agent which it engendered, or liberated.

All this may seem like so much trivia. But it is really quite significant and is relevant to the very core of our concern. For we need to bear in mind that at the time Freud made his pronouncements, the psyche, qua psyche, was officially nonexistent. Purely psychological forces were held to be inconceivable, and hence nonexistent, and he who played with such ideas was deemed to be either an ignoramus or a charlatan, and, most likely, a good deal of both at one and the same time. We need also to appreciate that neither Mesmer, nor Braid, nor Bernheim, nor Charcot, nor Janet, these being among the outstanding men to concern themselves with hypnoses, hysteria, and neurasthenia, postulated in their various theories the operation of purely psychological forces or mechanisms. They did conceive of subtle agents, such as immaterial fluidisms, animal magnetism, suggestion, neurasthemia, and so on. But these were not psychological dynamisms, as Freud's repression was.

In this connection, it will profit us to recall the conflict between the school of Nancy and that of the Salpêtrière. In the latter, Charcot demonstrated to his own satisfaction the existence of a "fluidium," for he was able, by means of large magnets, to transpose disturbances, such as paresthesias, contractures, and paralysis, from one side of the patient's body to the opposite side, or from some proximate to some remote part of the body. The Nancy school, however, discredited these demonstrations, for they proved that Charcot's patients were "trained performers," reacting exactly as was expected of them—and that the magnets were inconsequential, for a pencil in the hand of the hypnotist would prove just as effective if the patient but thought it was a magnet. Bernheim, the leader of the Nancy school, ascribed Charcot's, as well as his own, hypnotic influences to suggestion. Suggestion he described as the manifest influence of an extraneous idea (that of the hypnotist) on the brain, and hence on the behavior of the person who accepted the idea. According to Bernheim, suggestion though psychological in nature, operated as an exogenous force.

Freud, oddly enough, sided with Charcot against Bernheim. He had translated the works of both. This ambivalence, which is both interesting and significant, can be accounted for by the atmosphere in which he grew up. His psychiatric preceptor, Meynert, was an out-and-out organicist, and Brücke, the teacher who had made the biggest impression on Freud, was a partisan of that school of thought, elaborated by Helmholtz, DuBois-Reymond, and Ludwig, which militantly maintained that all vital phenomena, no matter how complex, and including also the mental and psychological, are ultimately explicable in terms of physics and chemistry. Brücke's teachings were Freud's point of departure in the elaboration of his psychoanalytic theories. But he did not follow them for long. The so-called "toxicological" theory of neuroses which Freud initially propounded he ultimately abandoned, and repression in the Freudian system acquired a pure and unadulterated psychological character.

I have gone to some lengths in elaborating the history of Freud's excursion into the field of psychosomatic medicine for two reasons—first, to celebrate his pioneering contribution, and second, to highlight the difficulties he experienced in freeing his own thinking of the materialist, organicist patterns which conditioned, and currently still hamper, so much of medical and biological comprehension and understanding. Also, my scruples as a medical historian would not allow me to gloss over the obscurities and paradoxes inherent in Freud's initial exposition. And while speaking in the guise of a medical historian, I think it of interest to point out that it was the Russian physiologist Pavlov who first demonstrated the purely psychological nature of the neuroses, albeit experimental, in his case. This field of study has been brilliantly and most profitably developed by a number of American workers, including Horsley Gantt and Howard Liddell.

To revert now to the main stream of our exposition: I had observed that the psychoanalysts were among the very earliest workers in psychosomatic medicine. It was they who postulated that disturbances in the psyche could, and frequently do, become manifest in somatic disorders. Initially this postulation was advanced as a protest to the prevailing organicist-mechanistic concept of the etiology of disease, a concept which held chemical-physical changes in the material structure of the body the essential antecedent to all manifest pathology. With time, however, the protest became *ein Ding an sich selbst*. It became, in other words, psychosomatic medicine. Now it was no longer just a protest; not merely the affirmation that hysteria, with all its protean symptoms and disorders, was not due to a "wandering of the womb," to animal magnetism, to hereditary debility, to some malign fluidium, etc., but was due, rather, to a purely psychological mechanism labeled by Freud "repression." Now indeed the initiative was with the psychiatrists, and they premised that a host of disorders, ranging from Dupuytren's contractures to psoriasis, were psychogenic in origin, or at least showed "evidence of being related to psychological stress." The list has grown with time, and currently it includes such morbidities as infantile cachexia, hyperinsulinism, diabetes, gout, hyperthyroidism, glaucoma, keratitis, asthma, hay fever, sinusitis, headache, peptic ulcer, ulcerative colitis, constipation and diarrhea, arthritis, backache, angina pectoris, hypertension, neurocirculatory asthenia, impotence, dysmenorrhea, hives, and eczema. This catalogue, compiled by Stanley Cobb, was drawn from a recent publication of the Association for Research in Nervous and Mental Disease (p. 9) (5).

In this array of disorders, it is maintained, not chemical and physical, but rather psychological, factors play the determinant etiological role. Thus has the Helmholtzean position been challenged. There seemingly is much more to life and to life's processes than chemistry and physics. There is also psychology.

So far so good. But when we look closer into the matter, we perceive that the victor has introjected the vanquished; or, to phrase it more simply, that psychosomatic medicine has incorporated within its own formulations some of the distorting concepts of organicist medicine. These, to name them promptly, are the error of specificity and the error of time-sequential causality. Let me hasten to make clear just what I have in mind. First, as to specificity. Organicist medicine has long maintained that every disease must have its specific causative factor: the tubercle bacillus in tuberculosis; the Pneumococcus in pneumonia; hypoinsulinism in diabetes, and so on. Psychosomatic medicine has seemingly not challenged this postulate. It has merely added a new morbific factor—the psyche, or, more specifically, emotional tension, frustrated drives, repression. Psychosomatic medicine, quite in line with organicist medicine, is patently that department of medicine which specializes in the psychogenesis of organic disease. It is concerned with the psyche as a morbific agent. Bunker has phrased it thus (6):

> The key question involved might be said to be that of "psychogenesis." That is, can psychological factors give rise to "organic"

disease? May they have a place in the chain of causative events which lead to "organic" disease? If so to what extent is this true, and what are the psychological factors thus involved?

The second gross error which psychosomatic medicine has incorporated is the fallacy common to all of etiological medicine. It is the fallacy of time-sequence causality. This formulation maintains that in a determinable time sequence it can be observed that factor A causes the eventuation of B, which, in turn, causes the eventuation of C, and so on—"till death puts an end to it all." Stanley Cobb has tersely phrased this issue: "One of the main tasks of psychosomatic medicine . . . is to study the sequence of events from stimulus to symptom (p. 18) (5). This is proximate to Bunker's "key question," cited before, namely the *position* of the psychological factors in the chain of causative events which lead to organic disease. According to Cobb, the position of the psychological factor is quite certain; the sequence of events is "from stimulus to symptom." The differential contrast between the organicist and the psychosomaticist thus becomes crystal-clear. For the organicist the somatic event precedes the psychological, or, as I recently heard it so aptly phrased, and with such enviable assurance, "the spirochetal infection is the inevitable and invariable forerunner of dementia paralytica." How blessedly peaceful it must be never to be troubled by such galling questions as to why the case in mind cohabited with infection, or why he did not apply prophylaxis, or adequate treatment to the syphilitic infection—in other words, never to be troubled by the psychological potential that must have anteceded the materialized event.

For the psychosomaticist, on the contrary, the psychological event precedes the somatic. The stimulus leads to the symptom.

Evidently, then, the time-sequence causality chain, as postulated in psychosomatic medicine, is but the mirror image of that postulated in organicist medicine. Thus, the evil has not been corrected; it has only been multiplied. And as long as it prevails, the conception of the "essence of psychosomatic medicine" as "the cooperation of practitioners of medicine, surgery, dermatology, etc., with psychiatrists—each doing his part and together helping the patient" Cobb (5) is neither encouraging nor promising. We have seen in other connections that the cooperation of specialists does not per se or per force, serve the best interest of the patient. In the absence of competence in comprehension, the opposite is more commonly the case. The patient, as an entity, is more likely to be overlooked and lost, the more numerous the cooperating specialists.

I cannot terminate the exposition of this part of my argument without bringing in witness Franz Alexander's labored efforts to deal with the incorporated faults which psychosomatic medicine has carried over from organicist medicine. In his definitive work "Psychosomatic Medicine" (7), we find the following categorical statements:

> With the recognition that in functional disturbances emotional factors are of causal significance, psychotherapy gained a legitimate entrance into medicine proper and could no longer be restricted exclusively to the field of psychiatry . . . (p. 43). Formerly every disturbed function was explained as the *result* of disturbed structure. Now another [sic] causal sequence has been established: disturbed functions as the cause of altered structure (p. 45).

The last is an unequivocal and a pertinent statement bearing on what I have termed the morbific potentials of the psyche and the mirror image of time-sequence causality. Alexander later reaffirms these views in the statement:

> The resistance to this concept is based on the erroneous dogma that disturbed function is *always* the result of disturbed structure and on a disregard of the reverse causal sequence (p. 46).

By the witness of these citations, it would appear that Alexander was unaware of and insensitive to the problems involved in "specificity" and of "causality." However, that such is not entirely the case is to be seen from the following citations:

> The term "psychosomatic" should be used to indicate a method of approach both in research and in therapy of somatic . . . methods and concepts on the one hand and psychological methods and concepts on the other. . . . Emphasis is placed upon the qualification "coordinate use," indicating that the two methods are applied in the conceptual framework of causal sequences (p. 50).

The obscurity of these sentences, wherein a plea is made for the simultaneous coordinate use of data in the conceptual framework of causal sequences, shows that Alexander is impaled upon the horns of a dilemma. On the one hand, he subscribes to the scheme of causal sequences; on the other, he would qualify psychosomatic medicine as a method of approach, distinguished by the simultaneous and coordinate use of data.

The time now has come to ask, What does all this add up to? Criticism is legitimate enough an exercise, but it is better received when it is, as they say, constructive. Unless one can perceive "a way out," expositional argumentation is bound to be anxiety-provoking, and at times exasperating. What, then, is the summation of the argument? What's to be done?

Actually the challenge facing us is clearly evident, and simple to formulate. We need to free ourselves of the naïve 19th century concepts of specificity and time-sequence causality. We need to pay more than nodding respect to the concept of holism and to the vision of man operating in an ecological setting. We need to eliminate from our thinking the concept of a causality relationship between psyche and soma.

Instead of reasoning that a patient develops a peptic ulcer *because* of emotional tensions, we need to understand that the given patient represents a dynamic aggregate, that he is affected by forces which alter his dynamic configuration, and that we witness such alterations in the totality of his being and in all of its relations. Similarly, instead of conceiving the sick person as having regressed to a lower personality level *because* of his illness, we need, rather, to understand that the interplay of forces which "makes" the patient sick, also, and at the same time, though possibly in different manifest degrees, effects that alteration in personality which we label regressive.

Medicine must needs become that science which studies the living organism, itself a dynamism, as it moves and is affected by the surrounding forces and continuously alters its own and the surrounding configurations. Force, in the patterns of matter and energy, has a common and basic character; yet in experience it is manifest in many guises—physical, chemical, thermal, electrical, psychological, and social. There are numerous distinguishable embodiments of force, and their dynamic effects upon the human organism are well known. These include such instances as parasites, bacteria, toxins, inorganic poisons, physical agents with high momentum, extremes in temperatures, etc. Some forces—for example, suggestion, ideals, panic—operate without corporeal embodiment.

The significant idea, then, is that the living organism conceived as a dynamism is continuously exposed to the effects of the multiform forces which surround it. The destiny of the organism, and its temporal configuration, is affected and determined by the very modification it experiences, as a result of the interaction of its own dynamism with the surrounding forces.

I have several times endeavored to illustrate this somewhat intricate concept by means of some analogical picture. The one that has served me best is that of a spinning top. There is a certain kind of top which carries on its upper surface a number of small discs of different colors. These discs are so geared to each other and to the top itself that, as the latter spins, the discs revolve and effect a continuous change in colors and hues. In this contraption the relation of the position of the colored discs to each other and the colors to be seen on the spinning top change simultaneously. The point to underscore here is that the colors do not change *because* of the change in the relations of the discs to one another. It is, rather, thus: The discs change *and* the colors change. A time sequence between the change in the position of the discs and in that of the colors is inconceivable; also, there is no causality relation between the one and the other.

You will, I am sure, recognize that what I have elaborated here is an instance of ecological relations. In this connection, I want to revert to Smith Ely Jelliffe, who, I believe better than any of the pioneers in this field grasped and understood the essentially ecological nature of psychosomatic medicine. Jelliffe was a prolific writer, and almost everything he wrote, whether it be on botany, on paleopsychology, or on the drama, affords profitable reading. From his many papers, I would commend two especially.* These papers do not spell out the principles of ecological medicine in full detail. But you will find therein the *Anlage,* the germinal thoughts, the ideas, and the vision of ecological medicine, related particularly to psychosomatic problems. Let me cite but two brief passages (9).

"Any deviation," wrote Jeliffe, "from object or aim threatens the harmonious action patterns within the machine" (p. 583) (9). And in elaboration of this somewhat cryptic dictum, Jelliffe wrote:

> When we refuse to get in line with nature, as registered in the faulty purposes of life, i.e., our mental states, even the kidneys, the blood pressure and urea, proteid, ionic milieu become involved and this is but one formula for many disease (9).

Many excellent research workers have labored, and are now laboring, to lay bare the "mechanisms" of psychosomatic disorders, and their labors have yielded good results. To the migraine sufferer it is no small matter that the attack can now be effectively aborted. It is ever of value to be able to intrude upon and effectively to interrupt and to amend the pathological processes operating in disease. But such interruptions, even when they succeed in removing the symptom, seldom correct the disease. In contrast to the many clinical and research efforts put forth, to lay bare the mechanisms of psychosomatic disorders, few have, or are, laboring

---

*References 8 and 9.

where Jelliffe first broke ground; that is, in the effort to orient the viewpoint and understanding of psychosomatic medicine holistically and ecologically.

So far as I am able to judge, Halliday, in England, and Grinker, in the United States, are the only ones to have cultivated this terrain with any intensity and perseverance. Halliday's excellent book (10) is holistic in viewpoint and ecologically oriented. Grinker's "Psychosomatic Research" (11) is a *capo lavoro:* a splendid exposition of the problems I have in part belabored here. I myself, in a much more modest way, have worked in this field, as witness my work "Social Medicine" (12). I would be remiss did I not mention in these associations the work "Recent Developments in Psychosomatic Medicine" (13), published under the editorship of our distinguished colleague Dr. Wittkower.

Having pointed out the task before us, which is to reorient our thinking radically, I am moved to phrase the question, which I believe must be in your minds. "How will all this profit us, and our patients?" Does it really matter whether we think as organicists or as ecologists, and whether we do or do not understand "the chain of causality?" Let us assume that we could bring relief to the migraine victims, to the asthmatic, to the hypertensive, to the ulcer or colitis sufferer; would not that suffice for them, and for us, too?

It probably would! But here there comes to the fore the range of one's vision, the embrace of one's understanding, and the magnitude of one's ambition to contribute to our science and to the ultimate good of people. It is a matter also of being intelligent and of anticipating the future.

The current ideological orientation of medicine as a whole, psychosomatic medicine included, will not do, for it does not meet the long-term needs either of the individual or of society.

In my paper "The Roots of Psychosomatic Medicine," I called attention to the fact that psychosomatic medicine drew its momentum not from psychoanalytic insight but from epidemiological necessity. Since the beginning of this century demographic disease patterns have changed remarkably. The infectious diseases have receded both numerically and in importance, while the functional and degenerative disorders have come to the fore. These last categories embrace many instances of psychosomatic disorders; indeed, I would venture the guess, for there are no dependable statistics on these scores, that the psychosomatic disorders outnumber all others.

The overwhelming question thus arises: How are we to serve these people? That indeed is the ultimate issue.

Candor obliges us to admit that the greater numbers are not served at all—at least not beyond the casual diagnoses of their immediate and superficial complaints, and the delivery of "a prescription for what ails them." Witness in this connection, on the one hand, our enormous consumption of anodynes, sedatives, analgesics, and other "pain and worry killers," and, on the other hand, that of the "picker-uppers," such as the amphetamines.

But on this occasion I am more concerned with the so-called psychosomatic patient than with the larger numbers that are not served at all, or that are treated superficially that is, symptomatically. The psychosomatic patient is all too often shuttled between clinician and psychiatrist. Generally, when the clinician comes to the end of his rope, he refers the case to the psychiatrist. The psychiatrist, of course, seldom refers his patients to anyone. A dermatologist, after a frustrating four-year tussle with an eczematous young man, referred him to me. Naturally, the young man wanted to be treated for his skin disorder. He did not quite grasp what I meant when I said I would be glad to treat *him,* but not his skin. However, my prize case was a young tuberculous woman, referred by an internist, with a unilateral pneumothorax, who suffered also from depression, anorexia nervosa, and mild paranoid ideas.

Cooperation of psychiatric and nonpsychiatric specialists in diagnosis and treatment of the psychosomatic patients is postulated as the high desideratum both by Alexander and by Cobb. Such cooperation is a widely fostered ideal in psychosomatic circles. It is, however, at best an ideal which is workable and feasible only in institutional settings. I am not even sure it is an ideal. I suspect that specialists are here to be employed, that is used, rather than to be cooperated with. One operates, rather than cooperates, with a tool or instrument. What I have in mind is this. By definition all psychosomatic issues are both clinical and psychological. But they are seldom equipotentially both. In reality and for effectiveness, one or the other must carry responsibility, the clinician or the psychiatrist. The other's services might be utilized in an interim. But the case must be treated within a definitive *Gestalt.* For this reason I cite, but do not subscribe to, Alexander's division of specialists into psychiatric and nonpsychiatric. At least I do not contemplate with satisfaction the existence of any specialty so devoid of psychiatric knowledge and insight as to warrant such designation. What I rather conceive of is the clinician, or general practitioner who, if you please, is so well indoctrinated psychiatrically that he is able to treat his own case competently, that is, with a full awareness of the psychologic components of both the patient's pathology and his therapy. Such a clinician, even when dealing with the so-called psychosomatic case, and what case is not such in some measure at least, is not likely to require the cooperation of the psychiatrist, except consultatively. If and when the patient's difficulties become predominantly psychological, he will, of course, be referred of the psychiatrist. Obviously, it is not expected that the clinician will also be a psychiatrist. Similarly, it is not expected that the psychiatrist will function also as a clinician. But it is to be expected that the psychiatrist will possess and will exercise more clinical acumen and awareness than is commonly the case today. Except for our institutional confreres, and a small group of psychologically oriented practitioners, psychiatrists in the main, and orthodox Freudians notably, seem to look upon the body as an appendage of the psyche, and hence they trouble little about it, at least clinically. All this might perhaps be phrased more charitably by saying that the psychiatrists appear to operate in the firm conviction that when all goes well with the psyche, all will be well with the soma.

I must dwell a bit longer on these scores to make sure that my point is clearly made. I hold that the clinician, contemplating the patient in the soma-psyche perspective, and the psychiatrist, in the psyche-soma perspective, each views the patient in a distorting tangent. I hold, further, that when you add up what they respectively perceive you thereby acquire, not a better picture of the patient, but, rather, a more distorted one. I submit that no view corresponds to the reality but the holistic and the ecological. I maintain that both the clinician and the psychiatrist, even when functioning in their separate fields, can operate holistically and ecologically. Their functions, however, are essentially disparate, for, even though psyche and soma are invariably involved and affected in health and disease, in the practical experience of man the case is generally "either-or."

Finally, I am persuaded that the historical function of the psychosomatic movement is not to add another to our Babel of specialties but, rather, to vitalize the whole of medicine, psychiatry no less than clinical medicine, with the holistic and ecological viewpoint. When that has been achieved, the psychosomatic movement will have fulfilled its mission and it will have been absorbed into medicine.

REFERENCES

1. GALDSTON, I.: The roots of psychosomatic medicine, *Canad. M. A. J. 70:*127-132, 1954.
2. MARGETTS, E. L.: Historical notes on psychosomatic medicine, in *Recent Develop-*

ments in Psychosomatic Medicine, edited by Eric D. Wittkower and R. A. Cleghorn, London, Sir Isaac Pitman & Sons, Ltd., 1954, pp. 41-68.

3. GALDSTON, I.: Biodynamic medicine versus psychosomatic medicine, *Bull. Menninger Clin.* 8:116-121, 1944.

4. FREUD, S.: *Gesammelte Schriften,* Vienna and London, International Psycho-Analytic Press, 1925-1934, Vol. I, pp. 332-333.

5. MILES, H. H. W.; COBB, S., and SHANDS, H. C., Editors: *Case Histories in Psychosomatic Medicine,* New York, W. W. Norton & Company, Inc., 1952, p. 9.

6. BUNKER, H. A.: American psychiatry as a specialty, in Hall, I. K.: Zilboorg, G., and Bunker, H. A., Editors: *One Hundred Years of American Psychiatry,* p. 500.

7. ALEXANDER, F.: *Psychosomatic Medicine: Its Principles and Applications,* New York, W. W. Norton & Company, Inc., 1953.

8. JELLIFFE, S. E.: Psychotherapy in modern medicine, *Long Island M. J.* 24:152-161 1930.

9. JELLIFFE, S. E.: Psychopathology and organic disease, *New York J. Med.* 32:581-588, 1932.

10. HALLIDAY, J. L.: *Psychosocial Medicine: A Study of the Sick Society,* New York, W. W. Norton & Company, Inc., 1948.

11. GRINKER, R.: *Psychosomatic Research,* New York, W. W. Norton & Company, Inc., 1953.

12. GALDSTON, I.: *Social Medicine: Its Derivations and Objectives,* New York Academy of Medicine, Institute on Social Medicine, 1947.

13. *Recent Developments in Psychosomatic Medicine,* edited by Eric D. Wittkower and R. A. Cleghorn, London, Sir Isaac Pitman & Sons, Ltd., 1954.

Part II:
FREUD AND FREUDIANA

11

The Place of Psychoanalysis in Modern Medicine

THROUGHOUT THE CIVILIZED WORLD, save only perhaps in that portion which lies behind the Iron Curtain, there will be celebrated this year the one-hundredth anniversary of the birth of Sigmund Freud. Even in those lands that lie under the shadow of the Soviet dictatorship and where the official psychiatric saint is Ivan Pavlov, it is not likely that the anniversary will go unnoticed. It will no doubt be made the occasion for the extollment of the dialectics of materialist psychology above what they will label "the bourgeois fictions" of Freudian psychoanalysis. And as they do so, all the great spirits, relishing their merited immortality in the Elysium, will rock in gentle mirth, for being great spirits they will recall that it was the sweet and gentle Ivan who ingeniously proved the basic validity of Freud's theses. Upon the sands of the Fortunate Isles they will draw circles and ovals and recount how Pavlov first induced an experimental neurosis in "man's best friend," the dog, by attempting to tax the animal's motivated discrimination beyond the limits of its innate competences. To them we must perforce leave further discourse on the foibles of men and scientists. We will do better to fathom precisely why so many among us will do honour to the memory of this great man on the centennial of his birth. For whatever one may think of his metapsychology, and however one may judge his system of psychotherapy, it cannot but be acknowledged that Freud was a great man, a great spirit—and that his thoughts, his theories, and his labours have had profound efforts not only in the special field of psychiatry, but upon all of contemporary medicine, and upon our intellectual and cultural life as well.

All this is the more remarkable since Freud, to use an American expression, was a medical maverick, a personage that bore the brand mark of no academic herd. The motto of his life could well have been that elected by Paracelsus, to whom, at least in the spirit of independence and Promethean courage, Freud was akin—*Alterius non sit, qui suis esse potest.*

Freud in every sense of the word was "a man to himself," a unique character. He had no lineal forerunner, and no contemporary runners-up. There was no Wallace to Darwin, no Colombo to Harvey, no para-personage to Freud. He had no co-discoverers, and in the beginning of his work no co-workers. However, it is not true that he was entirely an original thinker. He was an autodidact. But he also drew knowledge and inspiration from the past, and from a very few among his contemporaries —notably from Wilhelm Fliess with whom he stood in most intimate friendship during fifteen years of his young manhood (1). But all these stand in relation to his system of psychology as paint, brush, and canvas relate to the creation of a masterpiece. Still the uniqueness of his work and the profound and far reaching effects of his teachings cannot entirely be credited to his genius. The times, too, favored his enterprise. Had Freud lived and labored a hundred years earlier, or fifty years later, Freud would not have been *the* Freud whose historic magnitude we celebrate and marvel. Freud took time by the forelock.

This last affirmation imputes to Freud a great deal of volitionalism, of wilful, ambitious, calculating enterprise—far more than is common to the personalities of most outstanding scientists. The imputation is intended. Among the categories of those who are born to fame, those who have it thrust upon them and those who seek it, Freud belongs to the last. Freud was inordinately ambitious "to make a name for himself," to become famous. Long before he attained any measure of prominence, he earnestly spoke of his future biographers, and of the difficulties he was placing in their prospective labors—by periodically destroying his personal mementos. Anticipating his fame, he gloated over the travails of those who would attempt to reconstruct the story of his life and labors. "Let the biographers chafe," he wrote in a letter to his betrothed, "We won't make it too easy for them. Let each one of them believe he is right in his conception of the development of the Hero. Even now I enjoy the thought of how they will all go astray." That was written in 1885, when Freud was twenty-nine years of age. There is, of course, no inherent evil in ambition, nor aught discreditable in craving fame, unless, of course, they lead to evil ends, which in the case of Freud they signally did not. However, it is not possible to appreciate, nor to truly understand Freud's unique labors unless one is fully cognizant of, and takes into account, these dominant characteristics of Freud's personality. They are reflected in his compulsive need to be original, to be an autodidact, not to learn from others, but to think through his own thoughts first, and then to learn, if at all, what others had thought before him. "I do not want to read," he wrote to his friend Fliess (1), " . . . it stirs up too many thoughts and stints me of the satisfaction of discovery." And again: "First I want to get my own ideas into shape, then I shall make a thorough study of the literature on the subject. . . . So long as I have not finished my own work I cannot read" (2).

Nor can we appreciate Freud's relations to his disciples and co-workers, if we do not take into account his consuming ambitions. He welcomed co-workers—so long as they were disciples. He was gratified when his younger associates elaborated on his thesis, even when they did not always nor fully acknowledge the source of their initial inspirations. But he did not gladly suffer the presence of strong personalities, of actively critical, or ambitious co-workers. In summating the spirit of the Wednesday evening roundtable discussions which Freud inaugurated in 1903, and which were held at his home, Fritz Wittels wrote (p. 118): (3).

> "These evenings were not always interesting. Freud's purpose in the whole set-up was to drive his own thoughts through the filter of some informed, even though mediocre, brains. Strong individualities, or very critical and ambitious co-workers, therefore, were less acceptable to him. Psychoanalysis was the realm of his imagination and his will. He who accepted his sovereignty, was welcome. He wanted to look into a kaleidoscope which would multiply his own figures through reflection."

I fear that my insistence on the wilful ambitiousness of Freud's personality, his single devotion to the pursuit of his native thoughts, may give you a distorted and entirely erroneous picture of the man. There was nothing petty, grubby, or mean about Freud. He was rather a consecrated man, one who would not be deflected from his elected course, and his self-appointed mission. In his purview the world is wide and its highways many. Who chose to go *his* way was welcome, and he did not block the way of those who chose other paths. That the more spirited and the keener among his co-workers broke away from him is not to his discredit, any more than that among his faithful were many Lotus Eaters. Asked why Freud's followers exhibited so little originality, one of his favored disciples answered: *"Er hat uns alles vorweg genommen und nichts zu entdecken ubrig gelassen."* (He anticipated us in everything and left us nothing to discover). Wittells, who reported this incident

added: *"In dieser Hypnose lebt die orthodoxe Schule dahin."* The orthodox school labors under this hypnotic state (4).

It is not my intention to dwell at length on the singular, complicated,
and most interesting features of Freud's personality, nor to dilate on
Freud's relations to his disciples and co-workers. To those interested I
heartily recommend Fritz Wittels' biographic study of Freud. It is a more
judicious, more penetrating assessment of Freud's personality than is
Jones' adulatory biography, and it should be read in conjunction with
the latter.

I said the times favored Freud; I must now turn to the elaboration of
this somewhat cryptic affirmation. What were these times—what their
span, what their temper and mood, and what the burden of their faith
and beliefs. Freud began the study of medicine in 1873. In 1895 he
published (together with Breuer) his epoch-making work on *Hysteria,* in
1900 his work on *Dream Interpretation,* in 1904 the *Psychopathology of
Everyday Life,* in 1905 his *Three Contributions to the Theory of Sexuality,*
in 1909 his analysis of the anxiety states of little Hans, in 1912 his work
Totem and Taboo. These works may be taken as the incunabula of the
Freudian corpus. They appeared in the span of less than twenty years,
fifteen of which belong to the twentieth century. But Freud himself belongs to the nineteenth century. It was from that century that he drew
his scientific and philosophical nurture. It is to the science of that century
that his unique system stands as a reactive, piercing, and illuminating
challenge. Let us scanningly survey the world of science from, say, 1850
to 1900. Among its leading spirits, notably in the realms of biology and
medicine, were Rokitansky, Virchow, Claude Bernard, Helmholtz, Carl
Ludwig, Du Bois-Reymond, Cohn, Darwin, Haeckel, Ehrlich, Koch, and
Jacques Loeb. You may find this listing somewhat strange, more so because of those great names omitted, than because of those given. Let me,
therefore, hasten to explain that I have chosen from among those who are
distinguished for their influence on the *philosophy* of medicine rather
than from those who, like Pasteur, Lister, and Von Behring, achieved
great practical results. Those I have named were theoreticians in science,
as well as great performers in science. Even so I have not offered you an
all-inclusive nor exhaustive list. It is representative rather than definitive.
And what this galaxy of personages represents is the analytical, positivist,
materialist, school of thought which unreservedly held to the conviction
that "all the processes of nature, including those commonly called 'intellectual,' the whole physical and moral order of things, are reducible to
matter and motion and are completely explicable in terms of these two

concepts." Those who subscribed to this conviction dedicated themselves to the refined analysis of matter and to the explication of the ways in which motion and matter affect both the normal and the abnormal processes to be witnessed in life. The positivist-materialist scientists disallowed the possibility that any of the phenomena of experience, biological, social, and cultural, could not or would not in time be explained and accounted for on the basis of the interplay of matter and motion. This belief inspired not only the biologists, but equally such representative thinkers as the philosopher, Herbert Spencer, the sociologist, August Comte, and the economist, Karl Marx, each the founder of a populous school of followers. They also precluded the operations of any but materialistic factors.

The philosophy of positivist materialism was aggressively propounded in the manifesto of the so-called School of von Helmholtz, the most outspoken proponent of which was Emil du Bois-Reymond. "No other forces," he wrote, "than the common physical-chemical ones are active within the organism. In those cases which cannot at the time be explained by these forces one has either to find the specific way or form of their action by means of the physical-mathematical method or to assume new forces equal in dignity to the chemical-physical forces inherent in matter, reducible to the forces of attraction and repulsion." This was not solely the faith of the avowed followers of the School of von Helmholtz. It was the commitment of practically the entire world of science. The dissidents were few in number, and their influence nil.

I need not, I am sure, describe how much of life-manifest was indeed accounted for, made clear and understandable in terms of the interplay of matter and motion, nor yet is there any need to dilate on how great were the practical yields of this methodology in medicine, in animal husbandry, in agriculture, and in industrial technology. The greater part of the tale of modern science treats of the "miracles and wonders" that were effected by the followers of this school of thought. More pertinent to our concern is that segment of experience wherein the chemical-physical, and the physical-mathematical theories did not avail to explicate manifest events. Historically, and here we return to Freud, the singular crucial category of experience, the critical events, wherein the physical-chemical, the matter and motion hypothesis, proved miserably inadequate were those protean disturbances that carried the label of hysteria. The issue was really simple. One was called on to account how a limb can be "paralyzed" when it isn't paralyzed; how an organically and functionally intact eye can prove blind of vision; how one can sense on the intact skin, insensible sentations, or fail to "sense" what perforce must be sensible—

pinpricks and the like. How are these indubitable conditions to be explained, and how explain also their seemingly miraculous "cure." This, in a nutshell, was the issue, and on this issue the positivist, materialist, exclusivist matter-and-motion school of thought suffered overwhelming defeat. Defeated, it did not of course abandon its ground—it was, however, compelled to open its realm to the data and the theoretical formulations of depth psychology. The man who breached its stronghold was Sigmund Freud.

Interestingly enough, it was in the first of his significant psychiatric publications that the crucial issue was clearly set forth, and decisively settled. I have in mind the monograph on Hysteria which he published jointly with Breuer. I shall not belabor you with the rest of Freud's metapsychology—but I must solicit your close attention to the issue that divided Freud and Breuer, and which in the end, broke up a friendship of many years' duration. It is commonly asserted that Breuer, who first involved Freud in the intimate study of hysteria, broke away from Freud because he could not countenance or accept Freud's emphasis on sexuality as the primal cause of hysteria. Those who pretended to be "in the know" further hint that the decisive incident was an erotic gesture made toward Breuer by a young female whom he had jointly treated with Freud. But all this is small talk indulged in by those who would persuade us that Breuer was a prissy and prudish old maid of a man. We have it on the best of authorities, namely Freud himself, that all this is sheer nonsense. In his *An Autobiographical Study* (5) Freud affirms that he first learned from Breuer to suspect the role of sexuality in hysteria. It was Breuer who designated hysteria as referable to the *"Geheimmisse des Alkovens,"* that is the mysteries of the conjugal bed, and it was Charcot who referred to the condition as *"toujours une génitale."* Chrobak, a noted Viennese gynecologist, had a uniform prescription for hysteria. The prescription read: *"Rp. Penis normalis-dosim repetatur!"* Freud is no less clear and specific as to the issue that divided the two. It did *not* involve the matter of sex. This is what Freud wrote:

> "In answering the question of when it is that a mental process becomes pathogenic, that is, when it is that it becomes impossible for it to find a normal discharge, Breuer preferred what might be called a physiological theory: he thought that the processes which could not find a normal outcome were such as had originated during unusual, 'hypnoid,' mental states. This opened the further question of the origin of these hypnoid states. I, on the other hand, was inclined to suspect the existence of an interplay of forces and the operation of intentions and purposes such as are to be observed in normal life" (6).

The issue between Freud and Breuer, as we see, revolved about the problem "when and how do mental processes become pathogenic." Breuer advocated a physiological theory, and Freud a psychological. Freud, in his own words, postulated as the primary cause of pathogenic mental processes "a thwart in the operations of intentions and purposes such as are to be observed in normal life" (6). At first blush this may seem like a difference of trivial significance. But in effect it was, and proved to be freighted with enormous implications, fundamentally irreconcilable with the basic ideational commitments of the 19th century world of science. In the then prevailing scheme of biological dynamics there was no place nor currency, for "intention and purposes," nor could they be rendered in terms of physical-chemical, or physical-mathematical equivalents—the only terms acceptable in the realm of science. Breuer first, and after him the vast majority of the medical and psychological confraternity, rejected Freud's hypothesis.

That verdict has been largely reversed, and therein lies the essence of Freud's influence on contemporary medicine. How is that influence to be described? I believe it can be best summated under two headings, both of them foreshadowed and implicated in Freud's position vis-à-vis Breuer. The one can be labelled the Instinct Theory, the other Organ Projection. These labels are crude and not very informative, yet what they embrace is richly substantive and most significant.

Freud reintroduced into medicine *the function of meaningfulness in biological phenomena* in his words of "intention and purpose." Not only did he demonstrate that nothing in the operations of the individual is ultimately irrational—neither dreams, nor forgetfulness, nor slips of the tongue, nor errors, nor neurotic or psychotic behaviour—but that the whole of the individual's living experience is animated with purpose and intention. Man is not merely a congelation of sentient matter buffeted about by the arbitrary forces of the world he lives in, moving through life in the crazy pattern of a rudderless ship. Man is rather a creature impelled toward self-fulfilment, guided by an indwelling architectonic pattern, and conditioned by the effects of antecedent experience. Each one of us has an appointment with destiny, but ours is not the role of a passive sufferer. To the flat dimensions of matter and motion, of chemistry and physics, Freud added the dimensions of purpose and intention. Thereby he gave perspective to the vision of man in health and in disease. It is proper and common *now*, as it was not before Freud, to ask not only what caused an illness, but also what is its meaning to the patient, what purpose does it fulfill in his corrupted scheme of things. The question is neither valid nor answerable in every case. But that it can be asked is already a great good. More often than many among us suspect, the decisive clue to the remedy of a disorder can more easily be gained from an assessment of the *function* of the illness, than from the study of its specific causes.

It was not so long ago that the practice of medicine involved but two major operations, the making of a diagnosis, in terms of statistically established anatomic and physiologic norms, and the prescribing of corrective or supportive therapeutic agents. I am told that in some parts of the world this order of medical practice is still common. But where medicine is practiced in the more modern perspective, physicians are less hobbled by the statistical norms and are mindful of the variables of individuality. Anatomic and physiological data still serve as the basis for, but not as the ultimate criteria of, diagnoses. The clinical profile is projected against the psychological, the economic, and the social background of the patient, thus providing a better perspective on all that is involved, aetiologically, therapeutically, and prognostically. The elements for this panoramic picture of the patient are contributed by a host of para-medical co-workers, chiefly psychologists, social workers, and public health nurses. Therapeutically the clinician is supported and made more effective by nurses, librarians, hospital sociologists, occupational therapists, rehabilitation workers, and "follow-up" personnel. I am omitting specific reference to the operations of the psychiatric associate of the clinician—primarily because I will treat of that association later.

It would not be proper to "claim for Freud" all these noteworthy developments in the clinical practice of medicine. But it is more than a freak of history that most of the services which aid in the treatment of the whole man, rather than singly and exclusively with his illness, have either come into existence or have acquired telling dimensions and wide acceptance since the time of Freud's advent on the medical scene. It is most certainly true that his was the "leaven that raised the loaf." And the best evidence for this is the presence in the ideational orientations and para-medical vernaculars, of concepts and terms deriving from the early and now largely superseded or discarded Freudian formulations. Try discussing a patient with a social *case* worker, and you will promptly discover what I mean. But this is really quite understandable. Freud's metapsychology, his instinct theory, and his depth psychology penetrated into the cultural disciplines, into literature, the theatre, the plastic arts, anthropology, and even the law, deeper and sooner than into the bulk of medical thought and practice. Medicine was affected by Freud's ideas, collaterally and reflexly, as well as directly.

Neither time nor space will permit me to more than touch on the effects of Freud's theories in the fields of preventive and developmental medicine. To signal my meanings I need but point to the pediatricians, now so largely occupied with fostering the child's optimal development and progression, psychological as well as physical. It is currently expected that the pediatrician will serve also as a child psychologist, counseling parents on the "resolution of the Oedipal complex," on "sibling rivalry," on "manifest or repressed hostility," and so on. Nor is it feasible to trace the effects of Freud's ideas on educational procedures, industrial practices, criminal and domestic legal issues, and a host of other departments of social operations and relations proffering a variety of prophylactic occasions and opportunities.

I do feel, however, that we need to dwell longer and elaborate further Freud's Instinct Theory. He himself never fully, nor to my mind, satisfactorily, developed this theory. He largely took it for granted, and only parsimonously occupied himself with its exposition. In the end he postulated a bipolarity of instincts, Eros and Thanatos, the Life Instinct and the Death Instinct. Between them, in animated agitation, but pursuing a charted and purposeful course, life itself, made manifest in the individual, spins out its inherent meaning.

Freud's concept of the Death Instinct has fascinated me, and I spent some time and effort in fathoming its meaning and significance. The results were published under the title "Eros and Thanatos, A Critique of Freud's Death Wish" (7). In pursuing this theme I realized that Freud was less concerned with defining the variety of instincts made manifest in man's behaviours than with the ultimate goals for the realization of which they subserve as dynamic propulsions. Freud's Instinct Theory, in other words, postulated "an energy source," a source of libidinal impulsion, driving life toward its full eventuation. Given all this, the problems that particularly concerned Freud were—How and why is the eventuation of life, as witnessed in hysteria, in the neuroses and in the psychoses, impeded and deflected, and how are such untoward developments to be resolved and corrected?

The Instinct Theory of Freud had its counterpart in the Hormic Theory of McDougall (8), whose profound and illuminating study of the emotions and instincts of man is vastly superior to that of Freud, and does in fact corroborate many of Freud's fundamental postulates. McDougall did not, however, deal with psychopathology, nor was he interested in psychotherapy. But Freud was. He was a psychologist in order that he might be a psychotherapist, and he stinted the former, for the benefit of the latter. But even in psychology Freud's emphasis was singular. He was more concerned with the goal-striving character of the living process, with the paths and patterns of its fulfilment, than with the specific sources and nature of its dynamic energy. He was willing to lump "all of that" under the obscure and amorphous designation of the *Id*—the primal *It*. The *Id* he defined as the reservoir of psychic energy or libido. To the *Id* he ascribed all philogenetic acquisitions; the *Id* is the source of instinctive energy. But what concerned Freud first and last was "repression," that is the thwart in the operations of intentions and purposes to be observed in normal life. His contention was that intention and purpose, when blocked or repressed in their biologically legitimate avenues of execution, are not thereby undone and annihilated, but are transposed, and are then acted out in masked form, in illegitimate, that is destructive, patterns. The latter phenomena fall, of course, in the special province of the psychiatrist. But the first component, that of "the intentions and purposes such as are to be observed in normal life," concern all of medicine, and particularly the internist and clinician.

The commitment of my paper is expositional rather than exhortative. I am supposed to tell a tale rather than to draw a moral. Yet I cannot but observe that we are currently in great danger of missing out "on the intentions and purposes of life," so much are we taken up with and blinded by the effulgence of the phenomenal therapeutic whatnots that pour down upon us from the pharmacological and other industrial sources. The reversal of the untoward patho-phenomenal process being so very easy, why bother as to its cause or trouble as to its meaning? Here is a depression—a pill will reverse it! There is a psychosis—snap some synapsis, or convulse the gray matter, and lo—it is gone. Or is it? I shan't undertake to argue the issue, nor is it my intention to disparage the therapeutic and technical achievements of the pharmacological and other modalities. But I do feel that we are in some danger of losing precisely that illuminating interest and insight into the meaning of the living processes which Freud, more than any one, infused into medicine.

I conditioned my warning. I said we are in "some danger" of losing interest and insight into the meaning of the living process. The reason for my reserve derives from the second major influence which Freud's ideas have exercised upon modern medicine, that which I have labelled organ projection, and which will be more familiar to you as Psychosomatic Medicine. Few appreciate that psychosomatic medicine is itself a projection or a derivative of Freud's theories. Freud was, in effect, the first theorist in this "department" of medicine. And his initial, albeit indirect, formulation of the fundamental psychosomatic concept, he gave in the exposition of his difference with Breuer. In essence he opposed Breuer's physiological hypothesis with his own psychological theory which argued that the acting out characteristic of hysteria is in effect the somatic witness of psychological repression. This formulation carried two important implications: the first indissolubly conjoined psyche and soma, and the second rendered it possible to seemingly reverse the relational energic sequence between psyche and soma. Now it was possible to visualize not only "traumatic neurosis" but also "neurotic traumata." In a word, not only was somatic experience mirrored in psychic operation, but also the reverse.

I have on numerous occasions protested the corruption inherent in the term "psycho-somatic" (9). It perpetuates, despite the included hyphen, the dichotomy of soul and body, of psyche and soma. It also suggests, as I have myself phrased it, "an energic sequence" in which soma affects psyche, or psyche—soma. This is a misleading and erroneous formulation. Psyche and soma are in effect involved not sequentially but simultaneously, no matter in what order the results become manifest, physiologically, economically, or how. But, without at this point following up the protest to the term psychosomatic, and understanding its limitations, it can be affirmed that the psyche has been rendered more congenial, more familiar, more comprehensive to the clinician, in the formulation of psychosomatic than in any of the purely psychiatric representations—psychoanalytic, psychobiological, or otherwise. It is all to the good, and intending neither cynicism nor disparagement, I would add that it is of no great import whether the clinician does or does not have a precise grasp of the nature of the psyche and of its operation, so long as he understands and allows that it is a cofactor in anything and everything that he perceives and deals with in the human organism. There is a saying in the Russian that when a bear dances, the wonder lies not in how well he dances, but that he dances at all. To relate this to our theme—the wonder lies not in how well clinic medicine has "taken psychiatry to heart," but rather that it has countenanced it at all. And this, I would underscore again, clearly stands to the credit of Freud and to his ingenious psychological formulations.

Freud himself did not pursue the somato-clinical application of his theories. But two of his disciples did—the German, Georg Groddeck (10), and the American, Smith Ely Jelliffe (11). Both these men were exceptionally gifted. Both brought to psychoanalysis a breadth of instruction and a wealth of experience that singles them out among the followers of

Freud. Jelliffe was the more scintillating, the more mercurial personality, Groddeck the more solid, and the better organized. Yet both were poetic and romantic souls. It is a pity that the pioneering works of both these men are not better known and more widely studied. But the impetus they gave, following Freud's initial insight, to the study of the psychosomatic aspects of clinical medicine has carried it far. We now have more than a score of centres wherein psychosomatic studies are intensively and ingeniously cultivated and explored, and among the workers enlisted in these pursuits are to be found some of our very best clinicians, and our most painstaking and exacting research workers. Mindful of this we need also to bear in mind that whosoever labors in this field, or gains by its harvest, owes a debt of recognizance to Freud. This was beautifully expressed by Victor von Weiszacker of Heidelberg (12):

> "Looking at the history of medicine, and considering Freud's role in history, one, so to say, arrives at the distinction of 'before Freud' and 'after Freud'; and one then comes to the conclusion that there is no post-Freudian medicine that was not influenced by Freud. This conclusion will, of course, seem limited and negligible only to those who are altogether blind and deaf vis-à-vis Freud's magnitude and importance. For, if Freud is of such magnitude, this magnitude must have a meaning for medicine as a whole.
>
> "At present the situation is this. That what was initiated as the problem of the neuroses is now projected unto medicine in its entirety. Medicine as a whole, as can be perceived, has been affected by the impact of depth psychology. And we may also reverse this perception. Freud's psychoanalysis must then perforce appear as an important part, as a significant aspect of the progress of medicine as a whole. There occurred a reform of the art and science of healing."

At this point I must pay my respects to the title of my paper, which reads—The Place of Psychoanalysis in Modern Medicine. As you must have observed, I have referred but little and seldom to psychoanalysis as such, electing rather to treat of Freud's metapsychology, his theories, and his formulations. I am sure you appreciate that this was deliberate and intentional. Psychoanalysis means different things to different persons. It is frequently used as a designation for all that Freud contributed to psychology, psychiatry and medicine. In this sense Freud and psychoanalysis are deemed to be synonymous. But this equation is both unhistorical and uncritical. It is a lumping designation and a tricky one. If one subscribes to this formulation, one is perforce committed to an all-or-none position: you either take it or leave it, accept it or reject it. There is no alternative. This, incidentally, is the position of Freudian orthodoxy. But Freud himself affirmed that he was no Freudian, and in the spirit of his permissiveness I would limit the meaning of the term psychoanalysis to the therapeutic practices (not, mind you, to the theoretic formulations) developed by Freud, and now so staunchly defended by his orthodox adherents. Freud's therapeutic procedures and practices were historically warranted, but their unaltered perpetuation is indefensible and reactionary.

Let us inspect these matters more closely. At the time Freud began his work, the treatment of nervous and mental disorders had a very limited armamentarium (13). There was electrotherapy, overt or hypnotic suggestion, and there was rest and moral re-education. Electrotheraphy, as then practiced, appears to have been so much hocus-pocus, or at best a vague and crude form of suggestion. Rest proffered refuge, and the opportunity to recuperate from the fray, but no basic solution for underlying difficulties. Suggestion, overt or hypnotic, as well as moral re-education, constituted in effect, the imposition upon an already vulnerable personality of the ideational and affect patterns of a "foreign body." I think you will agree it was a miserably improverished armamentarium (13).

Taking his cue from Breuer, Freud began to treat his patients by the so-called "cathartic" method. The patient was hypnotized, but instead of receiving "suggestions," the patient was encouraged to talk. He did, and hence the therapy was frequently described as a "talking-out cure" and as "chimney sweeping." Later, Freud gave up hypnosis and instead encouraged the patient to tell of his problems and difficulties without restraint. This was the "head squeezing" stage, when Freud was not averse to placing his fingers on the forehead of his patient, encouraging him to recall—to remember. Finally Freud developed the "couch-and-free association" pattern of therapy now common to the orthodox analyst. The couch, we are told, was Freud's own refuge. He could not bear being stared at hour after hour. But free association was quite a different matter; it was crucial to his theoretical formulations. It was the reciprocate of repression. For to express the Freudian formula at its simplest the neurosis was in essence the acting out of repressed "purpose and intent"; the repressed was resident in the Unconscious; to the Unconscious the Conscious has no direct access. Dreams, slips of the tongue, and the errors of everyday life do offer, so to say, depth soundings of the Unconscious. But only prolonged and unhampered free association could in effect—like the pipes of Orpheus—bring Euridice back from the Stygian depths of Hades, that is, bring forth into awareness the repressed materials. There is much poetic meaning in this myth, illuminating both repression and the exhortative process of recall by free association. And only those who have had experience with free association, who have undergone or have witnessed the liberating, emancipating, effects of repressions brought into awareness, can appreciate the powerful psychodynamics operational in this process. These eventuations cannot easily be imagined, for they are outside the embrace of ordinary experience. Realization can come only by way of experience, but the experience itself is *not* hard to come by. What I mean is that there are no great tricks or mysteries involved in tapping the Unconscious.

Having stated all this, one must inquire more closely into the nature of the elements under consideration—in other words, we need to define what we understand by repression, the Unconscious, and by free association. The impulsion is there, but I'll not yield to it, beyond affirming that both repression and the Unconscious are psychological formulations to which Freud gave certain unique qualifications, but which were current and broadly appreciated long before Freud came upon the psychological scene. Free association, although also anticipated before Freud, by Galton among others, is more substantively his unique contribution.

But then, what is free association? Operationally it is the uncensored, uninhibited, verbalization of everything and anything that comes to mind. Psychologically it is the creation, intra-psychically and environmentally, that is, in the therapeutic situation and relationship of, as complete as possible, ideational and verbal permissiveness. Inner permissivenesses, rather than "endless jabber," is the touchstone of free association. But, be it noted, it does not follow that the more disorganized and the more inconsequential the patient's recitation—the more freely is he associating and the deeper is he reaching into his Unconscious. But this, I fear, is carrying us a bit too far into the esoteric technology of specialized psychotherapy. More immediate to our own interest is the historic verity that Freud, in his emphasis on free association and on the tacit passivity of the therapist, has taught us once again to appreciate the value and the importance of listening, of allowing and encouraging the patient to talk. Freud has *taught* us but I am not so sure we have *learned* the lesson. I have yet to see a clinical history form which begins with the heading "Present Complaint." All those I know of first drag the patient through the morass of past histories relating to grandparents and parents, to siblings and childhood ills, to accidents, operations, etc., and even when all these are duly asked, the patient doesn't really often get an ample opportunity to talk freely—to get things off his chest.

Another postulate of psychoanalysis, which has gained acceptance in current medicine, is the inherent meaningfulness of everything that the patient presents. The patient is not likely to be confronted, as he was but a short time ago, with the injunction—"Get it out of your head, it's all nonsense," nor with the cock-certain oracular affirmation—"It's all in your imagination—and you'd better forget it." To listen and to seek to understand, to listen attentively, receptively, sympathetically, in the conviction that what the patient has to say, even though seemingly meaningless, nay even non-sensical, *yet has meaning,* and that it is the bounden obligation of every therapist to search for and to fathom that meaning—is the vital burden of the instruction and inspiration which psychoanalysis brings to medicine.

I have treated of free association at some length because *it* and the *couch* are "brand marks" of the orthodox psychoanalyst, and distinguish him, witness the *New Yorker* cartoons, from all of his psychiatric brethren. But, instructive as Freud's therapeutic technique has been for psychiatry in particular, and for medicine in general, the technique itself is provincial and parochial to the broad realm of psychotherapy. Free association is effective in bringing into awareness repressed materials, and is emancipating *when the neurotic disorder is due to repression.* But, as experience has shown, and even Freud had to acknowledge, in the category of character neurosis not all neurotic disorders are due to conflict and repression, and those *others,* so very numerous in psychiatric experience, are not to be cured by tapping the Unconscious. As well expect a man to fatten by sucking on his own spittle, as that a defective, or distorted personality, or the victim of deprivational experiences, should grow into effectiveness and maturity by the endless audition of his own history and grievances. To effect a cure, in such instances, much more than free association is required. The total personality needs reorientation and re-education, and this implies much unlearning as well as much learning anew. This is a therapeutic enterprise in which both patient and psychotherapist must play calculated and active roles.

By the token of all this I am sure you will appreciate why I have taken pains to distinguished between Freud's metapsychology and theoretical formulations, and psychoanalysis as a psychotherapeutic procedure. While the latter will be, as it already has been, substantially absorbed into psychiatry, and will thus have no further warrant for a separate "apartite" existence, Freud's metapsychology and theoretical formulations will long sustain their historical identity and continue to catalytically affect both medical and cultural thought. This is not at all strange. Ideas are ever more viable, more potent, and more fertile than the technologies associated or derived from them.

In the realm of ideas, Freud is a colossus, and his stature will grow with time. The foibles of his personality, and the frailties of his system which we sport to point out will in the perspective of time be as nothing to the transcending significance of the insight he brought into a benighted world: a world drunk with the conceit of its sophistication, an ungodly and arrogant world. This man, who like the Biblical Joseph, was discountenanced by his brethren; this man, who also read the meaning of dreams, will be celebrated as the one who recalled to man his kinship with all of life, who in the modern vernacular spoke of man the microcosm, and of his relation to the universe, the macrocosm. It will be recognized in the future, even better than it is now, what it meant, and the courage it required, to make man mindful of the fact that life was more meaningful than the seemingly fortuitous, haphazard, interplay of matter and motion, that life had meaning eventuated in intention. He will be esteemed for his brillant—if at times erratic—protest against, his defiance of, the narrow and corrupting ideas of nineteenth-century science. Freud, who eschewed philosophy and espoused science, will yet be recognized as having greatly redeemed and vastly enriched the philosophy of science—and most notably the science of medicine. In the history of modern medicine, Freud and his psychoanalyses will have, as they currently have, a position of unique significance.

REFERENCES

1. FREUD, SIGMUND: *Aus den Aufangen der Psychoanalse. Briefe an Wilhelm Fliess, Abhandlungen und Natizen aus den Jahren.* 1887-1902. Letter 29. London, Imago Publishing Co., 1950.
2. *Ibid.,* Letter 86.
3. WITTELS, FRITZ: *Sigmund Freud,* p. 118. Verlag, Leipzig, Wien, Zurich, E. P. Tal & Co., 1924.
4. *Ibid.,* p. 115.
5. FREUD, SIGMUND: An autobiographical study, translated by James Strachey in *The Problems of Lay-Anàlysis,* New York, W. W. Norton Co., 1952.
6. *Ibid.,* p. 41.
7. GALDSTON, IAGO: Eros and Thanatos, a critique of Freud's death wish, *The American Journal of Psychoanalysis,* Vol. XV, No. 2, 1955.
8. McDOUGALL, WILLIAM: *Psychoanalysis and Social Psychology,* London, Methuen and Co., Ltd., 1936.
9. GALDSTON, IAGO: Psychosomatic Medicine, *A.M.A. Archives of Neurology and Psychiatry,* pp. 441-450, Vol. 73, 1955.
10. GRODDECK, GEORG. WALTHER: The *Book of the It.* New York and Washington, Nervous and Mental Diseases Pub. Co., 1929.
——: *Exploring the Unconscious.* London, C. W. Daniel and Co., 1933.

——: *The Unknown Self,* translation by V. M. E. Collins, New York, Funk and Wagnalls, 1951.

——: Internationaler Psychoanalytischer verlag, Wien, Schriften von Georg Groddeck, Wien, 1926.

11. JELLIFFE, S. E.: Psychotherapy in modern medicine, in *Long Island Medical Journal,* Vol. 24, p. 152-161, 1930.

——: Psychopathology and organic disease. *New York Journal of Medicine,* Vol. 32, p. 158-588, 1932.

12. WEISZACKER, VICTOR VON: *Diesseits und Jenseits der Medizin,* p. 254, Stuttgart, 1950.

13. GALDSTON, IAGO: Dynamics of the cure in psychiatry, in the *A.M.A. Archives of Neurology and Psychiatry,* Vol. 70, pp. 286-298, Sept. 1953.

12

Psychiatry Without Freud

IN CONSIDERING the subject of this essay, you night assume that I am indulging in a pious fraud. Actually, I favored the title for two reasons. First, because it is provocative—and then because it *is* a "pious fraud." Psychiatry, that is, present day psychiatry, without Freud, and without all that has been added to it by his disciples and followers, is difficult to conceive. A recitation that literally considered psychiatry without Freud would be of interest only historically—and most likely would be a confounding, if not a "lugubrious," story. Yet lest you also assume that I purchased your interest by a trick, I must add that, though the manner was something of a fraud, the intent remains pious, and that once beyond this point, I am, and shall remain to the end, very much in earnest.

Let me plunge into the issue directly, but by means of a tale, of which it may be said, with the Italians, *"Si non e vero, e ben trovato"*—"If it isn't true, it is well found." The story goes that when the Eiffel tower was erected in Paris it came to the mind of one bright person to set up a powerful arc lamp right at its very topmost point. In this wise he thought to illuminate the entire surrounding park. He tried it and it was indeed very beautiful. But it soon became apparent that, though it was truly brilliant, it did not work well. For those who came near were blinded by the light, and those who were at a distance were blinded by the dark. It had to be given up and the park about the tower has ever since been effectively illuminated by many lamps, none as bright as the original, but all of them placed at the dark spots all around.

If this tale is taken not too literally, and transposed not too exactly, it does have its application to the "state of illumination" in psychiatry. Freud is its brilliant arc at the topmost point of the edifice—blinding

162

when too near and obscure at the outskirts. Of course, the fault is not Freud's, and, like so much in human communication, the foregoing sentence is shot through with "scapegoat animism." "Galen retarded medicine for a thousand years," the historian writes. But it is hardly Galen's fault that for a thousand years none took courage to do by Galen as Galen did by others. It is, however, a fact that for too many, especially among the young psychiatrists, the brilliance of Freud is blinding, and blinding in many ways. They seem to labor in the belief that before Freud there was little or nothing worthy of the name psychiatry; that all antecedent psychiatric history was but the forerunner to a fulfilment achieved in Freud and in analysis. This is a sad delusion; yet its practical consequences are minor, since the past has its historic realities which persist despite neglect or misunderstanding. Of greater consequences is what happens now and in the future. In this relation we see far too many among the Freudians "stomping the treadmill of orthodoxy," to prove what has been proved, many times over. Far too few venture to reassess the formulations, to test the assumptions and to challenge the procedures by which they function. Yet there is a science in the asking of questions no less intricate and valuable than the science of finding answers, and empirical effectiveness unless hedged on all sides by challenge and question is like a desert, where for the want of gage marks one is easily lost.

There is, as you know, no dearth of psychoanalytic literature, but most of it is devoted to confirming what has been affirmed time and time again. I for one should like to see, not another instance spelled out in years of analysis, where the sight of the primal scene at the age of 2 is held to account for the vaginismus at the age of 20, but, rather, something new, and critical, and very pertinent.

I should be interested, for example, in a reassessment of the Oedipal cycle. Is the version now current fully adequate? Does it embrace the whole of the mythological tale and of the psychiatric experience? I have come to feel—and this by clinical experience—that the incest motif is but half the tale, that the real tragedy is derived from the fault of Laius, the father of Oedipus, rather than from Oedipus proper. For it was Laius, as you will recall, who craved a son, and it was he who sought to evade the fate foretold by the oracle, should he have issue. Who knows how the fates might have softened had Laius not bound the pierced feet of the child Oedipus and had he held him dear instead of exposing him on Mount Citheron. I am inclined to see in the tale of Laius and of Oedipus the embodiment of that primal wisdom which in the Hebrew is tersely versed in the phrase "The sins of the father shall be visited upon his children even unto the third generation."

I am not eager to advance these thoughts on the Oedipal cycle as otherwise than probationary; yet I think it more proper and more profitable to ask such questions than to repeat, in the adulation of a master, "The little boy seeks to possess his mother; the little girl, to displace her mother at the father's side," true though this may be. It were likewise profitable to study intensively the question of questions—the dynamics of the therapeutic result. How is the cure effected; when effected? Such study would involve a host of collateral inquiries. For example, how passive is passivity, and how free is free association? Much profit could be derived from the further, and critical, study of dreams. There appears to be not only a determinable meaning to the dream content, but meaning also in the pattern of the dream proper; there is, in other words, a morphology of dreams. Psychoanalysis has been called "ego" psychology; yet the ego per se has received but limited study in recent decades. Here, certainly, is a subject of nuclear importance. No less significant, since it is involved in so much of psychopathy, is the superego; yet there have been few studies devoted to its nature and derivation since Freud, first, and Jung, later, enunciated their respective theories and beliefs. All these matters are not essentially of an academic nature, worthy of pursuit in a leisure and fancy-free hour. The defense offered by one who was recently confronted by just these questions that "we are too busy doing things to be much concerned with how we do them" is in effect degrading. For these questions are vitally concerned with "the doing of things," and it is more than likely that in being concerned with how we do things we may be enabled to do them better. Considering the duration, the costliness and the not ever certain issue of psychotherapy, it would seem that any inquiry as to how we might function better should be not only welcomed but deemed the better part of discretion.

It was not my intention to set up a protocol for research and study in psychoanalytic theory and practice. In raising the few questions presented above, I meant only to illustrate where, and how, some of our younger men might leave off "stomping the treadmill of orthodoxy" and venture to illuminate those dark spots remaining.

The advent of Freud was one of the great historic experiences, and those who have compared him to Copernicus and Darwin did not indulge in spurious analogies. Freud "shook the world." He did what but few men in human history have done, that is, redirect human thought; create a new alphabet, a new vernacular and a new literature which not merely is corrective of certain segments of our inherited culture and credence, but, more, has opened up vast and new spheres of experience and learning. Freud has made available to us a new body of knowledge and also the instrumentalities by which that knowledge can be further extended. I think of him as I would of Loewenhoek, who not only uncovered the world of the infinite, but also shaped the tools for its exploration.

It is easy to apply superlatives to the name of Freud. One can do so without the hazard of contradiction, either now or later. But it is not so easy to specify just wherein particularly lies Freud's superlative merit. This is a most interesting and involved question, and whatever answer comes easily to mind by that very token may be considered wrong. Merely to hint at the intricacy of this problem, it is a fact that the greatness of such as Copernicus, Darwin and Freud is historically perceived to derive not from what knowledge they added, but, rather, from the influence they exercised. There is a relationship between the two, of course, but not in any sense commensurate. The knowledge, as in the case of Darwin, may even be grossly at fault; yet the influence, the impact, on human thought and destiny is, and remains, both salutary and enduring. I do not intend to expand on this theme; yet since it will advance my thesis, I want to offer this additional observation. Obviously, Freud's fame rests on his creation of psychoanalysis. This affirmation embraces all that entered into the genesis of the science of analysis—the discovery of the unconscious; the mechanisms of repression, the disguised emergence of the repressed; the identity and reciprocal interrelationships of the id, the ego and the superego; the function and meaning of the dream, and of everyday mischance and mishap; the technique of free association, abreaction and all the rest. But *all* of this does not account for *all* of Freud's fame. Nor does it account, on the other hand, for the enormous and intensive antagonism which Freud evoked among his contemporaries, and still does today among some persons and peoples. I do not presume to have the full or final answer to the sources of Freud's fame, or his defamation. For that, there would be need of a longer perspective than the present offers. But I would add to the accounts of his eminence one consideration too much neglected and too little understood. I should, however, confess that what I advance is one of my own and fond conceits, which, though propounded for some years, has not received the recognition it deserves. Freud shocked the world of science and of intellect in arguing and in demonstrating both the rationality of the irrational and the irrationality of the rational. The first of the two propositions was the less opposed; the second aroused frenzied resentment. It is this split with the formal rationalism of his age that distinguishes and separates Freud from his contemporaries in science and psychiatry.

I recently found an ally to my thesis in odd quarters, and I shall quote him briefly. Isaiah Berlin, fellow of New College and university lecturer in philosophy at Oxford, wrote a most interesting essay entitled "Political Ideas in the Twentieth Century" (1). Part of Berlin's thesis is that the twentieth century is sharply separated from the nineteenth by a barrier which "divides what is unmistakably past and done with from that which most characteristically belongs to our day."

> . . . The familiarity of this barrier must not blind us to its relative novelty. One of the elements of the new outlook is the notion of unconscious and irrational influences which outweigh the forces of reason; another the notion that answers to problems exist not in rational solutions, but in the removal of the problems themselves by means other than thought and argument (pp. 356-357).

It was the firm faith of the nineteenth century that *"la raison a toujours raison,* that memories and shadows were less important than the direct perception of the real world in the clear light of the day" (p. 360). These were the common assumptions of the rationalistic enlightened world. It is true that these assumptions were challenged and denied by a few isolated, "eccentric" thinkers—Carlyle, Dostoievski, Baudelaire, Tolstoi, Nietzsche. However, none of these was "a man of science," and hence none of them really challenged science. Such discomfiture as they caused to science could be neutralized by anatomizing them and exposing, as Max Nordau did, their "degeneracy."

Berlin counts Freud among the isolated and eccentric thinkers, who, "by giving currency to exaggerated versions of the view that the true reasons for a man's beliefs were most often very different from what they themselves thought them to be, being frequently caused by events and processes of which they were neither aware nor in the least anxious to be aware . . . helped, however unwittingly, to discredit the rationalist foundations upon which their doctrines purported to rest" (p. 369).

Freud, unlike the other isolated and eccentric thinkers, was a man of science. Though many a Nordau tried it, Freud could not be anatomized or his "degeneracy" exhibited for the pleasure and profit of the intellectual pharisees. He stood forth an obdurate challenge to the naïve rationality of the nineteenth century, and he endures as such to this day.

The antirationalism of Freud proffers some deep and challenging problems—in epistemology, in the dynamics of therapy, in esthetics and morals

—problems which few have braved, but with which we must soon come to grips. Fortunately, the "soon" is not now, and I am thus left free to further pursue my thesis.

The subject matter of psychiatry without Freud is Freud's psychiatric contemporaries. It is to them that we must now turn our attention. At the outset, it is worth noting again that these contemporaries of Freud, unlike him, were partisans of that rationalism which rested its faith on "the direct perception of the real world in the clear light of day." By bearing this in mind we shall be helped to understand much, both of their shortcomings and of their merit and worth to present day psychiatry.

The nineteenth century was much preoccupied with psychiatry. In this period lived and worked Caesare Lombroso, Jean Martin Charcot, Wilhelm Griesinger, Theodor Meynert, Richard von Krafft-Ebing, Moritz Romberg, Karl Wernicke and Emil Kraepelin, to name but a few of the most eminent. These men advanced enormously the nosography of psychiatry and contributed substantially to psychotherapy. They were engaged in passionate and long-enduring apposition of psychiatric theory and concept, some being somatocists and others functionalists. Their disputations are overshadowed by those waged today; yet one can with much profit return to them and perceive how keenly they dealt with the issues which, remaining unsolved, still trouble us. Prominent in their thinking and in their polemics is the issue of the so-called psychosomatic disorders. Seemingly, they had as fine a grasp of the matter as any current.

In relation to the nineteenth century Freud stands, at least professionally, in an anomalous position. He was born in 1856 and died in 1939. He bridged both centuries, "inherited" the psychiatry of the nineteenth century, but in effect initiated that of the twentieth; and, as I have noted above, the twentieth century is in essential respects discontinuous with the nineteenth century. Because of this, it is something of a puzzle to determine who properly should be counted as Freud's psychiatric contemporaries. Certainly, the calendar cannot be taken as the sole arbiter. I have breached this puzzle by selecting three persons, and I have chosen them not solely on the basis of the calendar, but also because of their professional and theoretical proximity—because they broach on Freud's thinking and work. I have selected them also because their respective works still have a vital bearing on psychoanalytic psychotherapy.

The three I shall consider are Pierre Janet, Pavlov and Adolf Meyer. Janet was born in 1859; Pavlov, in 1849, and Meyer, in 1866. Of the three, Janet comes closest to Freud, both in age and in his theoretical formulation of psychodynamics. With the latter this is so much the case that partisans, more passionate than informed, have charged both Janet and Freud with having "stolen" one from the other. There is, however, no evidence to support such charges of plagiarism; and, though there is great parallelism between Freud and Janet, they ultimately arrive at conclusions unmistakably and widely divergent.

Janet is in his own rights a remarkable figure. His erudition was vast; his accomplishments were enormous. He was well grounded in medicine in general and in neuropathology and in psychology. He was qualified in philosophy; he was a botanist of note. He was an indefatigable collector of data and of records. He wrote copiously and lectured widely. Yet, oddly enough, Janet is oftener condemned for his sins of omission than he is praised for the virtue of his achievements. Worse than that; he is badly neglected, at least outside the Latin countries. Freud contributed to this. His polemic against Janet falls short, both in justice and in objectivity. In his "Autobiography," he gives an inadequate summation of Janet's views on hysteria and then dismisses Janet as one who "behaved ill, showed ignorance of the facts and used ugly arguments" (2).

Janet is blamed for not "having been Freud," for not having discovered, despite his enormous labors, the theory of repression, which in psycho-analysis "is the foundation stone of our understanding of the neurosis." Janet rested his theory of the neurosis on the lack of an adequate psychic tension, on what he termed psychasthenia—on weakness of the psyche. There is, of course, no doubt that Janet not only failed to discover the theory of repression, but also that he never fully accepted it. In his "Psychological Healing" (3), Janet writes:

> . . . This conception of repression is undoubtedly one of the most interesting in the Freudian psychology. My own opinion is that the phenomenon must be explained in a different way, but it is none-the-less of great importance (p. 610).

What troubles Janet is "why the Freudians have extended the conception in this way, which is, to say the least of it, strange?" On this score, Janet ventures the opinion:

> . . . The reason is that they want at all costs to discover a traumatic memory underlying every neuropathic symptom, to disinter a more or less modified memory of an event which has stirred the subject's emotions. . . . Repression as we have described it, is not a normal phenomenon which, through clumsy handling, becomes the cause of subsequent disturbances; it is itself already a morbid disturbance (p. 646).

This opinion follows on one to the effect that "in normal life, repression leaves no traces." Here Janet touches on a provocative theme, for since repression is a normal function in normal life, why, then, does it engender neurotic behavior in some but not in others? The answer cannot entirely rest on the nature of the material repressed. Freud comes close to Janet in the judgment he advances:

> ... It may be assumed that neurosis hardly ever develops unless there are constitutional or congenital factors increasing the possibility for such a condition (4).

Despite their protestations, and Janet pokes a rather mordant wit at Freud and at psychoanalysis, there is much reciprocally illuminating in the works of Freud and Janet. I can subscribe to Mayo's statement:

> It is the fashion in these days to dismiss, somewhat cavalierly, the work of Janet as something that has been superseded by Freudian and other developments. . . . The outcome is unfortunate, for there is no real conflict between the observations of Janet and Freud. Indeed they work in different parts of the same field so that their researches are mutually complementary; and any one person trained in the findings of one only is probably committed to incomplete understanding (5).

There is a fiction current that Janet is a therapeutic pessimist, that he regards the psychoneurotic patient as a stigmatized degenerate for whom and with whom little can be done. Wittels (6) writes:

> ... Before Freud appeared on the stage the scientific explanation of neurosis was that it was all due to heredity and degeneration. The influence of heredity is undeniable, but the admission of this fact does not help us to cure our patient.

Actually, however, Janet is anything but a therapeutic pessimist, and his thesis concerned with psychological tension and psychasthenia is grossly misunderstood and misrepresented by many analytically oriented writers. Janet is pessimistic with regard to psychotherapy as a science. "Psychotherapy does not yet exist. . . . We are merely beginning to see what it ought to be and what in due time it will become (Vol. 2, p. 1206) (3). But it is otherwise with regard to the practical effectiveness of psychotherapy; on this score Janet affirms:

> Psychotherapy in the wider sense of the term, including within its scope all the methods of treatment based upon a knowledge of psy-

chological or physiological laws, has unquestionably done good service in a very large number of cases (Vol. 2, p. 1212).

However, no matter how badly Janet is misunderstood or misrepresented, the fact remains that there is a cardinal difference between the psychiatric orientation of Freud and that of Janet. To summate this difference in terms of repression and of psychasthenia is both correct and convenient. Dalbiez (7), who has treated the contrasting theories of Freud and Janet sympathetically and exhaustively, represents the difference in the following terms:

> Janet has emphasized only such sources of illness as arise from material causality, while Freud has studied only such as derive from efficient causality. . . . In metaphysical language, we may say that Janet's schema derives from the concept of privation; Freud's, from that of opposition (Vol. 2, p. 191).

In thinking on this, one is prompted to ask whether this difference in schemata did not derive from the nature of the material with which they, Freud and Janet, respectively dealt. In a passage which no doubt roiled Freud, Janet quoted approvingly the theory advanced by Friedländer and Ladame to the effect that there must be a peculiar kind of sexual atmosphere in Vienna—a sort of local demon, which, by epidemic as it were, takes possession of the population, so that in this environment the observer is foredoomed to overestimate the importance of sexual influences (Vol. 2, p. 620) (7). One need not agree that the Viennese "overestimated the importance of sexual influences" to appreciate that the cultural, and hence the psychological, atmosphere of Paris differed from that of Vienna at the turn of the century. It may very well be, therefore, that Janet saw many more cases of *deprivation* than of *opposition*, and Freud more of opposition or repression than of deprivation.

This matter is of more than historical interest to us, for it is a fact, reported on by many, that the types of cases widely seen today are not of the classic type first reported by Freud, but are more commonly mixed cases, in which deprivation plays an important etiological role. In the treatment of such patients it is necessary not only to uncover repressed material, but also to conserve, to reenforce, to redirect what Freud calls libido*, and Janet, psychological tension. This involves not merely the

---

* Libido—"the chief goal, purpose, pattern or wish of . . . conduct or behavior is the continuance of life. . . . That aspect of the transformed energy that pursues this creative goal, either within the body structures, as seen in growth or repair,

reintegration of such libido as is invested in the repressed material, or in "complexes," but often the addition to, or the increment of, the total libido available to the patient. Ferenczi, one of Freud's most able disciples and co-workers, came to this very conclusion and affirmed it to be incumbent on the physician, the psychotherapist, to reenforce, even to add to, the patient's libido. Few have followed Ferenczi's lead, at least among those who work outside the hospitals. It should be noted in this connection that a great deal of what is done in some of our better hospitals, independent of specific psychotherapy, is aimed at reenforcing and increasing the patient's libido.

In the mixed case, wherein etiology involves both repression and deprivation, it is frequently a question of which of the etiological factors should be dealt with first, and often it is better, indeed at times imperative, that before the repressed material is uncovered, the psychological tension, the libido of the patient, should be fortified. I recall a patient, a woman of 25, who, having tuberculosis, also suffered from anorexia nervosa, globus hystericus, vomiting, confusion and apathy. That she was suffering from a series of hysterical manifestations was clearly evident. That her neurosis derived primarily from "repression" could not be doubted. The sexual content of her symptoms was patent. This young woman had married some three years before, to escape her home. Her sexual experience was most unsatisfactory: coitus was usually per anum. She took the initiative in annulling her marriage and was encouraged by her parents, themselves rather inadequate persons, to return home. A futile and hopeless "asexual romance" filled the next year. That coming to an end, the patient reverted to her divorced husband, resuming her correspondence with him. He was serving at a military outpost. Her tuberculosis was discovered at about this time. When I first saw her, she was seeing her ex-husband two or three times a week, in the home of her parents. She indulged in some sexual play but not in intercourse. She accepted money from her ex-husband but was not certain that she wanted to remarry him. When she first came under my care, this young woman, standing 5 feet 8 inches (173 cm.) in stockinged feet, weighed 98 pounds (44.5 Kg.). It was painfully clear to me that in this patient's care I should

---

at biological levels, as seen in mating, or at socialized levels as operating for family formation, works of art, invention, civilization, and culture, has been called libido by Freud. Within the body it acts as a force, a tension, an impulse" (*Psychoanalysis Today: Its Scope and Function*, edited by A. S. Lorand, New York, Covici-Friede, Inc., 1933).

need first to deal with her deprivations, and only later with her repressed material.

I grant that the case cited is of an extreme nature; yet I am convinced that too little attention is generally given to the current libidinal dynamics of the patient, more thought and energy being devoted to the ferreting out of repressed, painful, distorted memories which, it is of course true, contribute to the genesis of the neurosis. Yet a strengthened ego, fortified by a rich libido, is better able to meet and to reintegrate repressed materials. I suspect that the task of dealing with the current libidinal dynamics of the patient requires closer study of the patient's needs and involves greater therapeutic initiative than some therapists are willing or able, to assume.

I would conclude my treatment of Janet by affirming that we cannot further neglect the thesis of objective energy, so ably formulated by him. Its incorporation in the conceptualization of the genesis of psychopathy not only will better illuminate the dynamics of disorder but should enable us to prove more effective, in terms of the economy of time and effort, in treatment. Certain it is that our experiences during the last war, both with the military and with the civilian populations, without in any way invalidating Freud's thesis on repression, has fully validated Janet's ideas on psychological tension and psychasthemia. It is revealing and pertinent that what was called "shell shock" in 1918 was in World War II renamed "combat fatigue." Without yielding aught to the mechanists, we can yet accede that all living organisms, from the lowest of plants to the highest of men, are transformers of energy. How much and how well man absorbs, transmutes and expends his energies is in part the concern of the psychotherapist.

From Janet, I would now turn to the second of Freud's "elected contemporaries," Ivan Pavlov. His work on the conditioned reflex touches but a segment of Freud's psychiatry; yet this contact is of great importance. Those who have a guardianship interest in psychiatry would do well to watch the resurgence of Pavlovianism, promoted in part by the authoritarian countries, but also by those whose predilections are for the concrete, the palpable, the directly mensurable. We are likely to dismiss Pavlovianism as a past movement which came to an inglorious end in behaviorism, and the ghost of which came to life here lately in a treatment for inebriety. Such a dismissal is unwarranted and hazardous. The simplicity of Pavlovianism has a fatal appeal, to which many of the unwary must succumb. The great ado about shock therapy and psychosurgery and all the recently developed physical and chemical modalities of treatment have given new life to Pavlovianism. Thus, for example, Masserman (8) takes a fling at psychoanalysis, stating:

> Even in relatively enlightened spheres of psychiatry there are relics of animistic thinking: *vide* the substitution of the Freudian terms of "Id," "Ego" and "Superego" for the gods that in ancient times were thought to be in control of man's passions and intellect; or the attempts by some psychoanalytic mythologists to use the Narcissus and Oedipus legends, not as poetic allegories but as proof of the supposed nature of man's unconscious conflicts!

Masserman is persuaded that his poor, bewildered cats, subjected alike to artificial conditioning, under artificial conditions, and then to arbitrary insult, will yield him better insight into the psyche of man than will the "mythology" of the psychoanaysts! It is not, however, the new behaviorists that need concern us here, but, rather, the bearing which Pavlov's work has on Freud's theories. Pavlov significantly confirms Freud's theory of conflict as a source of neurotic disorders. The classic demonstration of this is to be seen in the instance of the dog conditioned to distinguish and to respond appropriately to the exhibition of a circle and of an ellipse. All goes well as long as the two figures, circle and ellipse, are fairly distinguishable. When, however, the difference is reduced so that the oval is close in shape to the circle—ratio of axes, 8:9—the dog is thrown into a neurotic state. He becomes nervous, whines on the stand, twists and turns, and snaps at the apparatus. Pavlov accounts for these reactions as follows (9):

> . . . Broadly, we can regard these disturbances as due to a conflict between the process of excitation and inhibition which the cortex finds difficult to resolve.

Dalbiez writes:

> Pavlov's method will do us the service of bringing the problem of the etiology of the neuroses down onto the terra firma of experiment. It affords irrefutable proof of the existence of neurotic disorders due to a clash of opposed forces (p. 70) (7).

Dalbiez, however, does not, as Masserman does, naïvely equate the neuroses of the dog with the neurosis in man. Psychology cannot be reduced to physiology. "Pavlov only studies movements," Dalbiez writes, "whereas Freud analyses cognitive or affective states and movements, cognitively—affectively governed" (p. 83) (7). He quotes approvingly

Leibnitz' dictum to the effect that reflexology is true in what it asserts, and false in what it denies.

These considerations lead us back to the conditioned reflex. This is a physiological mechanism which subserves vital objectives, chiefly in the orientation of the organism toward the outer world. The conditioned reflex can acquire a psychological character when the stimulus which acts as the conditioner is of a psychological nature. Most pertinent to our deliberations, however, is the simple fact revealed by Pavlov that it is possible to "condition behavior," that is, to associate a stimulus (among humans, also an affect) with a motor, or behavior, pattern, in a causal relation. By the variety of stimuli utilized by Pavlov in his laboratory; it is evident that outside the laboratory the linkage of stimulus to behavior pattern is fortuitous; any combination is theoretically possible. Of course, as far as human beings are concerned, this theoretical possibility is never realized "in full"; human beings are not naturally "in harness on the experimenter's table," nor is the field as clear—too many conditionings are likely to be experienced simultaneously. Yet, as clinical experience shows, a good deal of psychopathy has the character of a "conditioned reflex," in the sense that a stimulus situation evokes a behavior reaction that is practically automatic and repetitive. It is also unsuited, ineffective and at times overtly destructive. The genesis of such a behavior reaction does not invariably derive from repression or conflict. It may be, and oftenest is, derived from a fortuitously determined association of stimulus situation with a motor or affect coincident. It may be, in other words, and in effect, an instance of malinstruction. of mislearning, or rather of learning what was valid as a particular but is not valid as a universal. The son of a harsh, domineering, brutal father will most likely associate the "father person" with unpleasant affects and react in a given manner— submissively, or cunningly, or aggressively, or in any combination or serial pattern. His conditioned behavior may have been realistic in respect to his "brutal father," but it will be neurotic when projected into his relations to the shop foreman, his boss or the traffic policeman. In such instances it must in part be the function of the analyst to trace back to its origin the coupling of the stimulus situation with the untoward behavior pattern.

Here a pertinent question arises: To what extent is the analyst's therapy operating as a "reconditioning" of the original "conditioned pattern?" In psychotherapy one of the least illumined chapters is that concerned with the dynamics of therapy. How the cure is effected and when it is effected are questions to which we can at best offer only partial and tentative answers. Of course, that is likewise true of other therapies. We know but little of the therapeutic dynamics of insulin, of the sulfonamides, of penicillin or of aureomycin. We know the end results, but not how those end results are achieved. In psychiatry, we speak in relation to the cure of abreaction, of transference, of a permissive atmosphere, of integration, of reintegration, of insight; these are useful and descriptive terms, but they do not afford us an adequate representation of just what is taking place while the patient is "being" cured. Probably personality and the psyche are too complicated in structure and function to permit us to trace the adventures, the progressions and the effects of a psychological element or of a psychological impact insinuated into their labyrinthine patterns. For that we may need to invent psychological tracer elements, akin to the isotopes, and the equivalents also of Geiger counters. All this being so, it is still appropriate and timely to inquire how much of the psychotherapist's therapy is in effect a reconditioning of the original, i.e., pathological "conditioned pattern."

This is a question which brings into awareness a large number of related matters—and some other pertinent questions. Thus, it is implied in modern psychiatry that memory is more deeply retentive of experience and knowledge than was ever suspected. Some neurophysiologists believe that every experience leaves its indelible engram in the involved neural unit and structure (10). In the light of this belief, it is interesting to speculate on what happens to the memories and experiences, repressed or otherwise, which are involved in the engenderment of psychopathy. Are they, like the evil spirits of olden times, exorcised? Is it possible to obliterate an engram? If not, what happens then to the memory? Without pursuing this involved matter further, it seems clear that if memory cannot be extirpated and completely undone, it should be possible to add to it and thus to alter its qualities. This process is implied in the reconditioning of conditioned behavior. Pavlov and Watson have demonstrated this possibility in the laboratory, and I am convinced that the reconditioning of conditioned behavior is the modus operandi of much effective psychotherapy. How could the son of the domineering, brutal father "unlearn" his original lesson gained in experience save by "learning" *in addition* that not all father equivalents are domineering and brutal; that some, indeed, are kindly and tolerant.

I am sure that you must by this time have anticipated the objectives of my excursion and know it to be the premise to a plea for freer activity on the part of the therapist. Passivity plays an important role in certain phases of psychotherapy. Passivity may itself have the quality of "action," but passivity is "orthodox," and too often the refuge of the bewildered, the insecure and the indifferent therapist. Activity in therapy is looked upon askance. Yet if the propositions I advance are valid, if much of psychotherapy involves the reconditioning of conditioned behavior, then purposeful activity on the part of the therapist is not only permissible, but to be expected, and indeed required. The caveat indicated is this: The therapist's activity needs to be illuminated by previously gained insight into the dynamics of the patient's psychopathy—an insight usually won by a passive attention to the patient's complaints and recitations. Unillumined by such insight, active therapy is likely to be bumptious, and fatuous.

There can be no doubt that the technique of "free association" is among the greatest contributions which Freud made to modern psychiatry; yet it is all too often forgotten that "free association" is primarily an investigative instrument, that it initiates and makes possible effective therapy but is not in and of itself therapeutic. Schilder (11) stated:

> . . . I might . . . formulate free association as a mutual effort between analyst and patient to bring the conflicts and problems of the patient into clear appearance. Thus, it is a directed effort and is based on a continuous inner activity of the analyst (p. 117).

The insight and the revelation which "free association" affords formulate in effect the therapeutic agenda which the patient, with the therapist's help, must then carry out and make operatively effective.

At this point, abrupt though it be, I must needs turn to the third of Freud's psychiatric contemporaries, Adolf Meyer. I doubt not that in the United States the influence of Meyer is as ponderable as that of Freud. Meyer was in every sense of the term a modest person. He was not "a fighter," either on behalf of his own or against another's point of view or theories. He was never diffuse in his thinking (though he was not particularly gifted as a speaker or writer); yet he never marshaled or organized his theories into a definitive text. He did give the name of "psychobiology" to his point of view, which he, in part, described as follows: "As long as there is life there are positive assets—action, choice, hope—not in the imagination but in a clear understanding of the situation, goals, and possibilities." By these positive assets, Meyer took his bearings, and by them he charted his therapeutic course.

Adolf Meyer, more sharply than any of his contemporaries, focused our minds and fixed our attention on the reality matrix, within which the sick and the well, the patient and the therapist, are fixed. Time and matter, opportunity and obligation, are of the essence of life and of living. We all muddle through as best we can and the mark of the therapist is that he muddles a little better and, by that token, can help those who muddle a little less well. Psychotherapists of every school, but particularly Freudians, are prone to forget all this. They operate as if time, means and opportunity were nugatory items, not to be given much weight in their accounts. But that is a false estimate, one that betrays both the therapist and the patient. We need to be mindful not only of the patient's effectiveness but also of our own. That often means compromise, or, more aptly and correctly, the trimming of dogma to the dimensions of reality. Paul Schilder was a man free of preconceptions and broadly experienced in every form of psychotherapy, and I subscribe warmly to his comments on psychotherapy.

> It is the important task of the physician to develop the patient's personality according to the capacities, endowments, and characteristics of the patient. He [the physician] will be better able to do so if he has the conviction that the other human being is an entity of its own and is valuable in so far as it is a definite person. . . . When the physician keeps the principle in mind that he has to respect the personality of his patient, he will not err too much. He has, furthermore, to keep in mind the specific social reality in which his patient lives. He should be further aware of the necessary limitation in his own point of view and should have, at the same time, a concept of his goals in life and the concept of the goals in life of the patient. The basic attitude in psychotherapy is that there is one human being who needs help and another human being who wants to give help. The attitude of the physician is the attitude of helpfulness and understanding. His aim is to relieve the patient from his suffering, and his conviction is that this aim can be reached by a better adaptation to the inward and outward reality, preferably by an increase in insight (pp. 170-171) (11).

Adolf Meyer's other term for psychobiology is ergasiology. This is an esoteric, and yet a fortunate, term, since it embodies the very idea of purposeful, goal-aimed action and underscores the second major component of Meyer's teachings. Ergasiology mirrors a purposeful organism that pursues immediate objectives, strung together in a long-term, but not always appreciated, pattern or trajectory. The human organism is always moving in a patterned direction, and even when the overt motion is irrational and contrary to the norm pattern one can assume that the overt abnormal only overlays and masks the normal. Irrespective of age and condition, there is, as long as life persists, a momentum, albeit at times rather weak, in the direction of the fulfilment of the goals initiated in the conjunction of the gametes, from which the individual derived. This realization is a therapeutic asset. It offers leverage by which the patient can be helped to regain well-being and effectiveness. This realization counterbalances the other, the one which dwells on the repressions, inhibitions, and impedimenta encountered in the past and shackling the patient. The reenforcement of goal-striving can be effected at the same time as insight is gained by uncovering of repressed, conflict material. The one need not always wait on the other.

Here I must wind up my argument. I shall not recapitulate the matters presented, save only as I offer an apology for their exposition. Freud ended his autobiographic study with the following words:

> Looking back . . . over the patchwork of my life's labours, I can say that I have made many beginnings and thrown out many suggestions. Something will come of them in the future. But I cannot tell myself whether it will be much or little.

I have attempted to indicate, in broad terms, something of what has come out of the "patchwork" of Freud's labors. That "something" is enormously important. But we who are Freud's inheritors cannot rest, but, rather, must strive to advance that discipline to which he and other great and good men devoted their best years and energies.

REFERENCES

1. BERLIN, I.: Political ideas in the twentieth century, *Foreign Affairs*, pp. 352-385, April 1950.
2. FREUD, S.: *Autobiography*, translated by P. Strachey, New York, W. W. Norton & Company, 1935, p. 57.
3. JANET, P.: *Psychological Healing*, translated by E. and C. Paul, London, G. Allen & Unwin, 1925.
4. FREUD, S.: *The Problems of Lay-Analyses*, translated by A. P. Maerkers Branden, New York, Brentano's, 1927, p. 169.
5. MAYO, E.: *Some Notes on the Psychology of Pierre Janet*, Cambridge, Mass., Harvard University Press, 1948.
6. WITTELS, F.: *Sigmund Freud: His Personality, His Teaching and His School*, translated by E. and C. Paul, New York, Dodd, Mead and Company, 1924, p. 122.
7. DALBIEZ, R.: *La méthode psychoanalytique et la doctrine Freudienne*, Paris, Desclée de Brouwer & Cie, 1936.
8. MASSERMAN, J.: Experimental neurosis, *Scient. Am.*, 182:38 (March 1959).
9. PAVLOV, I. P.: *Conditioned Reflexes*, translated and edited and edited by G. V. Anrep. London, Oxford University Press, 1927, p. 302.
10. RIGNANO, E.: *Biological Memory*, London, Harcourt, Brace & Company, 1926.
11. SCHILDER, P.: *Psychotherapy*, New York, W. W. Norton & Company, 1938.

13

Freud and Romantic Medicine

THIS ESSAY IS OFFERED as a contribution to the exegesis of psychoanalysis. It aims to lay bare some of the sources of Freud's ideas, and to specifically relate them to certain relevant ideas promulgated in Romantic Medicine.

I approach my task in the dual role of psychiatrist and medical historian. Both disciplines are requisite: psychiatry in order to understand Freud's own *élan vital,* and medical history to adequately appreciate the cultural setting and intellectual climate in which Freud grew up, matured, and effected his revolution in psychiatry.

Mine is not the first attempt to trace Freud's ideas to their sources of origin. Indeed there is a welter of such attempts. Many of them are concerned with uncovering so-called forerunners to, and anticipators of Freud. But there also have been some more meritorious attempts, such as were made by Dr. and Mrs. Bernfeld, Marie Dover of Darmstadt, and Louise von Karpinska of Poland. The most competent and the most penetrating efforts in this direction, however, stand to the credit of Fritz Wittels. His biographic study of Freud, together with his *Freud and His Time,* afford one valuable insight into the personality of Freud and into the relatedness of his ideas to those of his forerunners.

My own efforts at "tracing" Freud's ideas to their sources of origin are favored above those of my predecessors, including Wittels, in that I have, as they had not, access to the Fliess letters, and to the data concerning Freud's childhood, and young manhood given in the Jones biography. Of the two the Fliess letters are the more important.

In the exegesis of psychoanalysis three factors call for thorough study: first and foremost the person of Freud; second, the derivation and structuralization of his ideas; and third, the impact of those ideas upon the

179

realm of science and thought. This is patently a task of gigantic dimensions, and at this juncture I can pretend to no more than a modest enterprise.

What is to be noted relative to the person of Freud? Freud was a Jew, living in anti-Semitic surroundings. One of his earliest memories of his father revolved about an episode in which the father was insulted and could not, or would not, avenge himself, but swallowed the insult in a manner that seemed craven to Freud.

Freud was poor. He grew up in a home where want was not depraving but where it was an indwelling and abiding *Sorge*. Freud knew and suffered the hobbling effects of poverty for the greater portion of his childhood, his youth, and young manhood.

Freud grown into manhood was compelled by want to do that which promised him a living rather than what he wanted or would have preferred to do. His entire being was conditioned by these cruel and degrading determinants. The proverty that engulfed Freud was not simply economic: it was all-pervading, it was atmospheric. It is difficult to conceive the qualitative character of the poverty that engulfed a poor Jew living in Vienna during the latter half of the last century. It was not so much depraving in its effects as it was overwhelming and paralyzing. In such an atmosphere only those survive who have great endurance, and only those prevail who are gifted with an inordinate drive and with such competences as can lift them over the barriers of social insignificance, economic want, and racial prejudice.

Fortunately Freud was endowed with just such gifts and competences. He had an inordinate drive, great energy, and a superb intellect. But it must be understood that Freud's historical position is essentially the resultant of the interplay between his native qualities and the deprivational and provocative setting in which they operated. It is both conceivable and highly probable that had Freud not been subjected to the goadings of his manifold poverty he would not have risen beyond the relative mediocrity of an able man. Again, were Freud less gifted he would most likely have been lost in that anonymity of the *Kleinbürgertum* or the *Handelsstand* that embraced in its amorphous ambient the greater portion of Vienna's Jewry. But Freud was ambitious. That more than anything else is the outstanding characteristic of his personality. He was ambitious to avenge the Stygian nothingness of his origin, to more than make up for the insignificance of his patrimony and the devastating mediocrity, the undistinguished platitudinousness of the world in which he suffered his youth.

Given his goading resentment, his driving ambition, and his gifts, it can be predicated that Freud would have succeeded in any undertaking. He would have made his mark in any field. Whether it would have been so great a mark, so shining an achievement as that represented by psychoanalysis, is a moot question. For in the fruition of psychoanalysis are implicated certain fortuitous circumstances extraneous to Freud and his immediacies. Chief among these fortuitous and extraneous circumstances were the then prevailing convictions and patterns of scientific thought. And equally fortuitous and fortunate were the circumstances that brought Freud in contact with, and exposed him to, the influences and inspirations of a number of men—Breuer, Charcot, and Fliess. The last named, in my judgment, had the profoundest effect upon Freud's intellectual development—vastly greater than any of Freud's biographers have recognized or acknowledged (1).

Fliess has received but scant justice from Freud's biographers. Of course, Freud was their main concern and Fliess was but a side issue. In the Fliess letters, ingenuously labeled *Aus den Anfängen der Psychoanalyse* (2) (rather than 'Freud's letters to Fliess'), they sought for and found Freud, not Fliess. Of Fliess they were content to note that "he was said to be" charming and that he was some sort of crank about numbers. That and a few derogatory opinions quoted from among his disagreeing contemporaries and the picture is complete! (3). Fliess was not of Freud's stature, but he is treated by the Freudians as Freud was initially treated by his own uninformed contemporaries. From this general indictment I must exempt Fritz Wittels. Of Fliess he wrote: "[er] ist ein geistreicher und spekulativer Kopf, in mehr als einer Hinsicht Freud verwandt" (4).

I will return to Fliess later. For the present I want to revert to Freud's driving ambition to be preeminent—little matter in what—so but he be preeminent (5).

Freud was lapped in the myth of the hero. There is the apocryphal tale of his birth with a cowl, and the soothsayer's, in this case an old woman's, prediction that he would rise in the world and become a chancellor. Freud himself nurtured the aspirations of an heroic destiny. Long before he had any claim to distinction, Freud wrote seriously concerning his future biographers, and how difficult he was making it for them by destroying all materials bearing upon his intimate life.

Twice in his life he expunged his past. The first time in 1885, and the last in 1907. On two occasions he completely destroyed all his correspondence, notes, diaries and manuscripts (6). Writing to his betrothed in 1885 —Freud was then 29 years of age—he reported the destruction of his private papers, and observed: "I cannot leave here and cannot die before ridding myself of the disturbing thought of who might come by the old papers." "Let the biographers chafe; we won't make it too easy for them. Let each one of them believe he is right in his 'conception of the development of the Hero': Even now I enjoy the thought of how they will all go astray" (7). It is interesting to speculate why Freud was so eager to blot out the past.

There can be little doubt that Freud felt himself heroically predestined and convinced that it was up to him to eventuate this heroic destiny. For that Freud lacked neither energy nor enterprise. Describing Freud's three hospital years—1884-1887—Jones writes: "Freud was constantly occupied with the endeavor to make a name for himself by discovering something important in either clinical or pathological medicine" (8). Jones ascribes this drive to Freud's eagerness to marry "a year or two earlier." But this explanation is not convincing. The simple fact is that Freud was an ambitious man, even unto his old age, and it is quite consistent for an ambitious man to try to make a name for himself.

Before Freud turned to the treatment of nervous and mental diseases he ventured into a number of fields, seeking in each to make a name for himself. He experimented with pharmacological products, he worked in physiology, embryology, in neuroanatomy, dabbled in children's diseases, and tried his skill as a medical compiler, translator, and author. He was competent in each, came close to gaining distinction on several occasions, but attained in none the preeminence he sought and craved (9).

That came to him only after he had labored long in the treatment of nervous and mental diseases. And here we witness an instance of Freud's great good fortune, for at the beginning of this departure and for many years thereafter, Freud had for friend and mentor the gentle, generous, and ingenious Josef Breuer. The relationship between Breuer and Freud is too well known to require retelling, though it is worth noting that in later years Freud was privately hostile toward Breuer, though publicly he always spoke of Breuer in terms of praise and gratitude (10).

Freud not infrequently referred to Breuer as the Founder of Psychoanalysis. This, as Jones observes, is an exaggeration. It was an overassessment of Breuer's share, and it is to be seriously doubted if Breuer ever accepted the reference gladly or as a compliment. For Breuer was not sympathetic to Freud's "will speculations" (11). He was an orthodox scientist, an adherent of the school of Helmholtz, a devotee of Goethe and of Fechner. Yet there can be no doubt that by his participation in Breuer's famous case, Frl. Anna O., Freud was launched on a tangent of curiosity and interest which ultimately led him to the formulation of his theory and system of psychoanalysis. But Breuer disassociated himself from Freud long before the latter had gone far in these directions. And the reason for this was not, as it is commonly alleged, that Breuer became alarmed when Frl. Anna attempted to involve him in some of her sexual fancies, but rather that Breuer could not accept Freud's speculations.

It is this and not specifically Freud's emphasis on the role of sexuality in hysteria that estranged Breuer. Yet the common opinion holds to the contrary and Breuer is made to appear a shy, timid, prudish old maid of a man. Sexuality in hysteria was a secondary factor at issue—the primary one was in the nature of a broad philosophical difference. Freud himself described it clearly in his "Autobiographical Study" (12). The issue between him and Breuer revolved around the problem "when and how do mental processes become pathogenic." Breuer advocated a physiological theory and Freud a psychological. Freud, in his own words, suspected at the root of the pathogenic mental processes the operation of "intentions and purposes such as are to be observed in normal life." It was the thwart and repression of such intentions and purposes that, according to Freud, proved pathogenic. If one but granted that premise, it was incontrovertible that in our society the intentions and purposes of sexuality were subject to the greatest thwart and repression. But the premise was *not* granted, either by Breuer or by the world of science. The premise denied, all that was derived therefrom was likewise denied and rejected. One man in Freud's immediacy, however, did not reject the premise; that man, to Freud's great good fortune, appeared on the scene at just the right time, and that man was Wilhelm Fliess.

But before dealing with Fliess' role in Freud's intellectual development, it is imperative that we grasp in its full import what it was that Freud premised and why it was so grossly rejected and violently opposed. To state the issue bluntly and at its simplest—the imputation to life and to its manifold phenomena of intention and purpose was anathema to all the "best brains" in biology and medicine. Intentions and purposes smacked of vitalism, and reeked of teleology. Life, according to prevailing scientific belief, was to be accounted for in terms of matter and energy, in terms of molecules in motion. Purpose and intention had neither place nor meaning in the realm of science. Yet Freud postulated not molecules and motion but intention and purpose—"such," he added, "as are to be observed in normal life." Is it not understandable then why Brücke, Meynert, and Breuer, those closest to Freud in his student years and during his early manhood, were alienated and aggrieved? Freud had in effect betrayed them. He had renounced their common faith. Brücke, Meynert, and Breuer belonged to the school of von Helmholtz, a school whose adherents, embracing the outstanding biologists, physiologists, and physicians of the time, were bitterly and aggressively opposed to every theory of biology that posited any factor other than matter and energy.

The most outspoken and belligerent representative of this school of thought was not von Helmholtz, but Emil du Bois-Reymond, the Prussian patriot of French extraction. Brücke was a close friend of du Bois-Reymond. Bernfeld cites a letter written by du Bois-Reymond which contains the following affirmation: "Brücke and I pledged a solemn oath to put into effect this truth: 'No other forces than the common physical-chemical ones are active within the organism. In those cases which cannot at the time be explained by these forces one has either to find the specific way or form of their action by means of the physical-mathematical method or to assume new forces equal in dignity to the chemical-physical forces inherent in matter, reducible to the force of attraction and repulsion.' "

"Intention and purpose" did not belong to that order of forces deemed equal in dignity to the physical-chemical forces. Hence, Freud and his theories were not acceptable among the scientifically orthodox and respectable.

I have quoted Freud's own words on the differences between himself and Breuer, and underscored the word "intention and purpose." From this it might be assumed that in his own mind Freud was clear as to "where he stood and what he intended." But such an assumption would be grossly erroneous. Freud never made a clean break with the school of von Helmholtz, and I doubt that he ever, in the long span of his life, grasped the true issue that separated him from orthodox psychology. Freud was all his life, as Wittels named him, the Antiphilosopher, and "the issue" was in the last analysis philosophical. Freud, to use modern terms, was an ethologist, and an ecological and holistic scientist, *malgré soi*.

Therein lies the wonder and the tragedy of his association with Fliess— a wonder in the effect it had upon his thinking and endeavors, and tragic in the tawdry *finis* that was writ to that friendship. Tragic, too, is the disparagement and calumny heaped upon Fliess' person and memory by the adulating partisans of Freud.

Who was Wilhelm Fliess? Little was known of him before the Fliess letters came to light, and even now there is but scant information about him as a personage. Those who have commented on him, in his relations to Freud, tend to belittle him. Jones is frequently and overtly abusive in his treatment of Fliess. Hence, we not only know little of Fliess but that little which is published is patently derogatory and prejudicial.

The Fliess letters are but half a story. We do not have those written by Fliess to Freud (13). Freud destroyed them. Freud would have destroyed his own letters to Fliess, but fortunately they were saved. Unfortunately not all of them are published, nor are those published given in their entirety. Of 284 epistles only 168 have been made public. The explanation that some of the materials have been kept out because their publication would "be inconsistent with professional or personal confidence" leaves one, me at least, unsatisfied and unhappy.

Knowing so very little about Fliess, how are we to gauge his influence upon Freud? The answer is—by internal evidence, that is by the evidence we can gain in a careful scrutiny of Fliess' own thoughts and writings.

Were we to take our cue from Jones and Ernst Kris, Fliess would be written off as a fantastic numerologist, an otherwise gracious, informed, and charming man, but still, one who somehow developed a mathematical monomania. Neither Kris nor Jones have attempted to gain insight into the derivation of this so-called mathematical monomania, nor have they related it to Fliess' other preoccupations, to bisexuality, to right- and left-handedness, to the nasal reflex, to the periodicity of fertility and infertility. Had they troubled to do so in the framework of the requisite historical understanding they could have discovered that collectively all this has meaning and that from this meaning Freud drew deep insight and much inspiration.

What is the commonality, the embracing persuasion of Fliess' endeavors? I am not certain that he ever expressed it as such—but it is unmistakably that of Romantic Medicine. For in Romantic Medicine one finds not only precisely those concerns which Fliess pursued but also the exact counterpart of his own and of Freud's orientation to Nature and to Man. This orientation Freud derived directly from Fliess during the fifteen years of their intimate relation. Freud was not a student of philosophy and there is no evidence to show that he came under the tutorial influence of any one else as schooled and biased in these directions as was Fliess (14).

It is not possible to expound in this presentation the ample meaning and the historical as well as philosophical significance of Romantic Medicine. More nonsense has been written about Romantic Medicine, especially in the English language, than was ever contained in it. Yet though indeed Romantic Medicine embraced much flimsy and brain-fevered speculations, its fundamental assumptions, derived from the *Naturphilo-*

sophie of Schelling, were not only profound, penetrating and wise, but are finding validation and support in present-day science and biology (15).

Here I must content myself in merely highlighting the distinctions, the differences, the antipodal positions of Romantic Medicine, and the medicine so self-consciously triumphant in the days of Fliess and Freud. Recall the affirmations of du Bois-Reymond, who spoke not only for himself and for Brücke, but for the whole of the so-called school of von Helmholtz, that is for the whole of the modern world of science and biology. Du Bois wrote: "No other forces than the common physical-chemical ones are active within the organism." This affirmation, this pledge, made with the pugnacious overtones of a challenge—"and woe to him who does not do likewise"—was in effect but the reiteration of the pledged commitment of that science which came into being with the Age of Enlightenment. It was but the echo of the words and persuasions of Condorcet, of LaMettrie, of Holbach. These persuasions are tersely summed up by Ernst Cassirer in the following words: "All the processes of nature, including those commonly called 'intellectual,' the whole physical and moral order of things, are reducible to matter and motion and are completely explicable in terms of these two concepts" (16). In the purview of Lamettrie, the human body is an immense clock constructed with much artifice. In Holbach's *Système de la Nature* it is stipulated that no aspect of nature is to be introduced into the philosophy of nature which is explicable only in terms of man and his appetites and desires. It is the structure of the atoms that forms man, and their motion that propels him forward; conditions not dependent on him determine his nature and direct his fate. In this philosophy of science there is neither place nor acceptance for "intention and purpose," the two factors the misadventures of which are posited by Freud at the root of, as the *fons et origo* of, hysteria and the neuroses.

Lamettrie is usually assessed as an extremist among the philosophers of the Enlightenment, and that is correct. But in his postulates and premises he is in essential agreement with the leading philosophers of his age. The realm of philosophy, however, was not totally under their sway. There was also Leibnitz. And he stood athwart the philosophy of rationalistic materialism. Leibnitz was born in 1646 and died in 1716. Chronologically, therefore, he belongs to the 17th rather than to the 18th century. But the influence of Leibnitz's philosophy had the character of a delayed action. Its principal theatre of growth and operation was Germany and the Germanic countries, and the growth of German thought was guided by the influence of Leibnitz. The main trend of Leibnitz's thought gained recognition very slowly, but its penetration was nevertheless deep and effective.

What was the main trend of Leibnitz's thought? It can without distortion be summed up in one word, "appetency," which can in turn be translated as *desire, appetite, intention, purpose.* This stood in opposition to the rationalistic materialism of the French and English philosophies of the Enlightenment. Perhaps the terms "athwart" and "in opposition" do not correctly define the relation of Leibnitz's philosophy to that of the leading French school. For Leibnitz accepted, in the main, the Cartesian postulates of matter and motion. Where he departed from the Cartesian position, and this departure does in effect equate to an athwart position, amounted to this—Leibnitz endowed "matter" with "entelechy." Leibnitz's indivisible units of matter were named by him "monads." There is a tendency current to equate them to the atom of present-day physics. But the equation is not warranted. Leibnitz's monads were conceived of as units of matter possessed not only of the qualities of extension, impenetrability, gravity, etc., but also of desire, aversion, and memory (17).

"The monads," as Leibnitz envisaged them, "are the subjects from which all events originate, and the principle of their activity, of their progressive development, is not the connection of causes and effects, but a teleological relationship" (18). Teleology here implies purpose, inward form pressing for realization, and the specific, dynamic, process of becoming, as distinct from that of being.

The concept of inward form pressing for realization inspired a new feeling for nature and deeply influenced the intellectual history of Germany. Its finest form is witnessed in the *Naturphilosophie* that flourished during the latter part of the 18th and the first half of the 19th century.

The span between Leibnitz and Romantic Medicine is bridged by the philosophical contributions of Kant, Fichte, and Schelling. And Schelling was the Prince of the Romanticists. This may be given as the quintessence of the Romanticist's faith, a faith witnessed alike in *Naturphilosophie* and in Romantic Medicine, that the whole of the universe and that of being, human and all other, is bound together in an all-pervading, all-meaningful relatedness, and only in this relatedness is any portion of the total to be comprehended (19). This does not premise a static relatedness, but rather one of continued becoming. The relatedness of being is in a sustained process of transition toward newer states of being. In the light of this it is understandable how the idea of evolution crystallized in the speculative thinking of the Romanticists. Goethe who must be counted a partisan of the Romanticists, wrote on the metamorphoses of plants, and Lorenz Oken in the last issue of *Isis* (1835) (20), a publication which he founded, sketched a theory on the evolution of man which was substantially validated in Darwin's great work.

I doubt that Fliess would have relished being counted among the Romanticists. Yet it is a fact that in his preoccupations he stands in spiritual and intellectual kinship with the Romanticists. However, those who have treated of Fliess, notably the Freudian authors, would deny him even this much of recognition. They tend to write him off as a "mathematical monomaniac" a deluded numerologist. The derogatory opinions of Aelby to the effect that Fliess "was suffering from over-valuation of an idea" (a charge which could with greater warrant and in many more instances be levelled against Freud), Riebold's characterization of Fliess as "a player with numbers," and Frese's opinion that Fliess' nasal reflex neurosis "verges on the mystical" are cited with seeming relish in patent endorsement (21). It is not my intention to elaborate a defense of Fliess. But it is my intention to show how little those who are preoccupied with Fliess' so-called numerology understand what Fliess was attempting to establish. In the introduction to his major work *Der Ablauf des Lebens* (22) Fliess wrote:

> Very ancient is the question as to which laws determine the course of life. Manifold have been the answers. Belief and scientific notions have alternately ventured as solution. But be it a deity, be it the stars, be it cosmic forces that lie at the origin of the weather, be it finally the miracles of germination—in life, illness, and death they were ever *external* causes that influenced the living being in a so to say disturbing way. According to what pattern of inner organization life, not only human, but all earthly life, takes its course, how through this inner organization the generations are linked, and how with no less certainty than the hour of birth is the hour of death predestined —this will be demonstrated in these pages for the first time and in a completely new way. Not through any hypotheses; but solely by means of the most exact, mathematical analysis.

It must be granted forthwith that his "exact mathematical analysis" does not stand up under critical testing. But that does not invalidate his basic hypothesis that "nicht äussere Ursachen," but rather indicates that some "innere Ordnung" determine the evolvement and span of life. This is in effect a deep rooted conviction shared by all in the biological sciences. Nor is the possibility to be entirely precluded that some mathematical factor-formula may yet be derived which will prove statistically valid for the *hypothetical* individual (23).

Fliess' egregious blunder lies in his attempt to postulate a formula precisely applicable to every and any given individual. But Fliess' preoccupation with a mathematical formula to express the *Ablauf des Lebens* must be considered in conjunction with his other interests. Only thuswise can one appreciate his kinship with Romantic Medicine. Fliess was interested in bisexuality, in handedness, in sinistration and dextration, in the problem of mortality and death, in the periodicities of fertility and of sterility, in the relation of the nose to genitality. He anticipated what is currently termed the rhythm method of contraception. These items not only deeply concerned the partisan of Romantic Medicine but they were indeed at the very core of its dynamic philosophy. Lorenz Oken affirmed it as a cardinal principle—"Erstens liegt allen Gestalten der Natur der Gedanke der Zahl zugrunde" (24). Oken's primal figure was not an integer but rather zero. Rhythm and repetitiveness, the Myth of the Eternal Return, was an essential premise in the philosophy of Romantic Medicine. Novalis wrote: "Insofar as one envisages life as a complete whole, to that extent is it subject to division into periods and epochs. These periods and epochs of life must perforce bear a relationship to one another; for life must exhibit a *rhythmus* in its evolvement, and must express a harmony" (25). This thesis of periodicity is reflected in Fliess' mathematical calculations. Polarity, the relationship of apposites, was "die eigentliche Lebenslehre der Romantik" (26). This too is reflected in Fliess' theory of bisexuality. In the writings of J. J. Bachofen are to be found precise and specific references to *sinistration* and *dextration* and "die höhere Würde der linken Seite" (the greater dignity of the left side), identical with the ideas propounded by Fliess: The left side belongs to the female, the right side to the male. "In the morals and customs of civil and cultural life, in the peculiarities of attire and grooming, as also in folklore, and no less in the meaning of expressions, the same idea is repeatedly encountered, *major honos laevarum partium,* 'the greater dignity of the left side' " (27).

In citing these homologues to Fliess' theories in Romantic Medicine, I have no intention to suggest that Fliess plagiarized the writings of his predecessors. I intend only to define the framework of his thinking and to highlight its kinship with *Naturphilosophie* and Romantic Medicine. Whatever his specific preoccupations, they were set within the matrix of the philosophy of the Romanticists, and from this matrix, through the long enthusiastic and friendly indoctrinations of Freud by Fliess, Freud derived and nurtured his original ideas, which, in time, and *by dint of other labors* yielded his philosophy and system of psychoanalysis.

In the Introduction to the volume of the Fliess letters there is a chapter entitled "Psycho-analysis as an Independent Science." This is a paradoxical affirmation, for it lies in the very nature of a science to *not be* independent, otherwise it cannot be a science but only a mysterium, an esoteric discipline. Yet the intention of the affirmation is transparent. It but reiterates Freud's own claims—that he, and he alone, created psychoanalysis. Historically that is not to be doubted or questioned. But to grasp the full implications of this affirmation one must scrutinize it deeply. It is true that Freud created psychoanalysis but the question remains "out of what." Completely original, that is, virginal creativity is vouchsafed only to the musical and mathematical geniuses. Those in the plastic and graphic arts may in some instances be granted this supreme gift of inventiveness. But no one who contributes to science can be "virginally creative." He can only apply his creative genius to such singular insights as may come to him in the perspective of antecedent knowledges. The independence of Freud, the *Unabhängigkeit* of psychoanalysis, is meaningful and understandable only in the light of the fact that Freud was an autodidact. Freud vigorously intended to be original. He consistently abstained (to the extent possible) from acquainting himself with what others had done or had thought before him. He wrote to Fliess, "I do not want to read, because it stirs up too many thoughts and stints me of the satisfaction of discovery" (28). Reading, he discovered that "It is the oldest ideas which are the most useful, as I am belatedly finding out" (29). In another letter he wrote: "What have you got to say to the suggestion that the whole of my brand-new theory of the primary origins of hysteria is already familiar and has been published a hundred times over, through several centuries ago?" (30). Such discoveries disconcerted him. Freud preferred to think first and to "study" later. When he was working on his Dream Interpretation he wrote to Fliess: "First I want to get my own ideas into shape, then I shall make a thorough study of the literature on the subject, and finally make such insertions or revisions as my reading will give rise to. So long as I have not finished my own work I cannot read" (31).

Even so Freud did not and could not have made a thorough study of the dream literature, or he would not have written: "No one has the slightest suspicion that dreams are not nonsense but wish fulfillment." Certainly there were many writers, Novalis, for example, and even more significantly Gotthilf Heinrich von Schubert, who did not think that dreams were "nonsense." Schubert wrote a most penetrating work on dreams entitled *Die Symbolik des Traumes,* wherein he not only anticipated Freud's theories but affirmed that, among other functions, the dream served also that of wish fulfillment (32).

It is not my intention to set up a gallery of pre-Freudians, nor to challenge in any sense whatsoever Freud's claim to have been the sole and original creator of psychoanalysis. I do intend, however, to underscore the fact that he was an optative autodidact, and that he "discovered" by dint of great labor the components of his metapsychology, which components were already known, and defined, in many respects in superior ways, in Romantic Medicine. That includes his dream interpretation, the Unconscious, repression, the Id, Ego, and Super-ego, the concepts of Eros and Thanatos, and much else beside. I hasten to add, however, that while all these add up to a great portion of Freud's metapsychology, they do not add up to psychoanalysis as a psychologic system or as a therapeutic procedure.

Psychoanalysis could not have been conceptualized in Romantic Medicine, nor indeed at any time before the latter part of the nineteenth and the early part of the twentieth century. The reasons for this are not difficult to fathom. They are akin to those reasons which brought forth vitamin therapy in the twentieth century, and not before. Vitamin therapy, as is well known, provides the metabolic mechanism, in the second instance, with that of which it was deprived in the first instance. Until foods were subjected to refinements, that is to devitaminizing processes and to other corrupting influences, there was no compelling necessity for a science of vitamins nor for vitamin therapy. The metapsychology upon which Freud based his psychoanalysis was an integral component of Romantic Medicine, and there was no necessity to extricate it into a separate discipline. That necessity arose only when medicine was subjected to the dismemberment and disorientation it experienced under the influence of the French rationalistic science and in the so-called school of von Helmholtz.

I fear this argument may be misunderstood, that it may be taken for a value judgment rather than as it is intended as the exposition of an historical eventuation. I have a high regard for the philosophical framework of Romantic Medicine but I do not esteem the actualities, i.e., the practice of Romantic Medicine, nearly as high, nor in any respect of effectiveness even remotely proximate to the medicine of today. I am certain, however, that none of the leading personages of the Romantic period—Goethe, Schelling, Carus, Oken, Novalis, Grimm, or Schubert, to name but a few—would find himself otherwise than at home in the labyrinthine metapsychology of psychoanalysis. I do suspect they would find some of it naive, but still very familiar. And as for the neurotic and psychotic patient, I would feel quite secure entrusting his treatment, say, to Schubert or to Damrow.

But to revert to Freud: it appears quite clear to me that in his long and intimate association with Fliess he was indoctrinated in the ideational framework of a relatedness system—closely akin to that of Romantic Medicine—and that within this framework, which he singly and laboriously reconstructed, he worked out both the metapsychology and the operational patterns of psychoanalysis.

The break between Fliess and Freud, no matter how it may have been marked by overt events, took place when Freud, starting off from their commonly shared terrain of ideas and convictions, departed in his unique direction. Fliess understandably felt abandoned and denied, and he counted Freud an ingrate. Freud on his part was too feverishly preoccupied in the pursuit of his own concerns to allow himself the distractions of a friendship that had already given him its all. But that Fliess had indoctrinated and nurtured Freud in the philosophy of "world and man relatedness," there can be no doubt. Fliess' frustration was in a measure that of the hen that had brooded and hatched a duckling.

Freud, started on the pursuit of his metapsychology, could not and would not be deflected. In December 1897 Freud wrote that he was keenly looking forward to meeting with Fliess "and the fine things you will have to tell me about life and its dependence on the world process. I have always been curious about it, but hitherto I have never found any one who could give me an answer." And to this he added, and not in jest, "If there are now two people, one of whom can say what life is, and the other can say (nearly) what mind is, it is only right that they should see and talk to each other more often" (33). But in March of 1900 Freud was quite of a different mind. He declined Fliess' proposal that they meet at Easter, and gave a motley of explanations for his declinations. "Subtle resolution of contradictions," "inner reasons"—an accumulation of imponderables, which weighed heavily upon him," and so on—all of it adding up to the fact that he had no more use for Fliess. He was henceforth on his own.

There would be little profit in tracing Freud's psychoanalytic architectonics—the sequence in which he constructed his theoretical edifice—Jones has done that laboriously. It *is* of interest, however, to take note that his first, major, and in the opinion of many, his most significant work, was composed when he was still friendly with Fliess. The work was his *Interpretation of Dreams.* How did Freud come to make this study, to compose this work, so substantive in Romantic Medicine? In *Zur Geschichte der Psychoanalytischen Bewegung* (34) Freud states that he came upon dream interpretation "nachdem ich mich, einer dunklen Ahnung folgend, entschlossen hatte die Hypnose mit der freien Assoziation zu vertauschen." ("after I had resolved, following a vague inspiration, to substitute for hypnosis free association.") "My thirst for knowledge," he adds, "had not initially been directed towards the understanding of dreams. I do not know of any influences that directed my interest or gave me helpful expectation."

One is prompted to wonder—is this but another instance of Freud's amnestic slips? He did praise old Fechner for his understanding of dreams and Fechner, it should be noted, was a distinguished Romantic.

Two items remain to be dealt with: the reaction of the world of science to Freud's theories, and the phenomenal fact that despite great opposition they have substantially "prevailed," that is, they have received discrete, critical, but none-the-less effective acceptance in medicine and in psychiatry. As to the first, the fiction has been propagated that Freud met opposition chiefly because of his sex theories. Essentially this was not the case though it should be added that Freud's "sex theories," on their own, and apart from all other evocative factors, did arouse the sceptical derision of the scientific world. And well they might. The "sexuality" of current day psychoanalysis is quite different from that hypothesized by Freud in the 1890's and early 1900's. Much of that difference is glossed over in the psychoanalytical records of the reception given to Freud's early and initial formulations. But vastly more significant is the historic fact that Freud's theories were opposed and challenged on the score that they were not scientific, that they were wild to the point of being a "bad joke" (P. Janet). Wilfred Trotter wrote: "However much one may be impressed by the greatness of the edifice which Freud has built up, and by the soundness of his architecture, one can scarcely fail, on coming into it from the bracing atmosphere of the biological sciences, to be oppressed by the odour of humanity with which it is pervaded. One finds everywhere a tendency to the acceptance of human standards and even sometimes of human pretensions, which cannot fail to produce a certain uneasiness as to the validity, if not of his doctrines, at any rate of the forms in which they are expounded" (35).

Oswald Bumke wrote: "You may define science as you please. *Psychoanalysis is not natural science* nor any kind of science, nor is it a fairy tale. For unlike the latter, it does not spring from the heart, but rather from a coldly brooding and yet misguided intellect" (36).

Freud's system was indeed not science, as science was then known, but rather "reeked of humanity." It was not science for it dealt with imponderables lacking the accustomed dimensions of the accredited data of science. It reeked of humanity with all of humanity's ephemerities. It treated of hopes, aims, ambitions, goals, frustrations—the subjectivistic corruptions that encumber the operations of the undisciplined mind—the dross of human mentation which more than a century before had been fused off and discarded as so much slag in the crucibles of science.

Freud himself was cognizant of his scientific apostasy. In his *Introductory Lectures* (37) he warns his auditors that in order to grasp the burden of his intentions they will need, indeed will be required, to shed their indoctrinated and habituated patterns of thinking, perceiving, and testing, and that the very nature of proof in psychoanalysis will be such as must of necessity run contrary to their ingrained expectations.

Freud and his psychoanalysis stood forth as an offense against the objectivity and purity of science, and they were resented deeply and bitterly. And yet, they both prevailed. The many different elements which entered into the ultimate acceptance of psychoanalysis among the confraternity of learned disciplines, I cannot at this time undertake to catalogue or to describe. Two factors, however, stand forth above all others. Freud's personality, his Promethean drive and obdurate endurance, and the fundamental pertinence of the reorientation of man to himself, to the experience of growth and development, and to the intricate adventures of living, implicit in Freud's metapsychology, and in much of the technique of psychoanalysis.

It is most questionable whether psychoanalysis as we know it, historically and practically, would have come into being had there not been a Freud to bring it into being. But even at the time of Freud there was more than a nascent suspicion that matter and energy, substance and motion, physics and chemistry, and all the rest in accepted science, would not suffice to explicate all the phenomena and experiences witnessed in life. Indeed science itself had come under scrutiny and its basic assumptions were being challenged by science proper. It is relevant to recall that Michelson's crucial experiment on the velocity of light was made in 1881, and repeated in 1887 and 1905. Einstein wrote his initial work on Relativity in 1905, and the Curies conducted their unique studies on the pitch blende in 1898.

There was prevalent a valence of receptivity for the insight Freud brought to the realm of biology in general, and to psychology in particular. It is understandable that Freud and his partisans underscore the opposition he encountered. Historically, however, the acceptance of his ideas is even more noteworthy, and the acceptance was of no mean proportion. Holt spoke for many of his contemporaries when he said of Freud's work: "It is the first key which psychology has ever had which fitted." (*The Freudian Wish*). The "key that fits" is a happy phrase. It is the key we name by many names—ecological, holistic, ethological. It is in essence the key to the understanding of the universe and to man's relation to it— the crude blank of which was proffered more than a century ago—in Romantic Medicine.

I cannot terminate this presentation without speculating, however briefly, on what might have been the state of psychiatry today—had Freud never lived and never labored. I am persuaded that while we would not have had psychoanalysis as a discipline and movement, with all that this implies of good and bad, psychiatric knowledge, psychiatric theory, and psychiatric practice would in all vital essentials not have been any different from what they are currently. I am impelled to, but I am not happy, to thus commit myself. I am sure to be misunderstood, and likely to be abused. Oddly enough, I could with impunity and general assent say as much about other great personages in the history of science, of say Darwin, or Copernicus. But Freud is quite another matter! He stands unique! That is quite correct and it is precisely the point I want to make. Freud *is* historically unique—*in his personality*. None but Freud could have been Freud. But others could, and most likely would have done the fundamental work contributed by Freud. Freud has been compared to Darwin, to Newton, and to Copernicus. I concur in these comparisons. Yet to my mind there is but one man he truly resembles—not in any other respect —but in the signature of his personality: that man is Paracelsus. The motto of his life was: *Alterius not sit, qui suus esse potest.* Freud elected no motto, but the one he inscribed on the Frontispiece of his *Interpretation of Dreams* characterizes the passionate ambition that characterizes his life and his work:

FLECTERE SI NEQUEO SUPEROS, ACHERONTA MOVEBO. (Virg.)

("If I cannot influence the gods of heaven, I will stir up Acheron itself.")

It is my profound conviction that long after all that is sound and valid in his system of psychoanalysis has been absorbed and incorporated in psychiatry, Freud will be prized and celebrated above all else for the heroic dimensions of his being, for the valiance of his character, and for his Promethean spirit.

REFERENCES

1. I premise neither calculated neglect nor willful supression of any essential data. It is rather that Freud's biographers in the first instance were not aware of the quality and nature of Freud's friendship with Fliess, and Jones, who has written with the benefit of the Fliess letters, and much else beside, is either ignorant of, or too little concerned with, the philosophical and historical implications of the ideas so intimately shared by Freud and Fliess during the fifteen years of their association, years which confessedly were formative for Freud.

2. FREUD, SIGMUND: *Aus den Anfängen der Psychoanalyse. Briefe an Wilhelm Fliess, Abhandlungen und Notizen aus den Jahren 1887-1902.* London, Imago Publishing Co., 1950.

3. Jones vs. Jones—"Of more lasting assistance was that rendered by Dr. Wilhelm Fliess, whom Abraham got to know a few years later and for whom he conceived a great regard; it was Fliess who was mainly responsible for his treatment during his last illness," from Ernest Jones's Introduction to *Selected Papers of Karl Abraham*, p. 12. Leonard & Virginia Woolfe, Hogarth Press, London, and the Institute of Psycho-analysis, 1927.
    Again in Jones's *Life and Work of Sigmund Freud*, Vol. 1, p. 289 (New York, Basic Books, 1953): "Of those who knew him (Fliess), with the exception of the level-headed Karl Abraham, who was not impressed, everyone speaks of his 'fascinating' personality."

4. WITTELS, FRITZ: *Sigmund Freud*, Verlag, E. P. Tal and Co., 1924.

5. BERNFELD, SIEGFRIED: Freud's scientific beginning, in *The American Imago*, Vol. 6, No. 3, Sept., 1949.

6. JONES, ERNST: *The Life and Work of Sigmund Freud*, Vol. I, p. xii. New York, Basic Books, 1953.

7. *Ibid.*, p. xiii.

8. *Ibid.*, p. 78.

9. BERNFELD, *op. cit.*

10. JONES, *op. cit.*, p. 168.

11. FREUD, SIGMUND: *Aus den Anfängen der Psychoanalyse, Briefe an Wilhelm Fliess*, p. 18 (London, Imago Publishing Co., 1950): "In einem zufälig erhaltenenl Briefe Breuers an Fiess aus dem Sommer 1895, mehrere Monate vor dem Erscheinen der 'Studien über Hysterie' heisst es: 'Freud ist im vollsten Schwung seines Intellekts. Ich sehe ihm schon nach wie die Henne dem Falken.'"
    The above quotation is corrupted in the English translation to read, "Freud's intellect is soaring; I struggle along behind him like a hen behind a hawk." Fancy a hen struggling along behind a hawk!

12. FREUD, SIGMUND: An autobiographical study, translated by James Strachey in *The Problems of Lay-analysis*. New York, W. W. Norton, Co., 1952.

13. Only one brief note has survived.

14. And as Fliess observed with some pathos: "Mit Freud stand ich jahrelang in freundschaftlichem Verkehr. Ihm habe ich alle meine wissenschaftlichen Gedanken und Keime rückhaltlos anvertraut." *Der Ablauf des Lebens*, p. 583. Leipzig und Wien, F. Deuticke, 1906.

15. For a more ample treatment of Romantic Medicine, *vide* GALSTON, IAGO: The Romantic period in medicine, in *Bulletin of the New York Academy of Medicine*, Vol. 32, No. 5, May, 1956.

16. CASSIRER, ERNST: *The Philosophy of the Enlightenment,* translated by Fritz C. A. Koelln and James P. Pettegrove, p. 65, Boston, Beacon Press, 1955.
17. *Ibid.,* p. 88.
18. *Ibid.,* p. 83.
19. To study nature is to project one's self into, "to sympathize with nature, to trace the likeness between the inner life and the magnets, the crystals, the solar systems, the living creatures of the physical world." Royce, Josiah, *The Spirit of Modern Philosophy,* p. 175. New York, Houghton Mifflin and Co., 1931.
20. 1817-1835: *Isis; oder, Enzyklopaedische Zeitung,* Jena & Leipzig. Edited by L. Oken. Originally a political periodical until 1824, it changed title to *Enzyklopädische Zeitschrift vorzüglich für Naturgeschichte,* etc.
21. FREUD, SIGMUND: *Aus den Anfängen der Psychoanalyse, Briefe an Wilhelm Fliess, Abhandlungen und Notizen aus den Jahren 1887-1902,* p. 40. London, Imago Publishing Co., 1950.
22. FLIESS, WILHELM: *Der Ablauf des Lebens. Grundlegung zur exakten Biologie.* F. Deuticke, Leipzig, Wien, 1906.
23. Life expectancy at given ages is currently estimated, and accepted.
24. LEIBBRAND, WERNER: *Romantische Medizin,* p. 65. Hamburg und Leipzig, H. Goverts Verlag, 1937.
25. STENGEL, GERHARD: *Die Deutschen Romantiker,* Vol. I, "Die Zahl," p. 623. Salzberg, Verlag Das Berland-Buch, 1954.
26. HIRSCHFELD, ERNST: Romantische Medizin, in *Kyklos,* Vol. 3, p. 14. Leipzig, Georg Thieme Verlag, 1930.
27. STENGEL, *op. cit.,* p. 640.
28. FREUD, SIGMUND: *The Origins of Psycho-analysis, Letters to Wilhelm Fliess,* translation by Mosbacher and Strachey, p. 126, Letter 20. New York, Basic Books, Inc., 1954.
29. *Ibid.,* p. 157, Letter 41.
30. *Ibid.,* p. 187, Letter 56.
31. *Ibid.,* p. 249, Letter 86.
32. SCHUBERT, GOTTHILF HEINRICH VON: *Die Symbolik des Traumes,* p. 19, F. A. Brockhaus, 1862.
33. FREUD, SIGMUND: *The Origins of Psycho-analysis, Letters to Wilhelm Fliess,* translation by Bosbacher and Strachey, p. 238, Letter 79.
34. FREUD, SIGMUND: *Zur Geschichte der Psychoanalytischen Bewegung,* p. 16. Internationalen Psychoanalytischer Verlag, Leipzig, Wien, Zürich, 1924.
35. TROTTER, WILFRED BATTEN LEWIS: *Instincts of the Herd in Peace and War,* pp. 77-78, New York, Macmillan Co., 1919.
36. SACHS, BERNARD, M.D.: Bumke's critique of psychoanalysis, in *Mental Hygiene,* Vol. XVI, No. 3, pp. 409-427, July, 1932.
37. FREUD, SIGMUND: *Introductory Lectures on Psycho-analysis.* English translation by Joan Riviere. London, G. Allen and Unwin, 1922.

14

Freud's Influence in Contemporary Culture

THERE IS AN IMPLIED PRETENTIOUSNESS in the title of my paper which I am impelled to disavow. To treat amply of Freud's influence on contemporary culture one would need to possess both an encyclopedic intelligence—and, endless time. In 1936, when Freud's eightieth birthday was celebrated, Thomas Mann was called on to treat of a simpler theme, namely, Freud's influence on literature. He discharged his obligation in a singular way. Thomas Mann spoke about Thomas Mann. He did this both deliberately and apologetically—saying to his audience—"Perhaps you will kindly permit me to continue for a while in this autobiographical strain, and not take it amiss if instead of speaking of Freud I speak of myself" (1).

For a while I thought of using the same dodge, but then realized I couldn't get away with it. For while Mann could be identified with, indeed impersonate, Literature, I could hardly impersonate Culture— with a capital C. I did, however, resolve my dilemma in the sensible resolution to talk *about* rather than *on* Freud and contemporary culture. That shrinks my commitments to the dimensions of my competences.

Initially I must define the sense in which I intend to treat of culture, and more precisely also the meaning of "influence." Culture is that field wherein the anthropologists, and after them the sociologists, have the greatest fun—waging, like the knights in Valhalla, their daily and unending semantic and ideological battles. I for one have no intention to enter their lists. Even though the restriction is arbitrary I intend to treat of culture as the embodiment of the hopes, faiths, beliefs, convictions, and aspirations which give distinction to the realms and ages of man. And I will not deal with culture in the abstract, but rather in particular, with those media wherein and whereby culture, so defined, is preserved and

198

transmitted, and wherein its creativity is witnessed. You perceive that I am as wordy as the proverbial sociologist. What I intend to touch on is literature, the drama, some portion of the graphic arts, the vernaculars in general, and to top it off, Existentialism. This, too, may seem pretentious, but let it not discourage you.

I must also define the meaning of "influence." It is not my intention to delineate Freud's direct influence on any given medium or on any creative artists. It is my plan, rather, to show how greatly Freud's theories, and his labors, were effective in the creation of a pervading climate of opinion, of an embracing atmosphere of comprehension and insight, so that none that "drew breath" could escape being affected, in one way or another.

But to judge of this we must orient ourselves to some starting point, and I would select for simplicity the medium of the novel, in the time of the Romantic period.

The Romantic period followed on that of the French Revolution. It embraces essentially the last decades of the eighteenth, and the first half of the nineteenth century. The novels of this period have certain distinctive features—but the term "Romantic" does not describe them. Indeed, they were not romantic in the original sense of that term—that is they were not fancied extravaganzas represented, say in the Chanson de Roland, in the Arthurian Tales, or in Ariosto's *Orlando Furioso*. These were tales rich in fancy, ingenious in plot and counter-plot, and peopled with characters to which neither life nor experience affords a counterpart. They were magnificent creations—in the pure and uninhibited exercise of fancy. They were, in the pristine sense, Romances, and so labeled. For the term "Romantic" means: "Extravagantly ideal, sentimental rather than rational; fanciful and visionary." The Romances, in a word, had no relation to life as it is experienced. Now the novels of the Romantic Period were not of this order. They embellished but they did not violate reality. Their heroes and heroines—Goethe's Werther, for example, and Schlegel's Lucinde—were not at all ethereal, but rather earth-earthy. Their experiences and adventures were such as do not commonly, yet might perchance, fall to the lot of the common man. Furthermore the writers of these novels were sustained by a faith in the transcending meaningfulness of life. That above everything else distinguishes the novel of the Romantic Period, and for that reason the period were better named— the Transcendentalist Period.

This transcendentalism was, in a measure, pantheistic. It glorified nature and the natural. In that respect it was anti-classical, for the classical was artificial rather than natural. Rousseau is counted among the initiators of Romanticism. His *Nouvelle Héloise,* his *Emile,* and his *Contrat Social* represented, as Ford Madox Ford describes them, "a general revolt against the stifling conventions of the classicism of the eighteenth century" (2). But the transcendentalism which animated the Romantic Period was more than a movement of protest, and vastly more than the roseate, Arcadian *Schwärmerei,* which it is commonly represented to have been. It had its dreams to dream, but also its lessons to teach. For if life is meaningful, then its meaning must, like a correct equation, tally in either direction: or, to paraphrase it in its Greek equivalent—Character and Destiny must be two components in reality which bear a reversible relationship.

It were too much, perhaps, to claim for Romantic Literature, the fathomed grasp and the conscious exposition of this idea, yet it would not be, did we include in the ambient of literature not only the novel, but also poetry, the drama, and philosophy. Goethe's *Faust,* and particularly in its first part, is essentially an effulgent essay on Character and Destiny. But I feel more safe with the more modest claim. The Romantic Period, as mirrored in its novels, was naturalistic in the Rousseauist sense, that is, both realistic and romantic. Having withdrawn from the heroic and the palatial, the novelist could observe and treat of "life as is." This treatment of life is better witnessed in the Romantic writers of the non-Germanic countries: in the novels of Hawthorne, and Herman Melville, in Lermontov's, *A Hero of Our Times,* and in the novels of Stendhal and Flaubert.

It is among these authors that we first encounter the so-called psychological novel. Stendhal is credited with having initiated this order of novel with his *Le Rouge et le Noir* of 1831. But this, as most firsts, is simply the artifact of chronology. I mean, he did not originate the variety. Lermontov's epic appeared in 1836; Pushkin, counted a poet rather than a novelist, wrote *Eugeni Oneigin* in 1822-1829. Hawthorne's *Scarlet Letter* appeared in 1850 and Melville's *Moby Dick* in 1851. Each of these is preeminently a "psychological novel." Yet the point I want to make bears not on Stendhal's primacy. It is rather this: that as soon as the literary genius earnestly turns his competences to the perception, study, and description of man and his destinies, he must perforce psychologize.

In this connection it is of interest to note how many psychiatrists, notably psychoanalysts, have found among the authors of the Romantic Period, writers whom they relish to dub pre-Freudian. Thus, much has been made of Hawthorne's *Scarlet Letter* and Oliver Wendell Holmes'

Elsie Venner. These are in effect significant psychological novels, but they were not written in a clairvoyant anticipation of Freud and of psychoanalysis. Rather they were written in the spirit and the intelligence of their time. And the time itself was intensely preoccupied with psychology. Indeed, there was more of the pre-Freudian psychology in the psychology of the Romantic period than is to be found in its ample literature of novels and plays. Singly—Carus, Schubert, von Hartman, names preeminent in the history of Romantic Medicine, anticipated many of the elements that are to be found in Freud's metapsychology. Yet I must add, such anticipation does not make them pre-Freudians. Count these others, if you will, magnificent workers. Freud, however, was the sole architect and builder of his psychoanalysis.

Be that as it may, the Romantic Period, which eventuated as a protest against the classicism of the eighteenth century, itself experienced both protest and revolt, and came to an end circa 1850. It came to an inglorious end, and thereafter to be called a Romantic was tantamount to having suffered the worst of insulting disparagements.

Romanticism gave way to Realism. Not transcendentalism nor the ultimate meaningfulness of life, but the singular problems of singular individuals, the orphan, the factory child, the prostitute, the thief, the murderer, became the subject of the representative novel. The better known exponents of this school of Realism, in the English language, were Dickens, Thackeray, and Samuel Butler; in French literature, Emile Zola is the outstanding example, and among the Germans, Hermann Suderman and Gerhart Hauptmann. Both the Scandinavian and the Russian writers are eminently represented in this school—Björnson, Strindberg, and Knut Hamsun come to mind among the Scandinavians, and Turgenev, Dostoyevsky, Tolstoi, Chekov, Andreyev and Gorki among the Russians. This cluster of preeminent writers represents a broad spectrum of literary genius, and at first blush it may seem that they are too divergent, too singular, too distinctive in their respective creativity to be lumped under one category. In many respects, in literary style, for example, that is true indeed. And yet they do share in a common denominator. They treat of *problems* rather than of life transcendent. They are, if I be permitted to use the term, *typologists*. The problems they treat are those of social and economic adversity, of malignant heredity, of environmental stress, of political oppression, of personality defects. Their texts are not infrequently in the nature of social, economic, political, and cultural theses. Insofar as they *are* psychologists they mirror the effects upon the individual of poverty, ignorance, heredity, disease, social hypocrisy and repression. The Russian writers perhaps treat more deeply of the socio-psychological reticulum that ensnares the individual, though I doubt that Thomas Hardy, for example, would be found wanting, in comparison say to Gorki, or Dostoyevsky. But be that as it may, *this* fact is as true of Hardy as it is of Gorki and the rest, that the psychology of the Realist school was *deterministic*. The determinants are largely, if not entirely, *extraneous to the character,* and of a socio-economic, environmental nature. The prostitute is such because she was betrayed, abandoned, poor, or otherwise corrupted. The thief is avenging himself on society. The murderer has been brought to despair and driven to violence. Not that these authors overlooked *character*. They have not! Neither Strindberg, nor Dostoyevsky, nor Gorki, had been so remiss. But *character* was deemed to be native. One was born with a given character, and the story invariably begins with that assumption.

In this respect the Realistic writers were at one with the leading psychiatrists of their day—with Kraepelin, for example, and with Lombroso. Indeed they were in consonance with the emergent science of their age, which was in every respect, and in each department, belligerently deterministic. It was thus that the novel, and I might add, also the play, was *psychological in treatment, but not in insight.* Psychology mirrored experience, but did not illuminate it. There is a passage in Ford Madox Ford's *March of Literature* which I am moved to cite. It so well describes the deterministic psychology which animated the Realists. He is speaking of Dickens, Balzac, and Thackeray. "You always know beforehand," he wrote (3), "what Dickens will do with the fraudulent lawyer on whose machinations hang the fate of a score of his characters; you always know beforehand how Balzac will deal with the million-franc financial crises with which his pages are scattered; and you always know beforehand the sort of best-club comment that Thackeray in his own person will supply for every twenty pages or so of his characters' actions. There is no surprise." How could there be! Deterministic psychology, and determinism in general, *allow* for no surprises! It is thus that "given—a man has a cough, a hoarse voice, a black jowl and a wooden leg, not one of these novelists will let him take something to soften his voice, shave, or substitute a cork limb for the wooden peg that will stick out all over the story —ad nauseam." In brilliant contrast there is awakened in my memory the inspiring, the vivifying experience of Pirandello's *Six Characters in Search of an Author*, which I saw performed in my youth. There, as you may recall, the playwright who marshalled his characters, planning to manipulate them through his preconceived plot, finds himself taken over by the "characters." No less moving, as I recall it, was Sam Benelli's play, *The Jest,* in which both John and Lionel Barrymore shared the leading roles.

The dullness, the depressing aftermath of the Realist authors, both novelist and playwrights, are only now appreciable and comprehensible. They were not at the time when we were first exposed to them in our youth, or, as I might phrase it, in our pre-Freudian days. For they did arouse sympathy and passion, and we were persuaded that we were the witnesses of "life in the raw." Besides, their hearts were on the "right side," not anatomically—but for "liberty" and against "reaction," for "justice" and goodness" against "evil and corruption." Hugo and Ibsen; Strindberg and Zola; Tolstoi and Gorki! They still retain much of their magic, and no doubt *will* for many generations to come. But the rigging of their art is now perceptible as it was not in the days of our youth. And, would it be too much to say that Freud helped to clear our vision, and to sharpen our perception? I think not! He was not alone in this, but he became, for us, the embodiment of all the rest, the representative, the *Praesidium,* of that cultural emergence which cannot be named otherwise than Freudian.

It is not an easy task to define this cultural turn, even though the evidence of its effects is all about us. No small portion of the difficulty derives from the condition that it is so diffusely profaned. If a book or a play, a poem or a painting, treats of incest, homosexuality, a fetishism, or of a manifestly neurotic subject, it is more than likely to be labeled Freudian. Even those books distinguished for nothing but their superabundance of four-letter words are given this *affiche,* as if Freud invented pornography or opened the sluices of humanity's cloacal stream.

All this, however, is negative—it may clear the way for, but does not proffer insight into the nature of the Freudian impact upon contemporary culture. The problem must be treated affirmatively: and that is perhaps best done through a series of affirmations stated categorically at first, and defended later. Thus—Freud challenged the prevailing philosophy of determinism. The emphasis here is on the term *prevailing.* For Freud too is a determinist, but his embrace of factors that "decide the issue" extends far beyond that deemed acceptable by his contemporaries. Take for example the "irrational" factor. The positivists, among the scientists, philosophers and authors, allowed for no surprises. But Freud demonstrated that life is full of surprises, that dreams, for example, are meaningful, that slips and errors and forgetting are meaningful. Freud did not deny the validity of rationality or of logical deductions. He did, however, demonstrate that logicality is only one attribute of being and experience, and that the paradox is more native to man than is the syllogism.

His was not a system or a philosophy of the irrational, as some would make it out to be. He rather underscored the fact that the rational *does* embrace the irrational—that so-called error is meaningful and hence pregnant with rationality. He did all this not by simply playing with ideas born out of intuition as did the Romantics, but forged his conclusions in the travail of scientific research, study, testing and retesting.

Freud was no philosopher. He disclaimed all competence in philosophy and disavowed it. It is rather *we* who interpret *him* philosophically. Freud did not perceive, as we *can*, his position in the stream of cultural eventuation. Freud charted the trans-uterine emergence of character. He plotted the shores and shoals, the Scylla and Charybdis, that man must pass ere he reaches the haven of effective maturity, and *the ultimate* in self-fulfilment. Character, in the Greek sense, Freud demonstrated, is only partly given, the rest is attained in the adventures of living. There is a fatality that hangs over man, but, Freud proved, it is not implacable.

Freud was a psychiatrist, far more than he was a philosopher. Freud brought into our awareness the primal impulsions of life. In addition to the categories of time, place, and the immediacies of reality, there is a fourth category—that of life emergent. And it is the greatest of the four, and oft prevails even *against* the rest. The Romantics knew all this, and so did the ancient Greeks before them. But the Greeks knew it deductively, and the Romantics intuitively. Freud, however, not merely affirmed all this, but demonstrated it. He helped make the blind to see and the lame to walk. And as a result, derivative rather than direct, *since* his day all of our thinking and feeling and representation of life have been changed. These operations have acquired a new dimension: the dimension, not only of extension but also of depth. That Freudian psychology is called Depth Psychology is very proper indeed.

I must try to make my meaning more clear. Freud came upon a world that was naively sober and earnest. Truth, it held, was truth, and fact—fact. Relationships were patent, or were to be made so. There was, in other words, no hindside to truth, or fact, or relations. There they stood, stark naked and bold, for all who chose to see. Reality *was* reality, and neither ever was nor ever could be anything else. Reality for example could never be the symbolic, conventional representation of another reality standing behind it, which itself was but a symbol for something else, and so on ad infinitum. Everything was so very patent to the Victorians. Had not Herbert Spencer accounted for everything but the Unknowable? Nor was it otherwise in art, music, the drama, philosophy, philology, and so on. Not that everything was already known, but rather that the ways to knowledge had been amply mastered.

Into this all-too-cock-certain world Freud threw the bombshell of symbolism. Reality, he asserted, stood not monolithically by itself, but in a series of relatednesses, and was in effect but the latest symbolic representation of that relatedness. Dreams spoke in symbols, but so also do we, waking, for words have meaning and representations, far above and behind their explicit conveyance. So have art, and the drama. Things are not really *always* what they seem. They may be *that,* but commonly are *more beside.* Is it any wonder then that the Victorian world recoiled in horror? But fortunately not all of it. There were a few who also had heard the Siren song. They were not followers of Freud, at least not in the beginning. They rather shared with him in this deeper vision of being and reality. The Impressionist painters come to mind; Verlaine and Baudelaire, the poets, and Schnitzler, the dramatist and novelist. There were others too—Nietzsche, for example, but I cannot catalogue them all. The cardinal point to be noted is that Freud, so to say, *structuralized* his deeper vision of being and reality, organized it and communicated it so that others might share in it. This, may I add, Freud accomplished not in his system of therapeutics, that is in his psychoanalysis, but rather in his system of Metapsychology. Because he so effectively structuralized his understanding of being and reality, it is preeminently proper to speak of *Freud's* influence on contemporary culture.

These influences are readily perceived in literature, that is in the novel, drama, in poetry, in literary criticism, in biography, and in autobiography. They are to be witnessed no less clearly but in different respects in the graphic arts, and in what I term the vernaculars.

Freud's Metapsychology (what I have called his deep vision of being and reality) deals with the full spectrum of life, with well-being no less than with illness, with the normal as well as with the abnormal. But Freud was initially a therapist, one who treated the sick. He drew insight from his experiences with the sick. He was a psychopathologist *before* he became a psychophysiologist. Literature, for all-too-obvious reasons, seized upon Freudian psychopathology, and made it its own domain. This is, of course, in the best traditions of Aristotelian poetics. But as a result— Freudian psychopathology is better known to the public than is his metapsychology. Since there is so much pathology within and about us, this may not be at all bad. Indeed it must profit us to recognize and to understand psychopathology—as and when we encounter it. And to this end literature has made and is making its notable contributions. It is my impression that the playwrights are preeminent in this field—possibly because plays are generally compounded of action—while in the novel the author can dally on the scenery and soliloquize. But the contemporary novels and plays alike reflect the influence of Freud. They are not merely psychological as are those of Stendhal, that is psychologically descriptive —they are rather analytical and dynamic. They illuminate the operations of psychic forces within and upon the experiences and ultimate destinies of man—among men.

I have mentioned Schnitzler, the friend and contemporary of Freud. Two of his works are, to my mind, superb illustrations of what I have in mind. One is the play *Reigen,* the other his novel *Frau Beate und ihr Sohn.* The first is a kaleidoscopic *ronde* of erotic communion—between a number of pairs, each one of whom has shared the partner of another coupling. This superb work contains a minimum of prurience and of salaciousness, but it does profoundly portray how Eros is conditioned in the settings of varying interpersonal relations. *Frau Beate und ihr Sohn* deals with the motif of unconscious incest, but in such wise as to transfix one's soul with the humility of deep wonderment.

The other playwright who comes to my mind, as it must also to yours, is our own Eugene O'Neill, and among his many and truly great plays the one that I feel best bears on our theme is his *Emperor Jones.*

It is not possible in this space to cite other illustrative authors and playwrights. Beside there has been published a good book, badly named *Freud on Broadway* (4), which deals with this subject broadly and competently. I'll merely call this book in witness and stop there.

Of literary criticism, biography, and autobiography, there is no need to say much. You will recall, I am sure, the rash of debunking biographies which first appeared in the 'twenties, and which remained "in style" for a decade or more. These were, so to say, only weakly Freudian. They were rather reactive to the "stuffed shirt" patterns of the earlier biographers. But how deeply the writing of biography—in this instance autobiography—has been affected by Freud, one can perceive in that composed by Stanley Hall, who brought Freud to the United States in 1909, and in that written by Norbert Wiener.

I am aware that I have treated these items somewhat gingerly, but that is because I want to devote what little time is left me to the subject of *the vernaculars.* Vernacular is the term applied to a regional language. But it has a second meaning, of which the one I cited is derivative. It also means non-classical. The advent of the vulgar tongues, e.g., French,

Italian, Spanish—vulgar because they are not Latin or Greek—unbridled the intellectual and artistic potentialities of man. For all their glories, the classic tongues in time hobbled man's spirit, hedged in his creativity, and constrained his inventiveness. Since then every new vernacular, every new communication medium, has contributed to the greater growth and the more ample enrichment of the human mind and spirit. But while originally the vernaculars were only vulgar tongues, that is language in the pristine sense, they have since grown in variety. Thus there are new vernaculars in mathematics, in logic, in painting, in poetry, indeed in all the modalities of communication. You need but think of the motion picture, television, and most significantly of the animated cartoon, to perceive at once both the meaning and the enormous creativity of the new vernacular. And to these developments —by indirection—Freud contributed greatly and profoundly. Was it not Freud who challenged the naive objectivity and the plain rationalism of the nineteenth century? Did he not above all others reveal to us the function of the symbol? Well then, if the word stands but for the symbol, why not expound and expand the symbol in the word, and thereby come closer to indwelling meaning. The poet always endeavored to attain to indwelling meaning, hence his poetic license. His license is broader now since the time of Freud: witness in T. S. Eliot, E. E. Cummings, and Gertrude Stein. Schnitzler in *Fräulein Else*, and Joyce in *Ulysses* employed a new vernacular, that of the stream of consciousness. Patently this is related to, if not a direct derivative of, the Freudian "free association." O'Neill in several of his plays made his characters to speak out, and to experience, their repressed and unconscious thoughts and feelings. This, too, is in the nature of "a new vernacular." But it is in the graphic arts that we witness most clearly the enfranchising, emancipating, influences of Freud's emphasis on the symbolizing articulatedness of the psyche. The "humble contraption," the *mobile,* is in effect the limpid, animated, embodiment of the artists' hoary doctrines of masses, proportions, and relations. It is a multi-dimensional, shimmering exposition of the theory and philosophy of art that lies entombed in scores of musty volumes. The "mobile" is Freudian in spirit and speaks in eloquent witness of his impact on both painting and sculpture. The pointilliste painters, the Impressionists, the painters and sculptors of abstractions, and the Surrealists, are and have been creating new vernaculars, and thereby enriching the human psyche, and enlarging the dimensions of our cultural life. It matters little whether what they produce is Art— by your or my definition. Bethink ye rather that even Shakespeare babbled in his infancy. Nor should you misread the meaning of my words.

I know that the Impressionists predate Freud, even as did Schnitzler's *Anatol*. I am certain that neither Chagall nor Dali drew their inspiration from Freud. And I am persuaded that Freud, who surrounded himself with Egyptian, Etruscan, and Roman antiquities, was not partial to modernity in Art. But all this is really beside the point. Freud was not merely Freud, he was the embodiment, the realization, the exponential force of a transcending movement, "whose waves came awash upon the many shores." The impact of Freud upon Culture is akin to that of Darwin upon Science—no discipline remains unaffected by the concept of evolution.

And now comes my final salvo! I am persuaded that the philosophy of Existentialism shares the Freudian vision of being and experience. Existentialism is a loosely used *label*. It is affixed, to my mind, in gross error, to a good deal of degenerate and morbid literature. It is perverted by a coterie of craven and defeated souls, into a philosophy of swinish hedonism, and desperate permissiveness. It is not any of this that I refer to as Existentialism. I have in mind rather the works of Kierkegaard, of Heidegger, of Jaspers, and of Husserl. I mean that most illuminating treatment of the problem of "meaning and experience," of "purpose and achievement," the answer proffered by Existentialism to the vulgar query —"Of what good is life anyway?"

In Existentialism I perceive this answer, that "goodness apart from the experience" is a sham concept and a false query. The warrant for being lies in being, the meaning of existence is realized and achieved in existing. Freud too expounds this philosophy in his Metapsychology. It is embraced in his juxtaposition of Eros and Thanatos—in what he termed the life instinct and the death instinct.

REFERENCES

1. MANN, T.: *Freud, Goethe, Wagner.* New York, A. A. Knopf, 1937, p. 12.
2. FORD, F. M.: *March of Literature.* New York, Dial Press, 1938, p. 541.
3. FORD, F. M.: *Op cit.,* pp. 808-809.
4. SEAVERS, W. D.: *Freud on Broadway: A History of Psychoanalysis and the American Drama.* New York, Hermitage House, 1955, p. 479.

15

A Midcentury Assessment of the Residuum of Freud's Psychoanalytic Theory

TO OSLER IS CREDITED the division of the great in science into three orders: the Innovators, the Transmuters, and the Transmitters; understandably, Osler esteems the Innovators highest.

There can be no doubt but that Freud must be counted among the Innovators, among the highest ranking of the great in science. One needs only review the status of psychiatry in the pre-Freudian days to be convinced of that. And the nearer one approaches to Freud's own time, the more remarkable does his achievement appear. For if one goes back into the more *remote* past, one comes upon a great deal of comprehension and insight which, as an eloquent though not always intended tribute to Freud, is called—pre-Freudian. But then, we need to bear in mind that such insights were not strictly psychiatric in nature. For though physicians treated the mind and its illnesses since time immemorial, the science of psychiatry, and psychiatry as a special medical discipline, are of very recent origin, hardly more than 300 years old.

Psychiatry, as a specialty, had to wait on the development of the modern biological and medical sciences—on anatomy and physiology, on pathology and nosography, and on other divisions in medicine. Indeed, the very beginnings of modern psychiatry date from the time of the great innovations in modern medicine, and—until the advent of Freud and of psychoanalysis—psychiatry was heavily freighted with the theoretical bias of modern materialist science. It stands to the eternal credit of Freud that he breached the citadel of modern science, laying it open to the incursion of broader and deeper insights into the operations of the human psyche.

It is too great an undertaking to review in detail the position of psychiatry during the time immediately preceding Freud's development of psychoanalysis. Yet its main assumptions and its fundamental beliefs are readily summarized. In the main, the soul, the psyche, had been purged from the realm of science. Only philosophers, theologians, and a "crack-pot" fringe of men who claimed to be scientists, but who quite evidently were not, preoccupied themselves with the psyche. True scientists concerned themselves not with the psyche but with the brain, the organ of the mind, and with its functions and disorders. Disease of the mind was deemed to be, as disease elsewhere in the body, merely the attestation to, and the consequence of, disturbed function in the organ involved—in this case, the brain. The disturbance could be primarily organic or primarily psychologic. It could also be due to developmental defects, trauma, toxic agents, excessive fatigue, and such physiologic "upsets" as shock, grief, intense love, disappointment, ambition, masturbation, and excessive venery. The "upset" states were not deemed to be essentially psychologic, but rather physiologic: they were akin to the "dyscrasias" of the ancient physicians. Hence they were nominally reversible, and to be remedied by physiologic or pharmacologic means. Indeed, much of the psychotherapy practiced before Freud's time was of this nature, and we know of the rest cure, the fat cure, the retreat, hydrotherapy, the travel cure, sedation and stimulation cure, and the like.

It should be recognized that in these theoretical formulations and therapeutic practices not only was there a great deal of sound good sense and correct scientific understanding, but they also yielded most impressive results. One has only to consider the achievements in the treatment of "idiocy," of cretinism, and of the neurologic and mental disturbances associated with pellagra, to appreciate the persuasive and practical impact of organistic psychiatry. Nor can we doubt but that the physicians of this persuasion frequently achieved remissions and even "cures" with their rest procedures and the like. Time and the healing powers of Nature are, indifferently, allies to every school of therapeutic practice.

But granted all that and even more, it still remains quite clear that viewing "madness" as Chiarugi (1759-1820) phrased it, as "a primary injury of the brain" could not but greatly constrict the comprehension of those mental diseases which we now term the *neuroses*. It would totally disbar the holder of such views from access to the vast and profound sphere of psychologic medicine.*

---

* It is thus that we can explain and excuse the once very popular and now almost forgotten sensational work of Cesare Lombroso (1836-1909) *L'Uomo delinquente* (1876) wherein he ascribes criminality to innate constitutional factors, and sets out the stigmata by which the "born criminal" is to be recognized.

Illuminating of the nature and quality of psychiatric thought, even as late as the third quarter of the 19th century, is the classical text book of Griesinger's *Die Pathologie und Therapie der psychischen Krankheiten* (4th ed., 1876). Griesinger had no sympathy with "the moralising ideas that were held by bigots regarding the treatment of insanity" (1). Yet under the heading of the more direct moral action for the purpose of restoring mental health, he advised that morbid ideas which repress and conceal the former (healthy) individuality must "be uprooted and destroyed, while the old ego must as far as possible be recalled and strengthened" (2).

Most impressive though frustrating are the voluminous and truly splendid works of Janet who, better than any one before him, grasped and penetrated into the nosologic character and operational *structure* of the neurosis, but who never fully fathomed the dynamic antecedents, that is, the intra-psychic etiology of the neurosis. His was essentially a Cartesian orientation, an energy anchored theory, summated in the term "neurasthenia." It is against this background that we need to envisage the advent of Freud's psychoanalytic theories. It is against this background of belief and persuasion that Freud's achievements are to be viewed and understood.

But what, in essence, were they? Here again they cannot be given in detail, yet they *can* be characterized briefly. Freud stood out against the deepest convictions of the world of science, and affirmed that man's behavior, in health as in sickness, cannot be understood nor accounted for in the simple formula of "matter and motion," of "substance and energy," nor even in the terms of "pure anatomy and basic physiology." These terms were valid in themselves, but inadequate. Two other considerations must needs be included in order to understand man's behavior, and these are: man's innate drives, at times termed his instincts, and, the social milieu, the societal matrix in which he lives, and which both supports and inhibits him in his adventures in living.

Freud ascribed the neurosis to repression. "It is possible," wrote Freud "to take *repression* as a center and to bring all elements of psychoanalytic theory into relation with it. . . . The theory of repression became the foundation stone of our understanding of the neuroses" (3). Repression is, indeed, the crux of all psychoanalytic theory. All the rest, which is massive enough, is in effect ancillary to this core concept. Repression, be it noted, is not an anatomic nor a physiologic, nor even a pathogenic concept. It is, basically, a psychodynamic or, if you please, a Freudian *psychologic* concept. "Repression," Freud explained, "proceeds from the Ego, which possibly at the command of the Super-ego does not wish to be a party to an instinct cathexia originating in the Id" (4). Again, "The Ego feels a demand from an instinct which it wishes to withstand, because it suspects that satisfaction is dangerous. . . . The Ego undertakes a repression of these instinctual impulses" (5). It is not my intention to take you through the labyrinthine metapsychology, whereby Freud establishes the dynamic emergence of the neurosis from an initially effected repression. More significant, both historically and to our interest, would be a careful scrutiny of what is implicated in the concept of repression. Or to paraphrase this, it will profit us to inquire into *what* is repressed, *who* does the repressing, and *who* suffers thereby.

In Freudian parlance, the sufferer is the ego and, of course, the person in whom the ego is embodied. *What* is repressed, is some of the instinctual drives incorporated in the *id,* and the chief repressor is the superego. The *id,* according to Freud, "contains everything that is inherited, that is present at birth, that is fixed in the constitution—above all, therefore, the instincts. . . . (6). The superego represents, according to Freud, the internalization of the inhibiting forces of the outer world, initially encountered in the father, and thereafter in all who superintend the actions of the individual, notably during his formative years (7). Both the *id* with its instinctual drives, and the superego, in Freud's words, "represent the influences of the past—the Id the influence of heredity, the Superego essentially the influence of what is taken over from other people" (6).

For the moment it is not important whether we do or do not accept Freud's theory of the dynamics of repression. Of basic interest are the operational agents postulated, namely the id, with its instinctual drives, the superego, palpably of social derivation, and the operational ego, placed none-too-comfortably between the id and the superego. It may be asked—what is there so noteworthy about this trinity? Certainly it is an ancient vision of man-tripartite. Palpably, what is noteworthy is not so much the trinity as the timing of Freud's reaffirmation of this ancient knowledge and, also, the uses to which he applied it.

To appreciate this in full, we need to revert to the framework in which man was envisioned during the twin centuries of modern science, preceding the time of Freud. Man was perceived and contemplated in isolation —standing, so to say, by himself. Man was envisaged as a machine! La Mettrie's *L'Homme Machine* may well be "the extremity" of 18th century materialist philosophy and yet it reflects the essential tradition, and the basic faith of that age. In that faith, inspired by Cartesianism, it was held not only that the proper study of man is man, but that only in the dismemberment and scrutiny of *atomized* man, could man proper, and man's essential character be discovered and revealed. For two hundred years the greatest among the scientists labored in this faith, and progressively anatomized and atomized man in ever greater refinement and detail. And then Freud appeared; and what he said, in essence, was that science was wrong, that man does not "stand" in splendid isolation, is not a machine or a mechanism, and that neither his being nor his behavior can be understood save as they are envisaged in relation both to man's past, and to his future.

Psychologic man, reflected in his space-and-time-bound ego, is a being impelled by the vis-a-tergo of his id, and evocatively drawn by his superego and ego ideal. No machine can have an id, or an hereditary impulsion. No machine can aspire to become a more noble machine. No machine then is Man, and Man is not a machine. Man's behavior, neither in health nor in disease, can be understood mechanistically, even when "mechanistically" is spelled out in terms of chemistry and physics, electronic or otherwise. This is a shocking affirmation, and Freud reaped a full measure of scorn, disdain, and condemnation from the contemporary world of science for having made it. But time and experience have validated Freud's understanding of the nature of man, and medicine no less than psychiatry has increasingly abondoned its mechanistic orientation and has reorganized its data and its understanding, about the framework of ecology.

At this point, it would profit us to examine briefly the uniqueness of Freud. I have referred to him as one of the great innovators, and it is not improper to ask: How do innovators innovate? The easy retort—that they do so because they are possessed of genius—is nothing but a semantic circuit. They are innovators because they are geniuses, and geniuses because they are innovators. Galton credited the historically recognized geniuses with extraordinary intelligence, and that can hardly be disputed. Extraordinary endowment in intelligence is a prerequisite for, but does not in and of itself assure its possessor the historical status of genius or innovator. There are quite a number of negative instances on record. Norbert Wiener tells of two such in his autobiography. The innovator, I suspect, must be *a potential genius born at precisely the right time,* that is, at a time when his genius can effect an innovating revolution in thought. Thus favored the innovator serves as the instrument, whereby that which has long been incubating in the womb of the intellect is brought forth as a viable issue in the realm of the ideas. Such indeed was the genius of Freud, and this is the quality of his uniqueness (8).

I can treat this subject but briefly, and I do so because it will help us to appreciate to what extent Freud's basic concepts have been integrated into the larger and more fundamental biologic concepts.

Modern science was, since its initiation in the 17th century, largely rationalistic and mechanistic in its orientation. It was permeated with the spirit of the cartesian system, whose philosophy of science carried the motto "Give me matter and I will build you a world" (9). But even as no one religion ever gained the adherence of all mankind, so, too, for all its predominance, cartesian science did not hold sway over the minds of all thinking men. As a matter of historical fact, parallel with Cartesianism, there was current in modern science another school of thought, one that was not primarily analytic, but was rather holistic and ecologic. It didn't go by either of these names, for these are terms of comparatively recent origin. It was more commonly defined as the Transcendental. But this designation is not as informing as the anachronistic designations— holistic and ecologic. Yet both these terms are inherent in and are derivatives of Transcendentalism. The holistic and ecologic school of thought was primarily Germanic, even as the cartesian was primarily French. One may count among the great proponents of holism and ecology Paracelsus, van Helmont, Leibnitz, Kant, Schelling, and the entire host of the Romantic School of Medicine.

It is not fitting to venture here on a full exposition of the differences between the cartesian-analytic, and the transcendental-holistic philosophers; but one feature of the difference can and must be accented, for thus we are to be brought back to Freud and his psychoanalysis. I will cite the difference by a quotation taken from Ernst Cassirer's work, *The Philosophy of Enlightenment* (10). "Cartesianism never gained unlimited sway either in England or in Germany (as it did in France). . . . The growth of German thought was guided by the influence of Leibnitz. . . . Descartes simply rules out the life of plants and animals; he declares that animals are machines, thus sacrificing them to mechanism. . . . Opposed to this viewpoint is the doctrine of plastic natures. . . . We must attribute life to all those creatures which in the manner of their existence, in their external shapes as they appear to our senses, give evidence of forming forces working within them of which they are the embodiment. . . . The order and connection of the universe can only be grounded in these plastic natures, not in mere mass and motion."

Romantic Medicine espoused the philosophy of "indwelling forming forces" that shape the plastic being and destiny of the living creature and most notably that of man. Freud, deriving his inspiration from Romantic

Medicine, largely through his many years of friendship with Fliess, named the "indwelling forming forces" of the psyche the id, the ego, and the superego. It is thus that Freud fulfilled the requirements of genius and innovator; that he served as an instrument whereby that which had long been gestating in the womb of the intellect was brought forth as a viable issue in the realm of ideas. In the philosophic, psychologic, and medical writings of the Romantics one comes upon many concepts that are to be found in Freud's expositions. This is not to say that Freud "took them over" and gave them out as his own. Freud was no plagiarist. But Freud, drawing on experience, insight, and inspiration, arrived at conclusions quite like those of the holistic, ecologic, and transcendental thinkers and scientists last structured in Romantic Medicine.

I have allowed myself a somewhat longish historic excursion to demonstrate the why and wherein of Freud's uniqueness; to assess the significance as well as the disturbing impact of Freud's theories of conflict and repression in the etiology of the neuroses. It now remains for us to see what Freud did with his fundamental concept of repression, what issued from it. Here it would be well to differentiate between Freud's metapsychology, his theories on psychopathology, and his therapeutic system.

To highlight these distinctions, I will cite some fundamental examples. Freud's theories on the dynamic relations of id, ego, and superego fall into the category of metapsychology. Freud's postulate that the neuroses derive from the repression by the superego of id impulses falls into the category of psychopathology. His teaching that, by free association, the materials repressed into the unconscious can be brought into awareness, and are thus to be robbed of their pathogenic charge, falls into the category of Freud's psychotherapy. Of these three divisions in the *Freudian Corpus,* it is his Metapsychology that has fared best under the critical stress test of time and experience. Freud's theories on psychopathology, essentially monolithic in character, and in that respect quite like the germ theory, have been found to be (save of course by the orthodox) of limited validity. His psychotherapeutic theories, notably his emphasis on the role of "free association" in the orphean evocation of repressed materials from the limbo of the unconscious, can now be deemed only as an article of creed, which, even by the orthodox, is more honored in the breach than in observance.

I want first to deal with Freud's theories of psychopathology and psychotherapy, and lastly with his metapsychology. But a word of caution must be said in advance. Freud, like Ralph Waldo Emerson, did not believe in the fetish of consistency. Consistency, said Emerson, is the hobgoblin of little minds. Freud was never quite a consistent theoretician. In many respects he was only *consistently contradictory*. On some issues he couldn't ever make up his mind. Hence, when one says something fundamental concerning Freud, one can always be confronted with some passage from his writings which says or suggests just the opposite. Yet all that despite, Freud was not an amorphous thinker, and there is a distinctive pattern to his theoretical superstructure.

I intend to deal primarily with this theoretical superstructure and, therefore, we first need to look to his psychopathology. As already noted, this was monolithic in character, and was spelled out in terms of *repression*. The concept of repression is a very exasperating pathodynamic concept; for it is so very sound and good where it applies, and so utterly wrong where it doesn't. In other words, repression is a valid concept as applied to the economy of the human psyche, and is valid in the explication of some phases of psychopathology, notably those which belong in the category of hysteria, and hysterical, obsessive and compulsive reactions. Repression as a universal etiologic factor or an omnipresent mechanism in the psychoneurosis is little short of nonsense; but by and large, Freud did advance it as the universal etiologic factor and mechanism in the psychoneurosis. To support this vision, he had to invent a vast mythology, including that of the oedipal complex with its *infantile* incest wishes, and the castration threat. And he also found it necessary to particularize the unconscious processes of the mind and the psyche into *the unconscious,* thus creating within the psyche some Siberian-like region, into which the repressed was exiled beyond deliberate recall. Furthermore, to counter-effect repression, he invented the technique of *de-repression,* namely, free association, an uncensored vocalization of all that wells up into the conscious.

The rounded circuit of Freudian psychodynamics, psychopathology, and psychotherapy may, therefore, he sketched as follows: The ego, identified with the operational individual, is posited between the id and the superego. As long as the apposition of id to superego can be reconciled and compromised, so as to allow the ego, i.e., the individual, to effectively meet the reality situation, he is likely to remain *normal*. When, however, the impulses of the id are strongly repressed, the repressed material with its libido charge, while resident in the unconscious, will affect the operations of the ego, that is, of the individual, in distorting and pathogenic ways. Hence, to quote Freud: "All phenomena of (neurotic) symptom formation can be fairly described as 'the return of the repressed' " (7). To relieve this situation, de-repression by free association is utilized: the theory being that the repressed material is not accessible to the deliberate effort of recall, but will well up of itself, precisely because it carries the "compression charge" of the repressed.

It is in this connection, too, that Freud developed his dream analysis, holding that the dream is the royal road to the unconscious and, also, that every dream represents a wish fulfilment. As is well known, Freud changed his mind somewhat on the wish-fulfilling function of the dream.

One cannot but admire the subtle intricacy and the clever ingenuity of Freud's theories. And any one who has had experience in applying his theoretical concepts to given cases will acknowledge freely that they are frequently and remarkably most useful and effective.

But, when viewed literally and *in toto,* and judged as to universal validity rather than as fitting to given and particular instances, Freud's theories on psychopathology and psychotherapy must be adjudged as neither entirely proved nor entirely valid. Not all the neuroses are due to repression, not all of them are remediable by the recall and the integration of repressed material through the techniques of free association. Of course, the amusing thing is that no one confesses to taking Freud's theories literally and *in toto,* nor to believing in them as universally valid, not even the most orthodox of Freudians. But then I am persuaded that the true sign of Freudian orthodoxy is not subscription to the fundamental Freudian doctrines but rather anointment, that is, acceptance in the membership of the *official* Freudians.

The crucial element in the Freudian circuit of psychodynamics (psychopathology and psychotherapy) is—psychotherapy. In the minds of the public, and no less among some psychiatrists, that which distinguishes the psychoanalyst from the psychotherapist is, first of all, the couch and, secondly, the alleged passivity of the psychoanalyst who leaves all the talking to the free-associating, recumbent patient. Here again it should be observed that both the couch and free association are more in the nature of ritualistic symbols and instruments than of indispensable therapeutic prerequisites. The couch may be desirable and should be available, though in general is to be used sparingly. Free association should mean full permissiveness for the patient, and the beneficent exercise of listening by the therapist. I have used the term *should*—both in relation to the "couch" and to "free association." This term reflects not only my own experience and persuasions, but also that of numerous analysts whose judgment is summarized in a work too little known among psychiatrists. I have in mind Part II of Edward Glover's *The Technique of Psycho-Analysis,* a questionnaire research on common technical practices among analysts. There it is clearly revealed that a great divergence exists between what analysts are alleged to do, and what they actually do in the therapeutic situation. To sum it up then: neither Freud's theories on psychopathology, nor his theories on psychotherapy, have stood up "in total intactness" under critical scrutiny and cumulative experience. During the past quarter of a century both have been questioned and modified, in parts discarded, in others strengthened and developed, both inside and outside of the ranks of the psychoanalysts.

Thus far, we have considered chiefly Freud's theories on psychopathology and psychotherapy. There remains to be dealt with Freud's metapsychology. This is a distinctive division of Freud's psychologic doctrines. In his metapsychology Freud was concerned chiefly with defining the components of the human psyche, with sketching the stages of its developments, envisioning the relations of the psychologic individual to the psychologic mass. Freud, in other words, dealt with the embryology and with the developmental physiology of the psyche. He was an innovator in the realm of psycho-social anthropology and ethnography. His principal metapsychologic works are *Three Contributions to the Theory of Sex, Totem and Taboo, Moses and Monotheism, Civilization and Its Discontents, Beyond the Pleasure Principle, Group Psychology and the Analysis of the Ego.*

I would say here what I had said before in relation to Freud's positing of the id, ego, and superego, namely, that it is less relevant whether he is entirely correct in the details or in the development of his postulations, and more noteworthy and laudable in that he did make them at all. Freud's metapsychologic works are epoch-making, because they are sign posts, suggestive of directions to be followed, leading to terrains to be explored. They are not "the tax roll maps of suburbia." Others, less inspired souls, can accomplish that. Consider, for example, the work *Civilization and Its Discontents.* It is a raw work that treats of religion as an infantile delusion. Granted, Freud was a Jew living in a Catholic country, famous for its reactionary bigotry. It is not a "balanced work," and yet it is, and has proved to be, an evocative work, in that it has linked, in many ways, man's psyche and man's vision of the Father, in heaven and on earth. The point then is not that Freud is correct, but rather that his metapsychology is inspiring. He has suggested new departures in thought, even as Darwin suggested organic evolution, and Einstein relativity. But then, Freud's entire effect upon modern psychiatry can be properly summed up in the term "inspiring." Freud inspired new visions, new perspectives, new procedures.

Perhaps it were well now to summarize Freud's effects upon psychiatry. To begin with, he helped convert it from a static, anatomized specialty, into a dynamic integrative discipline. He rescued the study of psychologic man from the position of transfixed isolation, and set it back into the matrix of its social setting, framed by the derivations of the past and by the challenge of the future. He exposed and helped to discredit the over-reaching and arrogant rationalism of contemporary science. He helped to make clear how much of reason is shaped by emotion, and how deeply man's behavior is influenced by unconscious motives. He demonstrated most brilliantly the rationality of the irrational, in human behavior and in the operations of the psyche. He taught us how to appreciate the healing effects of an empathic relation between men, where one is troubled and the other is attentive and of good will. Freud summed this up in the term *transference relation*. He reaffirmed the self-healing power of the psyche. He taught us how to understand that the psyche has its developmental stages, and its developmental dynamics, no less than the soma, to which it is bound. He led us to rediscover the symbolic language of the dream, and of the untoward, the accidental, and the unintended, in every-day life. In the words of Roland Dalbiez, whose 2-volume work *Psychoanalytic Method and the Doctrine of Freud* (11) I would recommend to any one interested in a broad survey of the subject, Freud's work is the most profound analysis of the less-human elements in human nature history has ever known.

Psychoanalysis as a technique in psychotherapy will, with time, be ever more adsorbed into, and converted to, the broader uses of classical psychiatry. Many of the more esoteric, novel, and even bizarre theories of the Freudian system will pale in time, even as some already have; but historically, Freud's stature will grow to ever greater dimensions.

For the young aspirant in psychiatry, as for all of us, it can be affirmed that none can deem himself informed, unless and until he has acquired a penetrating understanding of Freud's metapsychology and of Freud's psychoanalysis.

BIBLIOGRAPHY

1. GRIESINGER, W.: *Mental Pathology and Therapeutics.* Translated from the German (2nd ed.) by C. Lockhart Robertson and J. Rutherford, London, New Sydenham Society, 1876, p. 59.
2. ———: *Ibid.,* p. 483.
3. FREUD, S.: *An Autobiographical Study,* 2nd ed., J. Strachey, Hogarth Press, 1952.
4. ———: The Problem of Anxiety (Chapter 2).
5. ———: The Question of Lay Analysis (Chapter 3).

6. ———: An Outline of Psychoanalysis (Chapter 1).
7. ———: Moses and Monotheism, Part III, Sec. II.
7. ———: Moses and Monotheism, Part III, Sec. II.
8. GALDSTON, I.: Freud and Romantic Medicine. *Bull. of Hist. of Medicine,* Vol. XXX, No. 6, Nov.-Dec., 1956, pp. 489-507.
9. CASSIRER, E.: *The Philosophy of Enlightenment, p.* 51.
10. ———: *Ibid.,* pp. 81-82.
11. DALBIEZ, R.: *Psychoan. Method and the Doctrine of Freud,* Longmans, Green and Co., 1948.

16

Psychoanalysis 1959

NINETEEN HUNDRED AND FIFTY-NINE was a celebrant year in the history of psychoanalysis. It is the 50-year anniversary of 1909, and 1909 was critical for Freud and for psychoanalysis. This was the year when Freud, on invitation from Stanley Hall, visited America and lectured at Clark University. This was the year that saw the birth of the first international psychoanalytic publication—the *Jahrbuch für Psychoanalytische und Psychopathologishe Forschungen,* with Bleuler and Freud as *Herausgeber,* and Jung as Editor. This was the break-through year which, according to Jones, marks the beginning of the international recognition of psychoanalysis.

Fifty years is a goodly span of time, one that lends the right perspective for the evaluation of historic, and notably intellectual, eventuations. Fifty years allows for the overlapping coexistence of three generations. Ortéga y Gasset (1), in his *Man and Crisis,* makes much of this. And indeed it is a profound insight. "The present," Ortéga wrote, "is rich in three great vital dimensions which dwell together in it, whether they will or no, linked with one another, and perforce, because they are different, in essential hostility one to the other. For some, 'today' is the state of being 20, for others 40, and for still another group, 60; and this, the fact that three such very different ways of life have the same 'today', creates the dynamic drama, the conflict, and the collision which form the background of historic material and of all modern living together."

I take it, our concern is with the historic background of psychoanalytic thought and development. In these relations we need recognize that ours is the generation of "twenty," to whom Freud stands as of the "sixty," and Brill, Jones, Ferenczi, and Jung, as the generation of "forty." Those

221

who come after us will have a different linkage. It will no longer be possible for them, or their descendants, to have known "the men who had known the man." Their vision, and I fear too, their understanding, while possibly more penetrating and expansive than ours, will lack that element of authenticity which is vouchsafed only to him "who was there when it happened." All of which is prelude to the affirmation that it is not only desirable that we should evaluate psychoanalysis in 1959, but that it is our obligation, our debt-to-be-paid, to those who by the accidents of later birth will not be able to know of these matters save only by hearsay. But how is one to assess Freud's psychoanalysis? It would seem most reasonable to review in brief the major postulations of psychoanalysis, to take note of those which experience and further study have validated, to catalogue those which in contrast have not survived close scrutiny and clinical trial, to see where the embrace of psychoanalytic thought has extended to other fields and disciplines, and conversely, how and to what extent psychoanalysis has been affected by concurrent developments in science and philosophy.

Confessedly, this is a most challenging and pretentious perspective, one that cannot be fulfilled in the limitations of an essay. Still, it may yet be useful to sketch the terrain, even if we cannot or may not fill in every detail.

I think it were wrong not to begin our evaluative venture with a full appreciation of the historic significance of Freud and his psychoanalysis. We must, as good historians, differentiate between the historic significance of an event, a personality, or an idea, and its ultimate, scientific validity or moral value. No one can deny great historic significance to Napoleon, though many will doubt his moral worth. Copernicus is historically no less a revolutionary thinker because his astronomical calculations have been proved wrong, i.e., inadequate. The impact of Darwin's teachings on evolution have had an historic effect on thought which is unaffected and independent of the questions raised on the correctness of his theoretical premises.

In that historical perspective, Freud and his psychoanalysis stand forth as preeminent in the dimensions of greatness, as do Karl Marx and his *Das Kapital,* and Charles Darwin and his *Descent of Man.* Freud, and those to whom he is compared, gave a new turn to the thinking of mankind.

Freud challenged the 19th century faith in man as a rational animal. This was a faith nurtured for some 300 years, and seemingly brought to a fine point of iridescent perfection just about the time (in the final decades of the 19th century) when Freud came forth to challenge it.

Nineteenth Century rationalism was *strictly* rationalistic, i.e., logically positivistic. It failed to perceive and could not recognize the rational function of the irrational. That is what Freud underscored, not precisely in this formulation, not with this implied self consciousness, but by indirection, in a piecemeal, clinical, empirical manner.

It were difficult to overestimate the significance, the import for human thought and destiny of the Freudian challenge. It is equally difficult to grasp its full weightiness, its fertility, its explosive potentials. Only the authoritarian states, the Communists, for example, appear to have some grasp of the transcending significance and the overwhelming surcharge of psychoanalytic premises and hypotheses. To them, Freud and psychoanalysis are anathema: an infamous adversary to be excoriated. *Ecrasez l'infâme.* The rest of the world, including also some of the psychiatric and the psychoanalytic portion, have, I would venture the opinion, only a vague and none-too-secure appreciation of the overriding significance, and the immutable validity of the essential premise of psychoanalysis. There are, of course, some exceptions among the psychiatric group, and for them this ventured opinion does not hold. But the group is not large. The rest are too easily made anxious by the advent of every new therapeutic modality offered for the treatment of psychiatric symptomatology. Many behave as if they feared that some new drug or combination of drugs would rob them of their specialty. They hasten, lest they be left behind, to get on the latest in the therapeutic caravan of bandwagons.

All of this is sad to behold, and yet it cannot but enhance our appreciation of the magnitude and significance of Freud's premise—the affirmation of the transrational nature of man.

Freud's psychology has been described as an "instinct psychology." The term "instinct" is currently in ill repute, and for very good reasons. For to the instincts have been credited all orders of motivations and behavior, from the belief in a personal God, to the loving graces of maternity. Call them instincts or not: Freud was cognizant that *before reason there was life,* and that life was impelled and regulated, and *is so even now,* by certain indwelling forces, not to be distinguished from life itself, which in a measure embrace, but most generally transcend that which the human mind recognizes as rational. Freud perceived, too, that the rational, and with it the moral and the social, often impedes the free play of the primal forces and drives of the living process, that their effective reconciliation fosters the rational, the moral, and the social, but that when left unreconciled, that is, in abiding conflict, ill health, in the physical as well as in the experiential and behavioral spheres, may, and commonly does, result. This, according to Freud, was the genesis of the neurosis. The neurosis, be it noted, need not be entirely absorbed in the overt pathology reflected in variant behavior, but may also turn upon the innate vital forces, that is, the primal drives. This is dramatically represented in anorexia nervosa, and more reconditely in certain forms of schizophrenia.

This most significant element of Freud's psychoanalysis, that which I would deem the most revolutionary and the most fundamental component of his system of thought, has not been effectively challenged in the past 50 years. On the contrary, it has been confirmed, validated, reenforced, and elaborated in many ways, and in numerous proximate and remote disciplines—in social anthropology, in animal psychology, in ethology, to name but a very few of the disciplines.

It is not possible to elaborate on this affirmation—space does not allow it. It is, however, desirable to define the essential quality of this "significant element in Freud's psychoanalysis." It amounts to the following: *Freud signalled the existence and the effective operation of a science of relations, as distinguished from the science of things.* How else could one account for the cure of an hysterical paralysis, since the count of things involved remains unchanged both before and after? It matters not that this science of relations had been known and understood in time past, and had been forgotten, or overlooked. It came as a revitalizing breath when it was advanced anew by Freud. Affirming this, I am aware that I seemingly credit Freud with more philosophical preoccupation and sophistication than is historically warranted. Freud was not interested in philosophy and conceivably, had he been confronted with the above formulation, he would have disclaimed it entirely. But that is of little matter; what one does may have little bearing on what one initially intended, and the effects yielded may not be cognizable to the one who effected them. Pavlov, in demonstrating the possibility of inducing experimental neurosis, little thought, nor later recognized, how much he thereby gave support to Freud's theory on the genesis of the neurosis. Pavlov never did recognize this, and yet that does not alter the fact.

Here I must round off this portion of my presentation, intended to attest to the historic significance and greatness of Freud and psychoanalysis. I have dwelt upon this at some length because I wanted to set down not only the acknowledgment of Freud's significance and greatness, but also more particularly wherein these dimensions of his significance reside. Many acknowledge that Freud is a most preeminent character in recent history. Not as many, however, know precisely how and why. Among the many literati and philosophers who have undertaken to treat of the greatness of Freud, only Isaiah Bowman has impressed me as fully knowledgeable. Of course I do not know them all, and some, I confess, I have read with a jaundiced eye. Yet the reason I am concerned with literati and philosophers is that the challenge voiced by Freud in the realm of psychiatry is one we face in every realm of being. How that challenge is met, how it will be resolved, will deeply influence the coming destinies of man.

From the basic premise of psychoanalysis we now need turn to some of its derivative formulations, bearing in mind that our concern is with how they have "stood up" in the intervening years, i.e., from the time of their formulation to the present. Without doubt the Freudian concept of the Unconscious is crucial to both psychoanalytic etiology and psychoanalytic therapeusis. The Unconscious is posited as the realm of the repressed, whence it, the repressed, can be evoked into the Conscious by the exercise of free association. Repression is effected by the Censor, whose represive operations are overcome, in the therapeutic situation, by the permissiveness of the atmosphere, and I would add, the evocative support of the therapist. No matter how "passive" the analyst may be, he still does insist that the patient withhold nothing and speak out everything that comes to mind. This evocation of the repressed from the Unconscious into the Conscious finds ultimate justification and presumed warrant in the postulation that the neurosis is fundamentally the resultant of repressed "material," material which will not stay repressed, but rather issues forth to embarrass the operations of the Ego and personality in devious and seemingly inexplicable ways. We see then that the major theoretical components involved in these operations are the Unconscious, the Censor, recall by free association, and the cathartic and curative effects of the recall.

Before treating of these theoretical components, it is desirable to observe that Freud linked all of them in what can only be described as a closed system. This was, according to Freud, the basic pathodynamic pattern of the neurosis. It likewise was *the* rationale for analytic therapy by free association.

In evaluating Freud's postulates concerning the Unconscious, *et al.*, one must therefore bear in mind not merely their individual validity and significance, but also that of their postulated interaction: thus it is quite possible that each postulate has its singular validity and yet, collectively, they may fail to add up to Freud's hypothetical summation. This, to

anticipate somewhat, is characteristic of the greater part of pristine analytical theory. It is seldom entirely wrong or in error, but it is likewise
not as correct, as inclusive, as broadly valid as it is pretended or claimed
to be. Thus, to restate and to amplify this affirmation, there can be no
doubt that the nonconscious is functionally a massive, and probably the
largest, component of the operational human psyche. The Unconscious
in the Freudian sense is unquestionably a component of that nebulous
terrain, the nonconscious. Where it is functionally located, at the core or
at the perimeter, and how close it lies to the realm of the conscious are
still unresolved questions. But of the existence of the Freudian Unconscious there can be no question, nor of the fact that its dynamic content
is provided by repression, nominally exercised by the Censor. All this can
incontestably be demonstrated experimentally in the phenomenon of
posthypnotic suggestion. However, acknowledging the existence of, and
the dynamic potentials of, repressed "material" contained in the Unconscious does not by any warrant commit one to the acceptance of Freud's
contention that *repression* is the sovereign cause of the neurosis. In fact,
it isn't, and probably is less so today than it was in the time of Freud.
The neuroses have many etiologies, and *repression* in the Freudian sense
is only one among them, and rarely so, in the pure and dominant form.

In this crucial reality, and in the fact that Freud was too much possessed
with his own ideas to welcome or to adsorb into his metapsychological
system those of his associates, particularly when they were divergent from
his own, lies the explanation for the emergence of so many "splinter"
schools of psychoanalysis. Unquestionably some of the splintering resulted
largely from the stresses of conflicting ambitions, nurtured by proud personalities. But even in the absence of pride and ambition, it could not
but become clear to the experienced and the studious that Freud's theories
on psychopathology and psychotherapy were far too narrow in their derivations and too restricted in their perspective on life's experience to
illuminate the entire field of the psychoneuroses. Many among Freud's
early associates ventured to ask if other dynamic combinations besides
repression, and other crucial segments of experience besides sexuality,
might not be involved in the engenderment of the neuroses. Those who
pressed their inquiries too far, too persistently, and too vigorously, found
themselves sooner or later outside the psychoanalytic pale, disparaged,
discredited, and denied. I am sure I need not read you the impressive
roll of the Freudian dissidents. What I would rather note here, for I've
never seen it treated, is the problem of those who were early drawn to
Freud and to analysis, whose names are listed as having shared in the

nascent stages of analysis, but of whom one hears little thereafter, who seemed to have vanished early and noiselessly. How many among these, I wonder, were also dissidents, unknown, because they did not choose to fight? And I wonder, too, how great, in consequence, was the loss for psychoanalysis. In these connections I recall the paper presented by Professor J. J. Putnam of Harvard, at the third International Psychoanalytic Congress, meeting at Weimar, in 1911. The title of his paper in German was *"Ueber die Bedeutung philosophischer Anschaungen and Ausbildung für die Entwicklung der psycho-analytischen Bewegung"* (On the significance of philosophical ideas and training for the development of the psychoanalytic movement). The burden of this exposition was a protest and warning against the monolithic theorizing and circular thinking that were patent in psychoanalysis. "Psychoanalysis," Putnam wrote, "is and should be recognized as being an instrument, not a doctrine. It binds us to no particular faith; it does not prevent us from holding any conviction as to universal truths. I doubt, however," Putnam continued, "whether psychoanalysis gives us all we need" (2). I am also moved to cite Sandor Ferenczi as the outstanding example of one who, having grown in experience and being natively studious, could not but perceive and react against the narrow and rigid formulations of Freudian theory and practice. Ferenczi did not merely protest—he experimented. He explored new theoretical formulations, and new procedures in therapy. Had he lived longer there is little doubt that he, too, would have "broken" with Freud, or more likely, would have been "disowned."

It is neither possible, in the time available, nor do I believe it would be profitable, to review here the distinctive academic and practical elements propounded and advanced by the factional schools of analysis. I would rather attempt to describe what seems to me to be their common accent. It is, I would say, an accent on the *extrapersonal,* in contradistinction to the *intrapersonal* factors, both in etiology and in therapy. This affirmation may at first sound a bit cryptic and, paradoxically, also too simple. Definitely, it requires explanation and elaboration. This I will attempt forthwith. Freud's theoretical formulations are concerned almost entirely with the intrapersonal operations and relations of the individual's psychic mechanism. Specifically, Freud's formulations revolve about the historic interrelations of the Id, Ego, and Superego—these interrelations being reflected in the individual's competences, adequate or otherwise, to deal with the reality about him. The psychoneuroses, according to Freud, were primarily the result of intrapsychic, or intrapersonal, conflict. The resolution of such conflict, according to Freud, would relieve the sufferer of his neurosis. This was uniquely the individual's task—to be worked out and achieved intrapsychically, that is, intrapersonally. The psychoneurotic individual could thus be said to carry *within himself entire* both the cause and the cure of his psychoneurotic disorder.

But it was not long before it became clear to some that conflict, with its consequent repression, was not the sole nor even the most important etiological factor in the psychoneurosis. Far more common were the factors of deprivation, and these derived most frequently from certain dimensions of the extrapersonal realm.

Allow me to paraphrase this in the form of a pat sentence. It became evident that "one's psychic being depended not only on how one reacted to *what* happened, but also on *that* which happened or *didn't happen!* Frequently that which should have, but didn't happen was the more important part of experience; hence the term 'deprivation.'"

This should be a concept easy to grasp. But it proved almost inconceivable to the generations who thought of disease only in terms of specific noxious agents. They could not conceive that the absence of a something essential to the economy of the being could also be the cause of disease. In fact, even in clinical medicine, this was not clearly demonstrated before 1912. In that year Casimir Funk, who the year before had coined the word "vitamine" (*sic*), showed that beriberi could be dramatically cured (and also prevented) by the administration of a crystalline derivative from rice polishings. This established the existence of what F. Gowland Hopkins of Cambridge, England, termed "disease with a minus sign."

In psychiatry, "disease with a minus sign" was not so clearly conceptualized nor so conclusively demonstrated as it was in clinical medicine. What did issue was the recognition that the psychological mechanism and man's psychic functions were deeply influenced by the individual's milieu-experiences, by his physical, economic, and cultural environment, by that which can be termed the "extrapersonal factors." As a result, some of Freud's associates and followers turned to the study of issues and matters beyond the Unconscious, the Censor, and repression. In accord with the common nature of historical developments, all this took place, not with conscious intent, but gropingly. The picture I have drawn is retrospective, it was not anticipated before it eventuated.

The interesting feature of this development is that different personages in the psychoanalytic realm chose to explore and to develop different segments of the milieu realm: Adler, the socio-somatic; Jung, the archaic-cultural; Wilhelm Reich and Franz Alexander, the immediacies of the external world and their constrictive influences. There were others who became involved in other pursuits, for the field of the extrapersonal is enormous indeed. One of the very earliest of the analytic deviants was Trigant Burrows, who dug into the basic psychologic consequents of the stereotypy of social organization and social communication. Burrows articulated some of the questions currently asked in existential-analysis: whether society itself is not one of the most significant pathogens in the realm of the psychic, impeding by its "socially sanctioned illusions" any essentially correct comprehension by the individual of his own actual being. Normal society, Burrows maintained, presents socially the same dissociations and image substitutions as are presented in the neurotic personality. "Normal social structure," he argued, "is not basic or fundamental in nature but, on the contrary, represents a secondary and substitutive fabric which, like the fabrications of the neurotic, is without direct biological or organic foundations" (3). Burrows was not a nihilist, nor an anarchist, nor antisocial. On the contrary, he envisaged a higher order of social relatedness, more consonant with man's essential, biological being. Burrows had few followers, and appeared to have made no impression at all on the psychoanalytic movement. Jones, in his biography of Freud, hardly notices him, and does not even honor him with one of those mordant sentences with which he spikes his comments on the other dissidents.

Better known, more widely recognized, and of deeper immediate effect, were the dissidents Karen Horney and Harry Stack Sullivan, both of whom gave rise to independent schools. Common to their separate orientations is this, that both Horney and Sullivan extended the theoretical encompassment of Freud's psychoanalysis to include the individual's contiguous *real* world, and also, those other mortals in it that impinge upon his own being. I have used the expression "to extend the encompassment of Freud's psychoanalysis." I must add that this is not intended to imply an initial total acceptance of Freud's formulations. On the contrary, much was discarded, sloughed off; only the core was retained and added to. But herein lies the difference between two orders of Freudian dissidents. One group sought to displace Freud's theories with their own "monolithic formulae." Among such I would count Adler, Rank, and Reich. The other group, including Jung, Ferenczi, Horney, Sullivan, Alexander, and Schilder did not seek to displace but to build upon, to extend the encompassment of Freud's psychoanalysis. In the end the results are at times hardly identifiable with the original, but if I may compound my figures of speech—"the foundations of large structures most often lie hidden."

I have thus far said but little about psychoanalytic therapy, concerning myself almost entirely with psychoanalytic theory. But, of course, theoretical changes must perforce be reflected in therapeutic practices. On occasions they precede theory. In "classical psychoanalysis" (the phrase is Ferenczi's), free association, including dream analysis, was the sovereign therapeutic means. It accorded very well with Freud's fundamental hypothesis that it was the repressed "material," resident in the Unconscious, that was animating the neurosis. In free association, and in dream analysis, the repressed material was likely to emerge into consciousness, for in both free association and in dreams the repressing censor is, to an effective extent, evaded. But, when the postulated etiology came into question, the therapy, too, could not but be questioned. And such indeed was the case, notably first with Rank and Ferenczi. Ferenczi is the more significant of the two. Ferenczi was one of the first to break into the traditional passivity of the analyst's role. He was not unwilling to confront his patient with blunt inquiries that called for deliberate responses, rather than a roaming over the Unconscious. Nor was he hesitant in proffering to the shy, anxious, or distressed patient, assurance, encouragement and affection. Ferenczi advocated, not a superficial and hasty, but rather an active analysis. He also recognized that many patients bring with them a history not merely of conflict, but also of deprivation, "that the origin of neuroses was to be found in definite traumas, particularly the unkindness or cruelty of parents. This had to be remedied by the analyst's showing more affection toward his patient than Freud thought proper or necessary" (4).

What was rather falteringly initiated by Ferenczi, who was ever loath to confront or deny Freud in anything, and did so only in pain and under duress, has been the consistent pattern of change in psychoanalytic therapy. This is perhaps best mirrored in Franz Alexander's therapeutic procedures (5) as well as in those developed by Frieda Fromm-Reichmann (6). The once rigid requisites and the paraphernalia of "classical analysis" (Ferenczi's phrase) now have historical significance rather than current pertinence. Glover (7), in his confidential study of the practices of British psychoanalysts, all of them members of the Institute, reveals "much unorthodoxy among the orthodox."

In all respects, and for the majority of psychoanalytically trained and oriented psychiatrists, there has been an adaptive loosening of therapeutic procedure—away from doctrinaire rigidity toward an objective effort to meet the multiphased challenge of the therapeutic problems and the patient's needs. Anamnestic depth is not sacrificed, but is attained more directly with a greater economy in time and effort. Insight, and its application to past and current experience, is favored by the analyst's more active participation in the therapeutic process. More effective, more courageous use is made of the transference-countertransference situation and relationship. The current reality problems of the patient are, when it is profitable or necessary to do so, accepted as legitimate therapeutic items and used as leverage for uncovering the past, as well as for the achieving of a clearer understanding which the patient may gain by ventilating them. The therapeutic relationship is not as exclusively confined to analyst and analysand as it formerly was, but may now, to varying degrees, be extended to embrace other persons intimately and significantly impinging on the patient's being. Not a few analysts are now "treating" both marriage partners, and will see, in analysis, or contiguously, child and parent, and/or siblings.

Of course there are some who will insist "All this is not analysis." But such a protest cannot be taken in earnest; and with such protestants it is profitless to discuss the issue. Of them it needs be said, in Virgil's words to Dante,

> *Non ragionam di loro*
> *Ma guarda e passa.*

I come to the end of my review of "Psychoanalysis 1959" with a sharp sense of frustration. So much that belongs within the scope of such a review is left untouched. So many points of issue remain undefined and unsettled. But that cannot be helped, for even if the requisite knowledge and scholarship *were* available, time, for certain, is not. This much, however, I trust has been made clear in this review: the grandeur of Freud's genius, and the revolutionary challenge of his analytical psychology; the expanding comprehension of the intrapsychic dynamics of the individual, and their, in part, derivative relation to the ecological setting in which the individual has his being.

Freud was, in the Oslerian categories, an innovator, that is, of the highest order among the medical greats. He will be remembered, as is Paracelsus, long after his "system" has been overlaid by the increments in knowledge and insight that are the burden of time. For, if there be aught that we who are the heirs of Freud are bound in the debit to our inheritance to comprehend, it is that we and all of mankind are currently in the adolescence of cultural development. Before us, in the person of our descendants, lies the prospect of a glorious adulthood, when mankind will culturally come of age. When that eventuates, Freud will be recalled and honored as one among the very few of whom it can truly be said—he was a *Wegweiser.*

REFERENCES

1. ORTEGA Y GASSET, J.: *Man and Crisis.* New York, W. W. Norton Co., 1958, p. 42.
2. PUTNAM, J. J.: *Addresses on Psychoanalysis* Vienna, Int. Psychoanal. Pr., 1921, p. 90.
3. GALT, W.: *Phyloanalysis.* London, K. Paul, Trench, Trubner & Co., Ltdr., 1933, p. 41.
4. JONES, E.: *Life and Work of Sigmund Freud,* Vol. III, The Last Phase. New York, Basic Books, 1957, p. 146 and p. 163.
   FERENCZI, S.: *Bausteine zur Psychoanalyse.* Leipzig, Int. Psychoanaly. Verlag, 1927-39, vol. 11, pp. 38-49, *Zur psychoanalytischen Technik,* and Vol. III, p. 380, *Die Elastizitaet der psychoanalytischen Technik.*
5. ALEXANDER, F. G.: *Psychoanalysis and Psychotherapy; Developments in Theory, Technique and Training.* New York, W. W. Norton Co., 1956.
6. FROMM-REICHMANN, F.: *Principles of Intensive Psychotherapy. Chicago,* Univ. Chic. Press, 1950.
7. GLOVER, E. G.: *An Investigation of the Technique of Psychoanalysis,* with the assistance of Marjorie Brierley. Inst. Psychoanal. London, Baillière, Tindall and Cox, 1940.

17

Eros and Thanatos — A Critique and Elaboration of Freud's Death Wish

IT IS MY INTENTION to propound and to defend the thesis that "those who fear to die lack the courage to live." This I advance not as an exercise in scholasticism, or as a proposition for dialectic fencing, but rather as a conviction derived from clinical experience. In other words I advance my thesis as a postulate in psychodynamics. But first I must define the two crucial terms involved: *to die* and *to live*. In the sense I employ them, thery are the equivalents of Eros and Thanatos. "To live" implies the dynamic process of "self-fulfillment." "To die" does not mean *"exitus,"* the instant of the final and irrevocable dissolution of the living process. In my usage, to die refers rather to that phase of Eros wherein the investments heretofore made in the immediate person of the individual are henceforth made in other personages and in the social organism. At first blush it may appear as if I had with some violence distorted the common meaning of the expression *to die* to suit my convenience. But a little reflection will suffice to correct that impression. The vernacular is replete with sayings that accord with my usage, as for example: "to die by degrees" and, even more pointedly, "to have given the best part of one's life." Furthermore, I want to relate my thesis—that *"those who fear to die lack the courage to live"*—to Freud's postulated death instinct. Thanatos in Freud's intention is also a something other than *exitus.*

I do not, however, want to entangle either you or myself in the briary wilderness of semantic subtleties. Even as Freud derived his theory of the death instinct from clinical experience, so do I base my thesis on clinical experience. And to these experiences I must refer, drawing from them, and not from semantics, such support and validation for my propositions as they will afford me.

233

I must begin with Freud's theory of the death instinct. Of all the theories which Freud postulated, this, I believe, is the one which has proved least acceptable to his disciples, even to those who by inclination and habituation are least prone to question the founder's words.

Time past "the death instinct" was discussed and disputed. Of late it has been neglected. It would seem as if the analysts shied away from it. And for that one can hardly blame them. For it is a knotty problem, and the more so because of the way in which Freud propounded his theory. "The goal of all life," so runs his crucial dictum, "is death." "The inanimate was there before the animate" (1), and to the inanimate the animate seeks to return. This retrogressive momentum Freud labels the death instinct. "Our speculation," wrote Freud in a subjoined note to clarify nomenclature, "then supposes that. . . . Eros is at work from the beginnings of life, manifesting itself as the 'life instinct' in contradistinction to the death instinct which developed through the animation of the inorganic" (2).

The quotations are from Freud's *Beyond the Pleasure Principle,* a work of paramount significance in analytical theory, but in itself a book of dismal pessimism. One is prompted to inquire what moved Freud to write this work. Ostensibly it took its departure from the observation that victims of "traumatic neurosis," more particularly soldiers returned from war who had suffered shocking experiences, repeatedly dreamt of the traumatizing events. Freud had previously postulated that the function of the dream was essentially wish fulfillment; the dream in other words was subservient to the pleasure principle and circumvented the *censor.* But the dream of the returned soldier, occupied as it was with most painful experiences and circumstances, did not accord with the wish-fulfillment principle. Freud then ventured a new tangent. "If," he wrote, "we are not to go astray as to the wish fulfillment tendency of the dream in consequence of these dreams of the shock neuroses, perhaps the expedient is left us of supposing that in this condition the dream function suffers dislocation along with the others and is diverted from its usual ends; or else we should have to think of the masochistic tendencies of the ego" (3). In effect, Freud does not much elaborate on the dislocation of the dream function, but pursues rather the labyrinthine problem of the masochistic tendencies of the ego. Granting that the dreams of the "traumatic neurosis" are "an exception to the principle that the dream is a wish fulfillment," he derives from this exception the concept of a prehistoric past for the wish fulfilling tendency of the dream, and "an insight into a function of the psychic apparatus which, without contradicting the pleasure-principle, is nevertheless independent of it, and appears to be of earlier origin than the aim of attaining pleasure and avoiding pain" (5). That principle Freud termed *repetition compulsion,* and he held it to be "more primitive, more elementary, more instructive than the pleasure principle which is displaced by it" (6).

By a very involved exercise in reasoning Freud arrives at the conclusion that "the goal of all life is death"; that the animate seeks to revert to the inanimate. Freud thus comes to the death instinct.

Freud is uncommonly apologetic in his exposition of the arguments involved in *Beyond the Pleasure Principle.* He terms this a work of speculation, "speculation often far-fetched, which each will according to his particular attitude acknowledge or neglect" (7). Most psychiatrists have chosen to neglect it. Freud's exposition of the death instinct is not only tortuous and labored, it carries a repugnant implication. One somehow senses that Freud here asks the question, Of what use is life and living? and then comes forth with the answer, Of no use at all: life is a trying interlude, a grievous rent in the blessed state of Nirvana.

Eduard Weiss in his paper *"Todestrieb und Masochismus"* (8) makes the observation that a psychological insight can also derive from an inner personal experience. *"Im Falle einer psychologischen Erkenntnis kann es sich auch um ein eigenes inneres Erlebnis handeln"* (9). One wonders what *eigenes inneres Erlebnis,* what inner personal experiences, may have contributed to Freud's bitterly pessimistic conclusions as to the purposes of life and of living. At the present we can only wonder. Perhaps the forthcoming volumes of Freud's biography will throw light on these matters. The future will tell. At present, even while rejecting his conclusions, we must affirm that Freud's preoccupation with the death instinct is genius manifest. Here, indeed, he has touched on a profound problem, one of the deepest that faces man, and the psychiatrist. As the Editorial Preface in *Beyond the Pleasure Principle* affirms, Freud expounds his thoughts on *the ultimate problems of life.* His exposition must perforce direct our own thinking to these "ultimate problems."

Let us first orient ourselves on the prehistory of the death instinct, for it does have a pre-history. To begin with we need to bear in mind that originally Freud postulated the pleasure principle as the *vis-a-tergo* of life. What motivated behavior in all its manifold patterns (so it was assumed), is man's desire to avoid pain and to gain pleasure. Freud refers to G. Th. Fechner's conception of pleasure and pain as psychic counter potentials, and affirms that in essentials Fechner's conception "coincides with that forced upon us by psycho-analytic work" (10). In effect, however, the pleasure-pain principle was commonplace to the thought of the eighteenth and nineteenth centuries. Rousseau gave impetus to this naive principle in his romantic picture of the uncorrupted primitive man.* In economic and social government it was advanced by Jeremy Bentham, the pioneer of the utilitarians (1748-1832). He applied the pleasure-pain principle to both man and the state, holding that the sovereign motive of the individual was the furtherance of his own ends. The policy of *laissez-faire* was founded on the assumption that each man knew his pleasures and would accordingly pursue them, and a good deal of Darwinian evolution and Spencerian sociology rested on the idea that the governance of all life, biological, communal and social, was piloted by the pleasure-pain principle. This principle is currently propagandized, though masked, in the Marxian concept of economic determinism as the decisive factor in individual and mass behavior.

Freud first propounded his ideas on the pleasure-pain principle in his *Three Contributions to the Sexual Theory*. That was in 1905. Shortly thereafter he ran into "academic difficulties." The *Ichtrieb* and the *Sexualtrieb* could not cover all the drives manifest in man's behavior. Love and hunger were not competent to explain narcissism, aggression, masochism. The original formulations were in consequence further elaborated by Freud and by a number of his coworkers. Out of these efforts came the concept of the superego, and some ingenious ideas on the derivation of melancholy by the conversion of sadism—that is, aggression—into masochism, and by the abusive predominance of the superego over the ego. Narcissism and sadism were not difficult to correlate with the sex instinct. Sadism, Freud argued, is but the aggressive component of the sexual instinct, and narcissism is but the investment of sexual libido in one's own person. The integration of masochism with the two postulated primary drives, in contrast, proved very difficult. And as we saw, Freud finally revised his scheme of primal drives, absorbed the *Ichtrieb* with the *Sexualtrieb* and postulated instead the two basic instincts—Eros and Thanatos—the life instinct and the death instinct (11).

I have compressed very much into very little, because the history of the development of analytical instinct theory is complex and labyrinthine, and also because only a part of that history, that which concerns masochism, is germane to my thesis. Those who are interested will find a competent review of the instinct theory in psychoanalysis in E. Bibring's *"Zur Entwicklung und Problematik der Triebtheorie"* (12).

---

* Vide *Rousseau and Romanticism* by Irving Babbit. Houghton-Mifflin Co., 1919.

Siegfried Bernfeld and Ernest Jones have also dealt with the instinct theory in psychoanalysis, Bernfeld under the title *"Über die Einteilung der Triebe"* (13) and Jones in a paper entitled "Psychoanalysis and the Instincts" (14).

To revert then to masochism, we find this the unreconcilable component in Freud's scheme of instinct drives. In "The Economic Problem in Masochism," Freud affirms the following: "We have a right to describe the existence of the masochistic trend in the life of the human instincts as from the economic point of view mysterious. For if mental processes are governed by the pleasure principle, so that avoidance of pain and obtaining pleasure is their first aim, masochism is incomprehensible. If physical pain and feelings of distress can cease to be signals of danger and be ends in themselves, then the pleasure principle is paralyzed, the watchman of our mental life is to all intents and purposes himself drugged and asleep" (15). But this affirmation is advanced only so that it might be promptly contradicted, for a bit further in this essay Freud draws the conclusion that, "A description of the pleasure principle as the watchman over our lives cannot be altogether put aside" (16).

He comes to this conclusion in a very simple yet rather ingenious way, namely, by arguing that the common clinical patterns of masochism, those which he terms erotogenic, feminine, and moral, are in effect the resultants of thwarted Eros. The first, the erotogenic, is "a condition under which sexual excitation may be aroused," the second is given as "an expression of feminine nature," and the third as a "norm of behavior" (17). But Freud's exposition does not end there, for even granting that masochism is the resultant of thwarted Eros, there still remains the problem of the nature and the dynamics of that thwart. In the effort to explore this phase of the problem of masochism, Freud developed the concept of the superego, and also postulated the existence of the death instinct.

There is no doubt that much of the masochism encountered clinically can be conceived of dynamically, as the resultant of thwarted Eros—the resultant, in other words, of the multiform inhibitions which society and neurotic elders impose upon the "id impulsions" of the individual. But I am certain that what Freud terms feminine masochism, and a good deal of what he labels moral masochism, cannot be accounted for as due to a thwarting of Eros, nor can they be explained on the basis of the death instinct *as postulated by Freud*. For be it noted Freud conceives the death instinct as diametrically opposed to the life instinct. In my view, Thanatos stands not in apposition to Eros, but is rather itself a phase of Eros. It is "the last for which the first was made." To quote my opening statement: "Thanatos is that phase of Eros wherein the investments heretofore made in the immediate person of the individual are made in other personages and in the social organism."

I intend to elaborate upon this thesis, drawing upon the data of biology and upon those of clinical experience. But I must first dwell a bit on Freud's dismal excursion into the realm of death. What moved Freud to treat the theme, and why did his exposition miscarry so badly? For miscarry it did, in the opinion even of some of his most devoted and enthusiastic supporters (see Jone's concluding comments in the article cited).

We can speculate more profitably on the second than on the first part of this query. Reading the confused and disjointed text of *Beyond the Pleasure Principle,* one cannot escape the impression that Freud was subjectively preoccupied with death, or better still, with the ultimate meaning of life. And in the background of that preoccupation one can discern the sphinx riddle of masochism: not the masochism of the "effeminate male" or of the self-defeating, accident-prone individual, but that of the mother woman, and of the altruist, of the idealist, and of the saint. Freud mentions that certain fish at spawning time will travel long distances to deposit their spawn in waters far removed from their usual habitats, and that birds will similarly fly great distances to nest in given regions. But he sees these merely as instances illustrative of the "repetition-compulsion instinct of all life." He seems to miss the point that it is only at spawning time that the fish will swim upstream to deposit their eggs, and to die; and that the birds migrate to nest and to hatch their young. In other words, he perceives the action but he is unmindful of its goal. In this connection it is pertinent to recall that Freud was never happy with the idea of teleology. Yet the very concept of instinct presupposes goal-directed behavior, that is, both *purpose* and *telos.* Siegfried Bernfeld acutely perceives this basic defect in Freud's version of the instincts. In his paper *"Über die Eintheilung der Triebe"* (13) Bernfeld observes, ". . . *Zielen handelt es sich in Freud's Trieblehre nicht."* All of the discussion concerning the instincts common to biology Freud rejects without even referring to them. From the very beginning Freud treated the instinct as an ordinary physical power stemming from the physical state of the individual and serving to cancel out, that is, to satisfy, another physical state or need in the individual. The problem of teleology is thus reduced to a minimum. It is equated to the concordance (*Übereinstimmung*) of the single functions of the organism, and similarly to a concordance between the behavior of the individual and the transindividual (19).

I suspect that this abhorrence of "teleology" accounts for Freud's gratuitous introduction of the following passage into the text of his essay "The Economic Problem in Masochism": ". . . but all those who transfer the guidance of the world to Providence, to God, or to God and Nature, rouse a suspicion that they still look upon these farthest and remotest powers as a parent-couple, mythologically, and imagine themselves linked to them by libidinal bonds" (19). Substitute "the guidance of the individual," that is, the course of his growth, development, and fulfillment, for "the guidance of the world," and Freud's intense negative reaction to teleology becomes patent.

It needs to be underscored, however, that living as he did in an atmosphere of benighted religious bigotry, in the Austria of the Hapsburgs, teleology, emotionally and conceptually, meant a something quite different to Freud from what we may understand it to mean today. Historical experience has shown that teleology is all too commonly a belief foisted by designing groups upon credulous man in order to make him more subservient and more pliable to their selfish schemes. But such experiences belong to the realm of social and political life. They have no bearing on biology. Here teleology, or if you will, morphologic and functional design and pattern, is universally manifest, from the purposive regeneration of the mutilated radial member of the starfish to the magnificent architectonic design realized in the normal growth and development of the human individual from "conception to the grave." Without an appreciation and full understanding of this teleological quality of the life of man it is not possible to understand the relation of Thanatos to Eros, nor the biological and psychological significance and role of masochism, both physical and moral, in the experience of man.

All of this can be referred to a small number of biological fundamentals. Human creatures, in common with all other living organisms, can be conceived of and are in effect, before they are anything else, metabolizing machines. They have the competence to a degree possessed by no other form of matter (crystalline or amorphous, for example) to absorb and to convert, store, and apply to their own uses extraneous matter and energy. This competence to metabolize is indeed prerequisite to life. It serves to sustain life, and it also makes growth possible. For the absorption of extraneous matter and energy is not limited to the sustenance requirements of the organism, but is commonly in excess of such needs. It is this excess that makes growth possible. What regulates the intake of the excess above the organism's sustenance requirements is an interesting question, but one which we cannot here pursue. Suffice it to observe on that score that such regulation appears to be a function of the cellular nucleus. It is in other words the function of the chromosomes of the elephant cell to regulate the growth of the elephant to the classical size, pattern, and proportions of the elephant.

But to revert to the mainstream of our argument, growth is essential to the vital process. In the experience of the individual the growth process is of two orders: growth by accretion and growth by "procretion." Let me hasten to add that the English language has no such term as "procretion." It has the terms "excretion" and "procreation." But both these terms are endowed with precise meaning and they do not express what I intend by procretion. Excretion signifies elimination and procreation means the reproduction of a new living organism. Procretion I intend to mean growth by investment in others than the self that does the "procreting."

Procretion is a growth process to some extent common to all multicellular organisms. But qualitatively as well as quantitatively it is most prominent and distinguished as a feature of human growth. How and why this is so will be clear as the argument develops. Here, and merely as an aside, I would affirm that while the laws of growth are basically common to and continuous in all life, some of the operational features of those laws are so distinguished in human experience as to be, for all intentions, unique. Procretion is such a feature.

But all of this is better expounded in the direct development of argument. Growth by accretion is the initial growth process. From the instant that sperm unites with ovum, the absorption of matter and energy is of such order as to provide a margin of excess over and above the quantities required for sustenance. That excess makes possible and is applied to growth. The organism thus increases in mass—and also in complexity. It not only grows but also develops. Again merely as a posited observation, and not as a something to be pursued further, we need to recognize that growth involves elaboration of relationships and proportions as well as increments in mass. The further pursuit of this concept would carry us too far from the subject of our main interest. Hence we can only touch upon it and pass on. Growth by accretion has its definite limits in many dimensions, but chiefly in bulk and in time. While the range in size both for the total organism and for its component parts is wide, limits within the encompassment of the so-called normal organism are fixed for both extremes. So too there are time limits for growth by accretion. The total organism is time bound, again in a fairly elastic range, but still time bound.

It is not possible for a given human individual to achieve at the age, say, of forty the growth by accretion which is ordinarily achieved in the years from six to fourteen and which for some reasons of deprivation he missed during those years in his life. Such an individual, if stunted, is likely to remain stunted.

A less involved exposition of what is implied in the affirmation that growth by accretion is time bound may be based on the well-known fact that longitudinal growth is deaccelerated and finally arrested when gonadic function takes on the proportions of maturity.

I underscore here *longitudinal* growth, for growth in other directions and in other respects, including growth by elaboration, continues. Despite that, it still is a fact that at a certain time, spelled out not in terms of a given hour on a given day, but rather in the range of months, growth by accretion is deaccelerated. The individual no longer grows by increasing in mass. Further growth is by procretion, by investment outside of the investing person. For be it noted it is not a part of the architectonic scheme of human development to reduce "intake" to the requirement limits of mere sustenance. To phrase it succinctly: "When growth ceases work begins, but the work is adult growth."

While this portion of my exposition has been made in terms of physical biology, I most certainly do not want to confine our deliberations to the physical-anatomical phase of the living process. The limitation was in the interest of simplicity. Once the general idea of what is implied in *growth by accretion, and growth by procretion,* is made clear we can securely move on to the examination of the other aspects of growth. As the human being is a social animal, living as an individual, set in a socio-cultural matrix, it is part of this architectonic scheme to grow in other ways as well as in mass and as well as in complexity. In these divisions growth is likewise witnessed: first, by the process of accretion, and later by procretion. All men, save of course the exceptions we each know, at some time cease to be students and turn teachers. Each man, again with the exceptions noted, on some occasions and in some respects ceases being a disciple and turns master, ceases being a mere copyist and turns inventor.

I recognize, embarrassingly and painfully, how easily one could take exception to the above statements and, indeed, make sport of their generalizations. But the "exceptions" and the "sport" would as much miss the mark as they are "easy to make." The criticism could only strike at the illustration and not at the essence of the argument which basically is this: that normal human growth in any division of being begins as a process of growth by accretion and at a certain stage—*if growth continues* —changes to the process of "growth by procretion."

This part of my exposition I have now labored sufficiently. I must hasten to tie it in with Eros and Thanatos. And I am sure you already surmise that Eros, pure and simple—for Eros after all is pictured as a handsome boy—presides over that phase of growth which I have labeled as growth by accretion. Thanatos takes over when growth is by procretion. Thanatos takes over when we cease to live mainly and primarily for and within ourselves. Thanatos becomes manifest when the pleasure principle undergoes elaboration to include also masochism. It is no mere accident, but rather a crucial feature in the architectonic pattern of man, that the epiphyseal cartilages are absorbed when gonadic function reaches mature proportions. As a longitudinal pattern the individual is now fixated and further growth is diverted in other directions.

The business of living takes on new meanings and new values. Life embraces Thanatos, the pleasure principle—masochism.

The masochistic feature of Thanatos is most patent in the diverted behavior of the female. She who was previously narcissistically bound, primping and pampering her own psyche and soma, now in the impulsion of the erotic drive, solicits and relishes the invasion of her being in a multitude of ways and manners. How great is the contrast between the meticulously groomed youngster standing on the threshold of womanhood, and the female big with child, blissful in expectation though swollen in proportions. The masochism of the birth ordeal and the masochism so picturesquely manifest in nursing and in caring for the infant child are attestations of the predominance of Thanatos over the innocent, narcissistic Eros that governed the early years of the individual's life. I said the masochistic component is most patent in the diverted behavior of the female. However, it is equally present but not as starkly manifest in the behavior of the male. This is more easily observed in the lower forms of life. I suppose the classical example is that of the males of certain species of spider *Avanea Diadema,* who after impregnating the female, yield to her also their little mite of matter and are thus immediately incorporated in the progeny. There are in effect many instances of overt-masochistic behavior to be observed among the male members of different animal species and these are commensurate in degree and quality, though different in pattern, with those characteristic of the *female of the species.* I underscore this in order to make the point that the masochism labeled *feminine* is in effect characteristic of both sexes. It is a feature of the living experience and not a prerogative exclusively of the female. It is to be borne in mind that both male and female salmon swim upstream to spawn and die. All of this is growth by procreation—and it is under the sway of Thanatos. It represents the investment of one's surplus, as well as of one's capital, in some being other than oneself. It is in effect a process in which attrition is also a significant feature. We wear ourselves out in living for others, and when we do it gladly and unmindfully we yield to that "death instinct" which is the fulfillment of life.

Thanatos in this sense is no figment of the imagination and no mere play on words. It is not death outright, nor yet a lugubrious "dying by degrees" such as the hopeless consumptive of time past might have portrayed. But it *is* a reversal of the earlier living process, that of pristine Eros. It is giving rather than taking, yielding rather than appropriating. It is growth by procretion rather than by accretion.

At this stage of our psychiatric knowledge we can better attest to the validity of the principles cited by the data of pathology than by those of physiology. Hence the warrant for the negative formulation of my thesis. "They who fear to die lack the courage to live." We have more data drawn from our clinical experience to support this negative formulation than we could muster in support of the positive affirmation.

The cases that illustrate the negative formulation are commonplace. These are the individuals narcissistically bound and egocentrically fixated. They may marry and even beget a child or two, very seldom more. Yet, they cannot yield of themselves. The male of this order is likely to be sparing of his seminal substance and yield it up grudgingly. One such whom I treated for a period, a man in his early forties, would have intercourse only on Saturday night. He required, so he claimed, all of Sunday and the remainder of the work-week to recuperate. He regarded his wife not as a partner with whom he formed an organic union, but rather as a separate but parallel being. He insisted on her working at a job, even after his own income was more than adequate to provide for both their needs and for their future security as well. Understandably he was the comptroller at a large bank. The couple had no children, by design. Fifteen years of such coexistence made a dipsomaniac of the wife. The husband elected for his mistress a young married woman, the mother of several children, whose husband was as dependent and narcissistic as her lover. It is pertinent to observe that my patient was the only child in a family disrupted first by the father's abandonment of the mother, and subsequently by divorce. When twelve years of age, and in a fit of hatred inspired by the mother, my patient armed himself with a revolver and set out to find and kill his father. Fortunately, he did not find the father. When the parents' divorce was granted, he sought and obtained permission to take the mother's familial name rather than his father's. His great ambition in life was to "make a million dollars."

Though characterologically he was repugnant, he was outwardly, that is, as a person, rather attractive. This, be it observed, is a common and seemingly paradoxical feature of this order of person. Probably because of their large narcissistic investment they give the appearance of inner security and of an affability the shallowness of which cannot be perceived until sounded for depth. These personages cannot, however, be classed with the psychopathic inferior personality. They are not really "rotten." They do not overtly cheat, lie, make vain promises, and are not parasitical. They are not psychotic and not even neurotic in the classical sense of the word, that is, they are not agitated by an inner conflict. As might be expected, their superego is not well developed or well defined, except in relation to the elementary phases of interpersonal relations, those taught to and generally acquired by the child, that is, factual truth and objective honesty. Not infrequently this type of personality is found to possess and to exercise a high intellectual awareness of social injustice. They may be "outraged" by the economic and social disabilities suffered by the "disinherited" and the "underprivileged," but their "outrage" is mainly intellectual, academic, and is freighted with little affect. The conviction seems warranted that with the intellectually gifted among this order of personality, preoccupation with the Masses is a compensation for the indwelling inability to invest in lover and child. The biographical data of many men and women famed as revolutionaries reinforce this conviction.

I have sketched the male example; now I would delineate the female counterpart. The task is a bit more taxing. A finer discrimination is requisite. Narcissism is in a greater measure the normal component of the female personality. It is a counterbalance to the primal masochism of the female. Veblen went astray, as do so many economists and economically oriented sociologists when they enter the realm of the psychological, in ascribing the exhibitionistic adornment of the female to the gesture of conspicuous consumption. The biological rationale of "powder and paint," of "jewels and perfumes," is more profound and more subtle than Marx or Veblen ever conceived. For all this it is more difficult to "spot" the *fixedly* immature female. Outwardly she may have all the stigmata of adult femininity. She may be well developed, enticing, flirtatious, and even seductive. But when put to the test of performance she is found to be wanting. She is frequently sexually frigid, but in an odd way, that is, not incapable of erotic tension or even of orgasm, but capable of these only on her own terms and on her own conditions. She is not responsive and conforming, but dictating and exacting. When she does not reach orgasmic climax, she is likely to blame her partner for not being "considerate" of her. When her partner initiates sexual play, she is prone to be unresponsive and to charge him again with being inconsiderate of her. Childbearing she is inclined to consider not as the fulfillment, but rather as the exacting price of marriage. As is to be expected, such a female frequently has difficulties in conceiving, is sickly during the period of gestation, and has a hard time delivering. She seldom can nurse her child, and when milk *is* abundant, soon acquires cracked nipples, mastitis, or other disabilities, which serve to terminate nursing. She seldom cares for her children in person, but rather turns their care over to a nurse, governess, kindergarten, boarding school, etc., acording to her economic status and the child's age. She is not averse to working in order, as she will affirm, to "help support" the home. However, as a "working woman" she is more likely to be an economic liability than an asset. This type of narcissistically bound female is most easily discerned in her rationalizations, in her philosophy of life. She will loudly protest that men and women are "equal," and will disparage as trivial the manifest differences between them. In the preceding generation she was a militant suffragette and a Lucy Stoner. Currently she is more likely to be "companionable" in that competitive spirit reflected in the popular song. "Anything you can do—I can do better."

As previously noted these persons are not neurotic in the classical sense of that term. But they are "people in trouble." As is to be expected, their difficulties generally become more pressing and more complicated the older they grow. They are embroiled with those who in a natural relation make demands upon them—principally their marital partners and their children. They are in constant competition with their mates, and yield little or nothing to their children. They make a virtue of staying young, of dressing like their children, of being one of the gang. Not infrequently they are the life of the party.

This type of case is difficult to treat. Brill used to designate them as "affect idiots." Fritz Wittels described the female specimen in his volume on love. Oscar Wilde mirrored this order of male personage in his novel, *The Picture of Dorian Gray.*

The etiology in this type of personality deficiency disorder is complex and multiform. It is not constitutionally determined, at least not in a negative sense. The bright, gifted, and attractive, other prerequisite conditions prevailing, are the more likely to suffer the retardation in development, and the fixation at a narcissistic level implicated in these conditions. Contributing factors are being an only child, being the oldest, or the youngest *and* the only member of the sex among the children; doting and indulgent parents, and particularly a soft, non-disciplining father; too great a disparity in favor of the child between the education and abilities of the parents and those of the child, or between one child and its siblings. The lack of religious commitment or its equivalent in ethical professions appears to be a contributing factor. So also is consistent economic security. Adversity, in these connections, would appear to have a something of the jewel about it.

The more ample description of this personality type, the analysis of its psychodynamic derivation and the problems involved in its treatment, though most desirable, would involve me in more of a task than I can at this point undertake. Besides it would distract us from the pursuit of the argument, which involves Freud's concept of the death instinct; to this the personalities described are illustrative but not central. For let me remind you, these cases are negative instances, witnesses in the sphere of pathology, of the psychophysiological principle I have advanced, to wit, that growth is first by accretion and subsequently by procretion, that this is the normal process, and that growth by procretion begins when Thanatos takes over from pristine Eros the governance of the living process. The pleasure-pain principle is modified by and compounded with masochism. It is thus that we find meaning in and justification for the dictum, "Those who fear to die lack the courage to live."

Two final observations need to be made. One concerns the prevailing socio-cultural climate. Currently it is dominated by a vitiated Eros. The emphasis is less on living than on enduring, that is, less on self-fulfillment than on the prolongation of existence. Aging, at almost all levels, except perhaps during the impatient preadolescent period, is regarded as an evil to be fought and to be opposed by every means. Conversely youth is at a premium. Death is regarded either as an unmitigated evil, even when it comes to the grizzly and spent geron, or perversely as an escape from life. In these respects the socio-cultural climate is sickly and sickening.

The other observation to be made concerns Freud's hypothecation of a disruptive, denigrating force which, he postulated, is operative in the organism to the end of bringing the organized matter back to its passive primary state. The existence and the operation of such a force is very doubtful, save in a play of fancy, as one might, for example, postulate a force of darkness indwelling in the candle's light which seeks to put it out, that is, to terminate the combustion. But, on the other hand, one can perceive an aversion to living, a pure and simple unwillingness to live, one that is not reactive but is rather an initial manifestation in some schizophrenics, and in some organically sick persons, notably infants and young children. Here the *vis-a-tergo,* the impulsion to live, appears weak or lacking. The disorder is, to my mind, organic and constitutional, and more frequently due to a disproportion in the components of being than to some specific pathology in a given organ or system.

Here I must summate the discussion: In the hypothecation of the death instinct, Freud broached on one of the profoundest problems embraced in life's experiences, that of masochism. The pleasure-pain principle which animates and governs living in the early years of existence, seemingly cannot account for the behavior of the mature healthy individual. It thus becomes necessary either to deny the sovereignty of the pleasure-pain principle during maturity, or to conceive of its elaboration to embrace masochism as well. The death instinct, such as Freud conceived of it, as a disruptive malign power, at war with Eros, cannot be validated in experience. But the death instinct as the fulfillment of Eros, Thanatos as growth by altruism, as investment in others, is to be witnessed in all of life's creatures, and most notably in man. In the cognizance of Thanatos it can thus be securely affirmed that the *who fear not to die have the courage to live.*

REFERENCES

1. FREUD, S.: *Beyond the Pleasure Principle.* New York, Boni and Liveright, p. 47.
2. FREUD, *op. cit.,* p. 79.
3. FREUD, *op. cit.,* p. 10.
4. FREUD, *op. cit.,* p. 38.
5. FREUD, *op. cit.,* p. 38.
6. FREUD, *op. cit.,* p. 25.
7. FREUD, *op. cit.,* p. 26.
8. WEISS, E.: *Imago,* Bd. XXI, No. 4, p. 393, 1935.
9. *Op. cit.,* p. 396.
10. FREUD, *op. cit.,* p. 3.
11. FREUD, S.: *An Outline of Psychoanalysis,* Chapter 2, New York, W. W. Norton, 1949.
12. BIBRING, E.: *Imago,* Bd. XXII, No. 2, pp. 147-176, 1936.
13. BERNFELD, S.: *Imago,* Bd. XXI, No. 2, pp. 125-142, 1935.
14. JONES, E.: *The Brit. J. of Psychology,* Gen. Sec. XXVI, part 3, pp. 273-288, 1936.
15. FREUD, S.: The economic problem in masochism, in *Collected Papers,* London, The Int. Psychoanalytic Library, Vol. 11, p. 255, 1924.
16. FREUD, *Collected Papers, loc. cit.,* p. 257.
17. FREUD, *Collected Papers, loc. cit.,* p. 257.
18. BERNFELD, S., *op. cit.,* pp. 136-137.
19. FREUD, *Collected Papers, loc. cit.,* p. 265.

18

Sophocles Contra Freud: A Reassessment of the Oedipus Complex

THE THEORETICAL edifice of Freud's psychoanalysis is resplendent with many conceptions and formulations. Freud was not only a master of the word, he was also skilled in the use of analogy. He was even more apt in the invention of provocative, startling, and suggestive terms and phrases with which to epitomize and to label significant components of his theoretical system. Thus, for example, Freud did not merely call attention to the sexuality of the child, but further described the child as a polymorphous, perverse little animal. The expression "anal-erotic" not only aptly described the compulsively fixated individual, but was calculated to stir and rattle the Victorian generation. What could better describe the Id than the term "Id": the elemental, the primitive, the *uralt*. And as for the Super-ego, how could you name it better? Certainly conscience is not its equivalent, for conscience is all-too-much the policeman and does not include, as Super-ego does, the aspiratory element. How apt is the expression "transference neurosis," and how suggestive and translucently illuminating is the term "counter-transference." *Abreaktion* is a harsh Germanic term, for which the more mellifluous Latin and Anglo-Saxon tongues provide no equivalent, but the very sound of that term is in itself suggestive.

Indeed, as one observes the superb skill with which Freud manipulated terms and expressions, one cannot but become suspicious that through this art Freud at times unwittingly seduces our reason. By the aptness of his terms he leads us to believe that there is vastly more of knowledge and certainty behind his verbal formulations than we do indeed find there, when in a less dazzled mood we soberly inspect their meaning content.

In affirming all this, I would not have you believe that Freud deliberately set out to mislead us, or that I would charge him with a kind of

248

verbal charlatanry. On the contrary, with deep respect for his genius, I intend only to underscore the fact that often there was more poetry than science in his expositions, and that frequently, even though his arguments were poor and his deductions faulty, his theme and thesis were of transcending import.

Contrary to the insistence of certain medical historians psychiatry is a very ancient discipline, in some respects even antedating clinical medicine itself. Yet despite the antiquity of psychiatry Freud's psychoanalysis stands forth as a unique achievement, as unique as Pasteur's germ theory, and Claude Bernard's homeostasis. Still, psychoanalysis did not spring like Minerva from the head of Zeus; it has its antecedents, or at least its antecedent components. Freud's psychoanalysis is a compact system,—logically, historically and clinically structuralized. But it is more singular in its formulation than in its elements. The Unconscious, which plays so significant a role in psychoanalytic theory, was known before Freud. The tripart constitution of personality, the Id, the Ego, and the Super-ego, though not thus named, was known to all psychologists since the time of Aristotle, and formed a prominent and integral part of the doxy of the Catholic Church. The significance and the function of dreams had been the preoccupation of many men, and in Plato's *Republic* one finds an illuminating reference to the upwelling, during sleep, of the uncensored cravings of the primal self from out of the depths of the Unconscious. Even the technique of free association was expounded by Galton, Darwin's cousin and the Nestor of genetics.

In tracing the building blocks of the Freudian system to the intellectual and scientific quarries from which they were derived, I do not aim to dim the lustre of Freud's originality. Quite the contrary! This exposition is but a prelude to my treatment of the most distinguished and the most original element in the Freudian system. I refer, of course, to the Oedipus complex. Though many before Freud treated of dreams, of the Unconscious, of free association, of the significance of slips and errors, one needs must go back to the days of Plato, and to the times of Sophocles to find the subject of the Oedipus complex expounded clearly and boldly.

Freud fully appreciated the pre-eminence of the theory of the Oedipus complex in the theoretical framework of psychoanalysis. In his psychoanalytic testament (1) he wrote: "I venture to assert that if psychoanalysis could boast of no other achievement than the discovery of the repressed Oedipus complex, that alone would give it a claim to be counted among the precious new acquisitions of mankind."

The analytic world concurs in Freud's assessment of the Oedipus complex, and holds it to be nuclear for personality development. Surveying the broad field of contemporary psychiatric thought, not only as it is formulated by Freud and his disciples, but also as it has been cultivated by the so-called Freudian deviationists and by those others who, though not disciples of Freud, are yet inspired and instructed by the data of dynamic psychiatry, one finds that the understanding and interpretation of the Oedipus complex is crucial to all systems of psychiatric theory, and to all the different patterns of their praxis. *Nolens volens* they each must take their stand on this score. This is indeed clearly reflected in a work recently published by Mullahy, entitled *Oedipus: Myth and Complex* (2). This work reviews and summates the different interpretations, the differences in accent and assessment which the more significant psychiatric schools of thought have accorded to the Oedipus myth and complex.

The Oedipus complex is indeed nuclear to personality development, and for that reason commands the most earnest, the most devoted, and the most penetrating study. I intend to contribute to this objective by reassessing the Oedipus complex. I want to counterpose Sophocles' treatment of the Oedipus Myth in the fifth century B.C. to Freud's exposition of it 2,400 years later. Since I have entitled this presentation *Sophocles Contra Freud* it is evident that I think there is some difference, and it *is* my intention to demonstrate not only that Freud misread the tragedy of Oedipus as represented by Sophocles, but that he has drawn certain psychological lessons from the Oedipal Myth which are not there to be drawn.

Freud dealt with only one of the three plays which Sophocles devoted to the Myth of Oedipus. He based his elaborate deductions on the single play *Oedipus Rex*. But Sophocles wrote three plays involving Oedipus —*Antigone, Oedipus Rex,* and *Oedipus at Colonus* and, be it noted, in just this order. For the contemporaries of Sophocles, the Oedipal Myth was not entirely embraced in the tragedy of *Oedipus Rex,* which mirrors but a portion of the "crimes and punishment" of the House of Labdacus. The incest of Oedipus was not the beginning of the tragedy of the House of Labdacus, but its mid-point. It highlights the Nemesis that followed upon the ubris of the House of Labdacus. The incest of Oedipus was not an initial crime but a consequent to the crimes of the father. *Oedipus Rex, Oedipus at Colonus,* and *Antigone* collectively portray the Greek version of the warning in *Exodus* that "the iniquity of the fathers shall be visited upon their children even unto the third and fourth generation." (Exodus, XX-5.)

At this point it is desirable to fix in our minds the essential plot of

Oedipus Rex. Laius, the father of Oedipus and the husband of Jocasta, was without issue. He consulted the Oracles and was informed by them that if a son were born to him, he, Laius, would die at the hand of his son. In due time a son was born to Laius and Jocasta. That child, later named Oedipus, was, on the third day following his birth, turned over by his mother Jocasta, to a shepherd with instructions that he be cast away to perish. But Oedipus did not perish. He was discovered by another shepherd and brought to the childless King of Corinth, Polybus, by whom he was raised as his own son. Then when Oedipus was grown to the stature of a man, stirred by doubt, he consulted the Oracle at Delphi. The Oracle revealed to him that he was fated to be "the slayer of the sire who begot him" and "to defile his mother's bed." Seeking to escape his destiny, and still believing that Polybus was his father and Merope his mother, Oedipus fled Corinth, hoping thus "to never see the fulfillment of the infamies foretold by his evil doom." But during his flight, at the meeting of three roads, Oedipus was rudely thrust aside by the herald of a man "seated in a carriage drawn by colts." In anger he struck down first the driver and then the old man who had assaulted him with his goad. This old man, unknown to Oedipus, was his very own father Laius, King of Thebes.

In his further wanderings, Oedipus encountered the Sphinx, that chimerical creature half woman, half tiger, who had besieged the land, and who destroyed all those who could not answer the riddle: "What is that creature that in its infancy walks on four members, in its maturity on two, and in its age on three?" Until Oedipus appeared none had unraveled her riddle and Thebes was sorely grieved. But when the Sphinx challenged Oedipus he made the right answer saying: that creature is man, who in his infancy moves on his four members, in maturity on his two feet, and in age supports himself with a staff. Her riddle solved, the Sphinx threw herself upon the rocks and perished. Thebes was liberated and to reward him the Thebans made Oedipus their King and gave him Jocasta for a wife. Out of this incestuous relationship four children were born, two sons and two daughters. Thebes prospered for a time but then a plague broke out in the city, and Thebes was once again sorely stricken. Oedipus consulted the soothsayers and was by them advised that the city was punished because the murderer of Laius had not been found nor was his death avenged. Hearing this Oedipus took an oath pledging himself to discover and to punish the murderer of Laius. Ultimately, by the witness of the shepherd to whom he was given as an infant, and by that of the other shepherd who brought him to the childless King of Corinth,

Oedipus is revealed to have been the murderer of his father and to have had incestuous relations with his mother.

Following on these catastrophic revelations Jocasta hanged herself, and Oedipus struck out his eyes. Led by his two daughters he went forth in exile.

This is the essential story of *Oedipus Rex*. The Myth itself is of ancient derivation. It was known long before Sophocles embodied it in his magnificent tragedy. There were several versions of the Myth extant in which the destiny of Oedipus was differently rendered. But these other versions need not concern us, for Freud took his line of departure from the *Oedipus Rex* of Sophocles. According to Freud, this Greek tragedy mirrored what he believed to be a universal phenomenon: the desire of the young child to have incestuous relations with his mother, and to destroy the father who stood in the way of their attainment.

Freud maintained that every child is fated to pass through the Oedipus complex. This is what Freud has to say on this score:

"When a boy, from about the age of two or three, enters upon the phallic phase of his libidinal development, feels pleasurable sensations in his sexual organ and learns to procure these at will by manual stimulation, he becomes his mother's lover. He desires to possess her physically in the ways which he has divined from his observations and intuitive surmises of sexual life and tries to seduce her by showing her the male organ of which he is the proud owner. In a word, his early awakened masculinity makes him seek to assume, in relation to her, the place belonging to his father, who has hitherto been an envied model on account of the physical strength which he displays and of the authority in which he is clothed. His father now becomes a rival who stands in his way and whom he would like to push aside. If when his father is absent he is able to share his mother's bed and if when father returns he is once more banished from it, his gratification when his father vanishes and his disappointment when he reappears are deeply felt experiences. This is the subject of the Oedipus complex, which Greek legend translated from the world of childhood phantasy into a pretended reality. Under the conditions of our civilization it is invariably doomed to a terrible end" (3).

Let me underscore the fact that Freud does not merely affirm that the child has a strong attachment to the mother. Freud specifically says that the little boy "desires to possess her [the mother] physically in the ways which he has divined from his observations and intuitive surmises of sexual life": in other words, that he specifically desires to have sexual intercourse with her. Freud ascribes to the young child what I would call *infantile* incestuous desires. These are to be distinguished from the incestuous desires of the adult.

Upon this basic assumption Freud then builds an intricate superstructure involving the so-called castration fear, the resolution of the Oedipus complex, and the concomitant flowering forth of the Super-ego. It is best to quote Freud's own words on these scores. After having described what he believes to be the universal infantile incestuous strivings of the young boy, Freud goes on to say:

"The boy's mother understands quite well that his sexual excitement refers to her. Sooner or later she thinks to herself that it is wrong to allow this state of things to continue. She believes she is acting rightly in forbidding him to manipulate his genitals. The prohibition has little effect and at the most brings about some modification in his method of self-gratification. At last his mother adopts the severest measures; she threatens to take away from him the thing he is defying her with. As a rule, in order to make the threat more terrifying and more credible, she delegates its carrying out to the boy's father, saying that she will tell him and that he will cut the penis off. Strangely enough, this threat only operates if another condition is fulfilled, either before or afterwards. In itself it seems quite inconceivable to the boy that anything of the sort could happen. But if when he is threatened he is able to recall the appearance of female genitals, or if shortly afterwards he has a glimpse of them—of genitals, that is to say, which really lack this supremely valued part, then he takes what what he has heard seriously and coming under the influence of the castration complex, experiences the severest trauma of his youthful existence" (4).

Whatever else one might say about Freud's primary and secondary elaborations on the Oedipus complex, one must grant that they are most ingenious! But their very ingenuity renders them suspect. Freud premises the sequential concatenation of many events, and one is impelled to wonder just how often this chain of events is likely to be linked in just that way. And what happens if one of the links is missing or is "out of order." What, if the mother does not adopt the severest measures to forbid the child to manipulate his genitals? What, if she does not threaten "to take away from him the thing he is defying her with." What, if she does not tell the father of the son's disobedience, and what happens when she does not threaten the child that the father will cut his penis off. What, if the child does not see the female genitalia until he is much older, or, seeing them is not shocked at all.

The more critically one studies the tortured formulations of Freud's theory of the Oedipus complex, the more inescapable is the conviction that in this instance Freud was traduced by his daring and betrayed by his ingenuity. Did Freud read aright the myth of Oedipus? Does the story of *Oedipus Rex* told by Sophocles really warrant Freud's deduction? Freud himself appears to be aware of certain difficulties, for he admits that the plot of the tale "constitutes a deviation from the analytical subject matter since Oedipus killed his father and married his mother unknowingly." But Freud, having noted these difficulties, seeks to evade them by propounding nebulous generalizations on poetic principles. Freud writes:

"One hears the objection made that the legend of King Oedipus has in fact no connection with the construction made by the analysis: the case was quite a different one, since Oedipus did not know that it was his father whom he killed and his mother whom he married. What is overlooked in this is that a distortion of this kind is unavoidable if an attempt is made at a poetic handling of the material, and that there is no addition of extraneous subject matter but merely a skillful employment of the factors present in the theme" (5) .

In the light of what we know of the Greek playwrights' ingenuity and of their boldness, one must wonder what warrant there may be for Freud's categoric statement that "a distortion of this kind is unavoidable in the poetic handling of the material." Freud was a great psychiatrist, but one must question his competences as a literary critic and as a dramaturge, the more so when one observes a footnote to the above cited paragraph, wherein Freud ventures the opinion "that the name William Shakespeare is most probably a pseudonym behind which there lies concealed a great unknown" (6).

Did Freud interpret the Myth of Oedipus correctly? My conviction is that he did not. Freud distorted the meaning of the Myth to suit his preconceptions. That is a great pity, for the Myth of Oedipus is pregnant with great meaning, and Freud, having misread it, perpetrated a double injury: the promulgation of his own errors and the blocking of a proper understanding of the meaning of the Myth.

Let us see how the Myth is treated by Sophocles. Sophocles wrote three plays which involve the parents and the children of Oedipus, *Antigone, Oedipus Rex,* and *Oedipus at Colonus*. These plays, be it noted, do not really constitute a trilogy in the traditional sense of that term. Sophocles did not pick up the theme at its beginning and follow it through its logical course. Actually he wrote on the last part first. He composed the tragedy of *Antigone* before he wrote *Oedipus Rex* and *Oedipus at Co-*

Ionus. However, in the three plays Sophocles portrays the bitter fate and the cruel destinies of the House of Labdacus.

To understand just what Sophocles intended to convey in these plays one needs to visualize the author and his plays in the setting of his land and times. One must appreciate the function of drama in Greek society. One must know the moral and philosophical bias of the contemporary thought. This would be a vast undertaking were we called upon to forge it for ourselves. Fortunately such is not the case for we can draw upon the knowledge and understanding of many pre-eminent scholars ranging from Plato and Aristotle, to Gilbert Murray and Werner Jaeger.

Sophocles was one of the three great dramatic poets in Greek culture. He stood between Aeschylus who was thirty-five years his senior, and Euripides who was fifteen years his junior. He lived in the golden era of Greek culture in the fifth century B.C. He was a contemporary and friend of Pericles. He was by the witness of those who knew him an extraordinary person, wise, temperate, and a sober observer of human beings. It was said that Aeschylus wrote of man as he ought to be, and Sophocles of man as he was. Here it is proper to inquire what was the function of the dramatic poet in the Greek society of the fifth century. To understand that we must needs know what it was that troubled the minds of the Greeks of this period.

Werner Jaeger (7) offers a direct and succinct answer to this question. "The Greeks of the sixth and fifth centuries," he writes, "had long been brooding on the great religious problem: why does God send suffering into the life of man?" During the preceding centuries it was commonly believed that man was the plaything of the gods and that man's destiny reflected no more than the caprice of the Olympians. When Aesop was asked what was Zeus engaged in, he answered: "In humbling the exalted and in exalting the humble" (8). In the purview of Aesop, the gods were jealous of man, and they smote him at will to keep him humble. But in the fifth century B.C. this common and primitive viewpoint was challenged by the dramatic poets. Aeschylus expounded the moral thesis that each man fares according to his deserving, that even the individual life, viewed in its happiness and misery, is long enough to justify the ways of God to man. In the tragedies of Aeschylus, Nemesis or divine justice displaces divine jealousy (9). Not the gods but man himself is the ultimate arbiter of his destiny. For the exposition of this lesson on the selfhood of man the dramatic poets chose as vehicles the great myths of Greece. Werner Jaeger phrased it thus: "Tragedy was the first type of poetry to apply to mythical tradition a regular structural principle—the conception of the inevitable rise and fall of human destiny, with its sudden reversals and its final catastrophe" (10).

The theatre was the great teaching institution of the Greek populace. The dramatic poets taught the man of the Greek polis to recognize the tie between crime and punishment. Instead of thinking of man as the helpless plaything of the Gods, he came to see him as the arbiter of his own destiny and hence the begetter of his own misery.

This newer persuasion raised the stature of man. It imparted dignity to his person, and provided him with the foundation for a sound morality. But it also made more acute the problem of fate and of free will. It brought to the fore the soul-stirring questions of corporate guilt, and of long deferred punishment. Most of all it evoked that most troubling query—"Wherefore are the innocent children guilty and punishable for the transgressions of the sinful father?"

This was a problem that no less agitated the Hebrew prophets than the dramatic poets of Greece. For it had been said among the descendants of Abraham that the sins of the father shall be visited upon his children even unto the third generation. True, it was not entirely clear whether the children were to be punitively afflicted for their father's sins, or whether the children of the transgressing father would perforce suffer the inevitable consequences of their father's sins. The prophet Ezekiel (Chapter 18) rejected the first interpretation and freed the notion of moral responsibility from all ties of blood relationship. "What mean ye, that ye use this proverb, The fathers have eaten sour grapes, and the children's teeth are set on edge? . . . The soul that sinneth it shall die. The sons shall not bear the iniquity of the father, neither shall the father bear the iniquity of the son."

According to Plutarch, Euripides also boldly accused the gods of grave injustice in visiting the sins of the parents upon the children. The moral indignation of the prophets is noble and inspiring. But the sobereyed poets were troubled by the witness of that which could be construed only as the unassuaged operations of a malignant hereditary curse. Life and legend told of numerous families in which, because of some ancestral crime, the taint of guilt was transmitted in the blood, and generation after generation was visited by the anger of the gods.

This was the problem that stirred the souls of the dramatic poets, and to this problem both Aeschylus and Sophocles devoted their genius and their skills.

Aeschylus appears to have been the less clear in his mind on these issues. He argued that not actual guilt but the tendency to guilt is inherited. He deemed man the master of his own fate, for a man could foster the tendency to guilt, or he could resist it. An act of will, said Aeschylus, is necessary to wake the curse into life (11). But in his dramatic presentations Aeschylus for the most part portrayed "the natural continuity of guilt." In *Agamemmon* (Lines 758-60) Aeschylus affirms: "The impious deed leaves after it a progeny, all in the likeness of the parent stock."

The main burden of the tragedies of Aeschylus is "that as crime engenders crime in the individual heart, so in a house the guilt of the fathers tends to lead the children into new guilt and to extend itself over a whole race" (12).

This torturing problem, the weight of the sins of the father upon the destinies of the children, lies at the core of the Sophoclean plays. This is the issue about which revolve the tragedies of Oedipus. *Oedipus Rex, Oedipus at Colonus,* and *Antigone* set forth in majestic proportions the calamitous interplay of sin and suffering in parent and child. From this purview it is patent that the incest of Oedipus was not an initial crime but rather a derivative punishment, and that this punishment gave issue in turn to other crimes.

Freud appears to have completely missed this. In *Oedipus Rex* Sophocles exhibits the utmost depths of degradation, patricide and incest, to which the son may be reduced whose father and mother are unmindful of their moral obligations.

Let us look more closely at the tragic destinies of the House of Labdacus. We begin with Laius, the father of Oedipus. He was childless and had inquired of the Oracle as to the prospects of issue. He was told that if he had a son, he would lose his life by the hand of his own child. There is in this prophecy of the Oracle a something of transcendent depth and meaning, for if the prophecy is understood not in its literal but in its symbolic sense, then it becomes clear that every father is consumed in his parenthood and that every son "displaces" his father in the love of the mother. But that aside, and even assuming that the prophecy is to be understood in its literal rather than in its symbolic meaning, then still Laius the father and Jocasta the mother of Oedipus are guilty of murder. For on the third day after his birth Oedipus, bound in foot, was given to a shepherd, to be cast away to perish.

Here then is the initial crime. It engendered a progeny of other crimes. It led to the destruction of Oedipus, of his parents Laius and Jocasta, and of his progeny.

To grasp the full import of the tragedy of *Oedipus Rex*, we need to ask, as Sophocles appears to have asked, what might have happened if, despite the prophecy of the Oracle, Laius and Jocasta had rejoiced in the birth of their son, and had nurtured him in love and care. Might not then the fates have been mollified? Might not the transcending goodness, and the enduring virtue of Laius have served as an all-encompassing shield against the dire menace of the outrageous prophecy?

I have advisedly said that Sophocles *appears* to have asked these questions, for Sophocles was not an Isaiah. He wrestled with, he defined and clarified, but did not resolve the moral issue expounded in his tragedies. Yet even though he does not give a clear nor ultimate answer to the Why of Oedipus' fate, he pleads his partial innocence. When, in the play, *Oedipus at Colonus,* Oedipus is taunted by the Chorus he defends himself passionately and with pathos.

To the Chorus Oedipus says:

"I have suffered misery, strangers,—suffered it through unwitting deeds, and of those acts—be Heaven my witness!—no part was of mine own choice."

When Creon, the brother of Jocasta, names him "a patricide,—a polluted man,—a man with whom had been found the unholy bride of her son," Oedipus speaks this soul-searing speech:

"O shameless soul, where thinkest thou falls, this thy taunt,—on my age, or on thine own? Bloodshed—incest—misery—all this thy lips have launched against me,—and all this I have borne, woe is me! but no choice of mine: for such was the pleasure of the gods, wroth, haply, with the race from the old. Take me alone, and thou couldst find no sin to upbraid me withal, in quittance whereof I was driven to sin thus against myself and against my kin. Tell me, now,—if, by voice of oracle, some divine doom was coming on my sire, that he should die by a son's hand, how couldst thou justly reproach me therewith, who was then unborn,—whom no sire had yet begotten, no mother's womb conceived? And if, when born to woe—as I was born—I met my sire in strife, and slew him, all ignorant what I was doing, and to whom,—how couldst thou justly blame the unknowing deed?" (13).

And yet though Oedipus was not knowingly guilty of the crimes of patricide and incest, he was guilty of obdurate impiety—of what the Greeks termed *nosos phrenoon,* a frenzy of the spirit that hastened his destruction. This is witnessed in numerous passages but nowhere more forcefully than in *Oedipus at Colonus.* When Antigone, the daughter of Oedipus, pleads for her brother Polyneices who has come to beg for

Oedipus' blessings, Oedipus refuses to see him. Antigone, addressing her father, says:

"Thou art his sire; so that, e'en if he were to wrong thee with the most impious of foul wrongs, my father: it is not lawful for thee to wrong him again.

"Look thou to the past, not to the present,—think on all that thou hast borne through sire and mother; and if thou considerest those things, well I wot, thou wilt discern how evil is the end that waits on evil wrath; not slight are thy reasons to think thereon, bereft, as thou art, of the sight that returns no more" (14).

Oedipus yields, but instead of blessing Polyneices, he curses him and his brother:

". . . begone, abhorred of me, and unfathered!—begone, thou vilest of the vile, and with thee take these curses which I call down on thee—never to vanquish the land of thy race, no, nor even return to hill-girt Argos, but by a kindred hand to die, and slay him by whom thou hast been driven out" (15).

In this curse lies the doom of his sons and also the seed of the fatal tragedy of Antigone.

Tempting though it is to pursue further the destinies of the House of Labdacus, I must limit myself to the exposition already made: and *that*, I feel certain, fully supports the conclusion that Freud failed to grasp the meaning of the Sophoclean play *Oedipus Rex*. I will not reargue the argument, but merely cite the conclusion. The patricide and incest of Oedipus were not *his* crimes, but the dire consequences of the guilts of Laius, his father, Jocasta, his mother, and of Oedipus' own *ubris*. There is nothing in *Oedipus Rex* to justify Freud's contention that the play expounds the universality of the infantile incest wish. This play, and the other two, teach quite another lesson, one that reflects on the father rather than on the son, that has to do with moral fortitude, with love, with charity and with mercy, rather than with sexuality in general, and with infantile incest longings in particular.

But here another problem comes to the fore. Granting that Sophocles does not support Freud's theories on infantile incest, may it not be that they are yet valid—even without Sophocles' consent? Perhaps Freud's only error was to call on the *Oedipus Rex* for witness. This query transposes the problem of the infantile incest wish from out the realm of the Greek tragic poets into that of a clinical psychiatry. Now we need to inquire not what Sophocles said and meant, but rather what experience teaches. But here again we are confronted with the witness of the side effects of

Freud's ingenuity in coining terms and phrases. His inventions are like some highly polished objects which, because they are so very scintillating, render it difficult to discern their contours and to define their borders. Freud's terms, Oedipus Complex, Castration Fear, and Penis Envy, are so convenient and suggestive that in wide usage they have outrun the confines of the meaning originally given them by Freud. Thus many psychiatrists who do not at all subscribe to Freud's ideas on infantile incest, employ the term Oedipus Complex to describe the sensually determined affect bond between mother and child, and between child and father.

Castration Fear, and Castration Complex are very apt terms wherewith to describe psychological emasculation. Yet their usage does not bind one to the literal meaning of castration. Penis Envy hardly means the subjective wish for the objective virile member, but describes rather discontent with, fear and rejection of, femininity and in consequence an envy of male prerogatives, most often without any real comprehension of what those prerogatives imply.

In canvassing the experience and judgment of psychiatrists it is imperative that we should be alert to the fluidity in meaning with which many psychoanalytic terms in general, and the Oedipus Complex in particular are used.

It is correct to say that only the devout and worshipful disciples of Freud still accept his dicta on the Oedipus Complex in their pristine form. Most others, as Mullahy (16) has clearly shown, differ from Freud, some few in minor, and the greater number in major respects. Neither Alfred Adler nor Jung accept Freud's version of the Oedipus Complex. Otto Rank obfuscates it with his theories on the Birth Trauma. Erich Fromm, who has devoted much thought and study to the Oedipus Complex, sees it "not as a symbol of the incestuous tie between mother and son, but as the rebellion of the son against the authority of the father." Sullivan, while assigning a determining role to the parents and especially to the mother, in the "shaping of the child," rejects the idea that the role is a sexual one, even in the wide sense in which Freud conceives of sexuality. Karen Horney is even more outspoken; not only does she reject Freud's formulation of the Oedipus Complex but argues further that Freud's classic formulation can have dangerous consequences. For while we are preoccupied with the alleged infantile incest wish, we are prone to overlook the most important of all of the child's needs—interest in, and respect for, the child, and the necessity for real warmth, reliability and sincerity by the parents.

The consensus of clinical psychiatric experience does not support

Freud's contentions that every little boy desires to physically possess his mother "in the ways which he had divined from his observations and intuitive surmise of sexual life." Freud's formulation of the Oedipus Complex as the universal and specific infantile incest wish, must be rejected as unproved and in error. And yet, this does not quite dispose of it. The curtain is not thus to be rung down on Sophocles—nor on Freud either. We are impelled to temper the finality of our judgment with Galileo's immortal phrase: *E pure si muove*. This concept *is* vital: it stirs and is stirring, if not with the vision of Freud, then with that of Sophocles. Yet Freud cannot be counted out, for it was *his* inspiration to link the Sophoclean tragedy with the dynamics of the child's psychic growth, with its maturation and with the growth of its Super-ego. Moses, with whom Freud nurtured a deep identification, did not enter the Promised Land, but it was he who led the enslaved hordes through the wilderness to the very gates of the Promised Land.

In the Oedipal Myth there is embodied the concept of the parental matrix within which the nascent personality and the psyche of the child are nurtured and fashioned. Where there is love of parent for parent, and yet so much free scope as to include in the embrace of affection also the child, there the child will effectively learn how to fulfill the tasks and to meet the challenges of its own growth and maturation, and reciprocally will bear affection for the parents. But where the parents themselves are immature, and encumbered with neurotic reaction and behavior patterns; where the father knows not how, or is unable to function as male, husband and father, or the mother will not or cannot play her reciprocal roles, there indeed is the child most likely, nay, bound to suffer.

It is this simple yet vital validity that lies at the core of the Oedipal Myth—and not the fancied incest wish of the child. Whosoever, day in day out, treats with those troubled in spirit and mind, with the sick that come to the psychiatrist for help, cannot but recognize that he confronts in his patients not the sins of the children but "those of the fathers." And he must be mindful also that the problem with which Sophocles wrestled confronts him likewise this day, for when he has helped the patient to lay bare the past, to gain insight, he must further help him to act upon his insight. Thus the psychiatrist is at one with Sophocles in holding that the individual's destiny is fashioned not alone by what happens to him but also by what he does about it.

REFERENCES

1. FREUD, S.: *An Outline of Psychoanalysis.* New York, W. W. Norton & Co., 1949, p. 97.
2. MULLAHY, P.: *Oedipus: Myth and Complex.* New York: Hermitage Press, 1948.
3. FREUD, S.: Reference 1, pp. 90-91.
4. FREUD, S.: Reference 1, pp. 91-92.
5. FREUD, S.: Reference 1, p. 95.
6. FREUD, S.: Reference 1, p. 96.
7. JAEGER, W. W.: *Paideia,* translated from the 2nd German edition by Gilbert Highet. New York, Oxford University Press, 1945, Vol. 1, p. 251.
8. BUTCHER, S. H.: *Some Aspects of Greek Genius.* London, Macmillan & Co., 1904, p. 107.
9. BUTCHER, S. H.: Reference 8, p. 109.
10. JAEGER, W. W.: Reference 7, p. 254.
11. BUTCHER, S. H.: Reference 8, p. 116.
12. BUTCHER. S. H,: Reference 8, p. 117.
13. MULLAHY, P.: Reference 2, p. 437.
14. MULLAHY, P.: Reference 2, pp. 443-444.
15. MULLAHY, P.: Reference 2, p. 448.
16. MULLAHY, P.: Reference 2, chapters 6-11.

19

Job, Jung and Freud:
An Essay on the Meaning of Life

THE NAME of Job is not to be found in any of Freud's writings and he has seemingly never concerned himself with this most precious and evocative book. And yet there is ample warrant for linking Freud with Job, and both with Jung. The latter is the more obvious, for Jung (1) has published a tortured work which he offered, substantively and by title, as an *Answer to Job*. Freud, too, proffered an answer to Job, but by indirection only, and under several titles: *Totem and Taboo* (2), *The Future of an Illusion* (3), and *Moses and Monotheism* (4).

It must prove immensely interesting and profitable to analyze the answers to Job given by Freud, the skeptical Jew, and by Jung, the ambivalent Protestant and believing Christian. It must prove even more illuminating to explore, in its entrancing profundities, the problem of Job—in the light of the answers given by Freud and Jung.

But first *it is desirable to define* what *is* the problem of Job. At its simplest it can be stated as "the problem of evil" (5). Why is there evil in life? Why does evil befall the innocent, the young, the blameless, the just, the virtuous? Why are not the wicked ever and always and in the measure of their wickedness smitten with evil?

But this is the problem of Job phrased at its most elementary and most primitive level. The problem of Job concerns also the relation of man to God, and of God to Man. Can and does God love and favor the man Job, whom he freely exposes to the malevolent trials of Satan? And can Job persist in his devotion to God, despite all his unmerited affliction? Why does not Job follow his wife's counsel—to curse God and die—since that would so obviously "square accounts" with his Creator, and bring a final end to his torturesome afflictions?

263

The problem of Job involves much more. It embraces the all-encompassing problem of "what life is about"—What is its meaning? How can the sentient man meaningfully relate himself to its puzzling, paradoxical, frustrating adventures, and to its inevitable terminus in death?

The Book of Job is a post-exilic masterpiece, and its composition is dated circa 400 B.C. It has engaged the interest of innumerable scholars throughout the ages, down to our own times. One of the very finest expositions of The Book of Job was published in 1920 by Morris Jastrow, Jr. of the University of Pennsylvania (6). His analysis of the text as given in the Hebrew and in the King James version of 1611 leads him to the conviction that in both versions the original Book was altered and corrupted by the inclusion of commentaries and addenda of later origin. In an appendix to his work Jastrow gives the redeemed version of the Book of Job.

The misadversions of the Job text are significant and meaningful to us over and above their exegetic burdens. They reflect some of the early efforts to include in the Book of Job an answer to, as well as the statement of, the problem of Job. Thus it is clear that the four speeches of Elihu represent, as Jastrow phrases it, "an endeavor to find a solution that might save the day for orthodoxy" (6). And the happy ending of the story of Job, wherein Jahveh restores everything to Job in double amount, and prolongs his days on earth to twice the biblical span of three score and ten, argues for the immediacy of the rewards which the Almighty allegedly grants to the worthy this side of heaven. It pleads that all the plaints of Job to the contrary notwithstanding, not evil but justice reigns supreme in life, and in God's relation to man. That, too, is the later-day "answer" proffered by orthodoxy. In the original, the problem of Job remained unanswered, an open question propounded by one of heroic dimensions—a man to challenge God.

The Book of Job, universally acknowledged as *the* masterpiece of the Old Testament and as one of the great creations in world literature, suffers from its celebrity. It is more famed than known; more praised than read. I think then it might be the better part of discretion to treat ourselves to a resumé of the story of Job.

Job is described as a man living in the land of Uz. He is a "perfect" and upright man, one that feared God and eschewed evil. He possesses great wealth and a large family of sons and daughters, on whose behalf he is continually offering sacrifices, to guard against the consequences of some possible secret infidelity on their part. On a certain day, when Satan appears with the Sons of God before the Almighty, the Patriarch is instanced as a perfect man. Satan, however, suggests that his piety is dependent on his wealth, and that if he loses this he will renounce God. Accordingly, Satan is allowed to put him to the test. But even after he has stripped Job of all his possessions and slain all his children, Job says: 'The Lord gave, and the Lord hath taken away; blessed be the name of the Lord.' Still Satan challenges Job's piety; so long as the man himself escapes unscathed, he still has something to fear, and he worships God to save his skin. "But put forth thine hand now, and touch his bone and his flesh, and he will curse thee to thy face." So Satan is allowed to go to any lengths short of actually killing the man. He smites Job 'with sore boils from the sole of his foot unto his crown.' Even Job's wife now fails him, and counsels him to 'curse God and die.' But Job rebukes her saying, 'Shall we receive good at the hand of God, and shall we not receive evil?' Three friends then appear, and for seven days sit by him in mute sympathy. At last Job breaks out in bitter lamentations over his undeserved fate. For this Eliphaz rebukes him, declaring that misfortune is never undeserved. Job answers him, and each of the other accusing friends in turn. But the more he persists in upholding his righteousness, the more vehement his friends become. Job then appeals from man to God. Would that he could find the seat of the Almighty Himself, and there make his defense, and hear the Almighty's words. A fourth friend appears, Elihu, who insists that the power of God silences all question of his justice. Job, he says, is wrong in appealing against the sentence of the Almighty and the Inscrutable. God can have nothing to lose or gain by Job's actions, he cannot be motivated by a vindictive spirit against him, and can only be influenced by pure justice. There the great climax of the drama is reached. The Deity himself appears in the whirlwind and charges Job with presumption—overwhelming him by the tale of his power and wisdom in Nature. Finally, Job confesses his folly and repents 'in dust and ashes.' The friends are rebuked, while Job is approved. After this Job is restored to greater prosperity than ever, and becomes the father of seven sons and three daughters, as before.

Told thus, we have the skeleton but none of the flesh, the beauty, and the inspiration, of the Book of Job. In beauty and sublimity it matches the best ever written by man, from Homer and Aeschylus to our own time. But for the present we are less concerned with the sublimity of the form than with the profundity of the problem which the Book of Job expounds. On this score, however, we must first formulate a certain basis of agreement—agreement as to the essence and nature of the problem.

It can be argued, as indeed it has been, that the Book of Job embodies not one but a host of problems. One can, so to say, find in Job whatever issue in ethics and religion one has a mind to discover. That, however, is not a criticism but rather an attestation to the inspirational fertility of the Book of Job. This is indeed a great work and one may read into it, and draw from it, a variety of meanings and insights, even as one can from its distant homologue—Goethe's *Faust*. Still we must define what *in* and *of* the Book of Job concerns us initially and predominantly. In a measure that has already been affirmed in the very title of this essay. Our initial concern with the Book of Job is psychological. We are interested in discovering to what extent the story of Job represents the story of everyman; how deeply the problem of evil, so sharply brought into relief in the tale of Job's afflictions, corresponds to the problem of evil inherent in the living experience of everyman—this day as in the days of Job.

To begin then, we must agree that the Book of Job is not the unique tale of a mythical personage, but rather the parabolic, or allegorical statement of a timeless issue that darkens man's existence, expressed with moving eloquence and deep passion in the name of Job. We can find its counterpart among the dramas of the Greek playwrights, in the Oedipus trilogy of Sophocles and in the *Medea of Euripides,* for example. Job is patently everyman! What happened to Job is a large scale representation of what typifies the human lot. True, it does not fall to everyman's lot to be bereft at once of fortune and family, to be afflicted with loathsome disorders, and to be upbraided and made suspect by the very friends who had come to console him. But then the Book of Job is composed with the accents of genius, transmuting the prosaic misadventures of life's experience into epic revelations.

Any one of the several misfortunes that befell Job would have sufficed to try his patience and to test his faith in God's justice and mercy. But stark and overfreighted as the tale of Job's afflictions may be, its wholeness, its totality, its cumulative impact, brings it closer to the actuality of human fate than would have the exposition of a singular misfortune. For in its larger sense the Book of Job treats of human destiny and not merely of the caprice of misfortune.

The bereavement of age falls upon all who senesce, and Job was 70 when put on trial. The aged uniformly are bereft of their possessions, be they fortune, kin, friends, peace, or well being. Death is the crowning outrage. No man then can find pristine or ultimate justice this side of heaven, and some suspect that heaven itself was invented to provide the promise of an equilibration of justice and injustice, beyond the ken of the living. Each thoughtful man is faced with Job's problem—Job is everyman.

Here a minor digression is indicated. It is easy and tempting to read into the Book of Job a multitude of preconceptions, and to find in its texts the requisite supporting evidences. But if one were, by an excess of caution, to abstain from every attempt at interpretation, which always involves preconceptions, one would be deprived of all poetic creativity. Thought and experience were then indeed arid and prosaic. The symbol is the soul's vernacular, and the symbol cannot be understood literally, but only transliterally, that is, by being interpreted.

I posit as an interpretation of the Book of Job that it is primarily concerned with the meaning of life, that the issues of evil, and of the relationship between God and Man are implicated issues which, if abstracted from the primary concern with life's meaning, would themselves become meaningless.

And I am persuaded that this conjecture, this preconception if you please, can be validated by much solid, internal evidence. The Book of Job, I hold then, is not primarily a theosophic work. The central figure is neither Satan nor Jahveh, but Job, and the issue is between Job and Job, not between Job and his Creator. Jung is seemingly of the same conviction, but he is brought to it by totally different considerations. Jung perceives in Job "the man who triumphed over Jahveh." "The victory of the vanquished and oppressed," writes Jung, "is obvious: Job stands morally higher than Jahveh. In this respect the creature has surpassed the creator" (8). But we are not yet in a position to take up Jung's *Answer to Job*. I must rather touch on what I consider to be some of the internal evidence justifying the opinion that the Book of Job is primarily philosophical rather than theosophical. I mean that the significance of the God figure is encompassed in the meaning of life, rather than the reverse. Historically, of course, the relation between the two is circular, but in the Book of Job the relation is magnificently fixed, contemplated, and expounded. Job's affirmation "Though He slay me, yet will I trust in Him," is an election, an attestation of will and not a confession of impotence. It is still meaningful, though never as sublime an affirmation when, in the credo of the Existentialist, Life displaces the Almighty. "Though life slay me, as indeed it inevitably must, yet will I trust in it. It also will be my salvation." Job exempts his Creator when he rebukes the foolish counsel of his wife "to curse God and die" with these simple words: "What shall we receive good at the hand of the Lord, and shall we not receive evil?" Palpably Job intended life no less than the Lord, for is not the will, the intention of God made manifest in and through life? And yet, as I shall show later, God cannot be equated to the immediacies of life, and Job never intended such an equation. Job was not an Existentialist.

It is of interest that Job was tried when the days of his life were approaching the end of their biblical allotment. Job was three score and ten years of age when he was afflicted. Granted he was a most righteous and God-fearing man, but surely in the Land of Uz there were other pious and prosperous souls, younger men whom Jahveh might have given over to the sport of Satan. A younger man would have had greater hopes, higher ambitions, and hence deeper frustrations. His afflictions would have been greater, and his lamentations louder. Such a one might indeed have cursed God. Why then did the lot fall upon an old man? Plainly because it *is* the lot of every aging mortal to be so afflicted, but only rarely that of the young. For the young man affliction is misfortune, but for the old it is destiny. By the same compelling reasons it was not a single affliction that tried Job's body and soul, but all of Cassandra's lot, including a shrewish wife and a triplet of unctuous, righteous, and garrulous friends. Job was a man keen in mind and sharp in perception, who had outlived his years and the transient pleasures of the early ages, and who in his lamentations reflected the tragic denouement of life's experience.

In the perspective of his long life Job perceived, as every reflective man must perceive, that there is no indwelling justice in life. Those trivia that are enacted by the occasional men of honesty at the counting tables of the mart or in the magistrates' courts are not justice, but only the exercise of governance in the traffic of man's everyday affairs.

He perceived, as every reflective man must perceive, that Evil indwells in life: Was it not recognized even in humanity's infancy that Father Chronos eats up his own children? Was it not said long, long ago, "only that man is fortunate who was never born?" It was upon these problems that Job brooded. The problems are symbolized in his particular bereavements and afflictions, but they are, in effect, not singular to Job's life but common to everyman's. It is obvious then that the Book of Job is essentially a philosophic work, one that is rooted in life's experience, that seeks to abstract from life's experience the meaning of life, and that seeks to relate both experience and meaning to the all-embracing vision of God. Jastrow, to whose study of the Book of Job I have referred several times, also treats the Book of Job as philosophy (9). According to Jastrow, Job's philosophy was one of protest: one that raised questions, questions that bear upon the meaning of life. "It [the Book of Job] is the protest of profoundly religious spirits," wrote Jastrow, "who seek to unravel the mysteries of life and decline to content themselves with the repetition of meaningless phrases, or to be lulled to rest by a false view of conditions" (10).

To unravel the mysteries of life, not to content oneself with the repetition of meaningless phrases, not to be lulled to rest by false views of actuality, has been the inspiring devotion that motivated the labors of mankind's elect. It was Freud's inspiring devotion, as well as Jung's. But how radically different are the fruits of their respective labors.

Freud, seeking to unravel "the mysteries of life," achieved a great deal in laying bare the mechanisms of the psyche, but in the end he not only found no answer to the meaning of life, but was persuaded that the question itself is meaningless. Life, Freud appears to affirm, is to be experienced, not to be understood. And in life both Men and Nature are malign. "The masses," Freud wrote, "are lazy and unintelligent, they have no love for instinctual renunciation, they are not to be convinced of its inevitability by argument, and the individuals support each other in giving full play to their unruliness" (11) . Nature, according to Freud, traduces us, she "does not ask us to restrain our instincts, she lets us do as we like; but she has her peculiar effective mode of restricting us: she destroys us, coldly, cruelly, callously, as it seems to us, and possibly just through what has caused our satisfaction" (12). In the purview of Freud individual man is on all sides hedged in by malice and malignity. Not love but dread binds man to his fellow men, and the resulting union has the essential character of an armistice 'tween man and man, and a united front of "All against Nature." Insecurity of life, an equal danger for all, Freud affirmed, unites men into one society (13) and it is the principal task of culture, its real *raison d'être,* to defend man against nature (14).

Freud was not a gentle cynic. It is an enticing vision to picture Freud in the circle of Job's friends, sharing in what is called the Symposium, but which, indeed, was rather a lamentation for man and a dirge for life. I can fancy the cynical counsel that Freud would have proffered Job: to resign his childish expectations, the projection into senescence of his infantile wishes; to be stoical in the face of cruel nature which spares no man, and is indifferent to all; to die in the hopeful expectation that some remote generation of man would by the science of probabilities, inspired by the roulette wheel, formulate subtle schemes to insure the Jobs of the future against financial ruination resulting from the loss of their oxen, she-asses, camels, and sheep. In similar vein I can picture Freud consoling Job on the untimely death of his sons and daughthers, and reffecting in sober spirit on the probability that this misfortune will inspire the scientists to discover ways to reinforce human dwellings. And

270 Psychiatry and the Human Condition

to crown this vision, I can fancy Freud commiserating with Job over his plague of boils, and offering consolation in the forecast of the antibiotics, which surely would prove specific against every variety of boil. What I cannot and would not conjure up in fancy is the withering scorn with which Job the Patriarch would respond to Freud's shallow cynicism, and to his naive faith in science.

In this presentiment it is not my intention to be flippant, nor to be disrespectful to the memory of a great man. After all, it was Freud who taught our generations to appreciate the dynamic reality and the potency of the Super-ego. And yet Freud *was* shallow in his cynicism and naive in his Science. Otherwise, could he have failed to understand the full implications of the closing sentences of his *Future of an Illusion,* and understanding them could he have allowed them to stand as published? He wrote: "No, science is no illusion. But it would be an illusion to suppose that we could get anywhere else what *it* cannot give us" (15). This can have but one meaning: "What science cannot give us, cannot be gotten." This must include faith, hope, love, and charity.

Let me further quote Freud. His god is neither Jahveh nor Elohim, but *Logos* (the primacy of the intellect), linked to its twin, *Anaghe* (external reality) . "*Logos,*" Freud affirms, will realize those of our wishes "which external nature permits, but he will do this very gradually, only in the incalculable future and for other children of men. Compensation for us, who suffer grievously from life, he does not promise." *Logos,* Freud's god, is seemingly no more just nor merciful than Job's Jahveh. The problem of evil remains unsolved.

Moses and Monotheism (4) was the last book written by Freud. At the time of its composition he was 82 years of age. It calls for no great perspicacity to recognize that in this exposition Freud identified himself with Moses—even Ernest Jones appreciated it. There is a something sibylline in this identification. Be it recalled that Moses led the Jews to the Promised Land—but did not himself enter it. For Moses had broken faith with the Lord at the Waters of Meribath-Kadesh in the desert of Zion. "Because you did not pay me due honor among the Israelites," said the Lord, "accordingly you shall view the land from a point of vantage; but you shall not enter the land which I am giving to the Israelites." (*Deuteronomy,* 32: 51-52.) Freud led us to, but did not "enter upon" the promised realm of the Super-ego. That remains for his followers and his inheritors to achieve.

The case is otherwise with Jung; but then, Jung is no Moses. This affirmation, I fear, may be a bit cryptic, but it will soon become clear, I trust.

Jung wrote an essay on Job with the title *Answer to Job* (1). The title is without the article "an" or "the." This is a tortured book, involved, discursive, of varying compactness and clarity, now diffuse and misty, now projecting clear and suggestive apparitions, like the face of a beloved one discerned in a cloud or in a fog. It is a distressing work. It irritates and angers. And yet it is so earnest, so groping, so babbling in its effort to articulate profundities, that one cannot cast it off, nor yet reject it.

Jung was 76 years of age when he ventured to catechize himself "as to the nature of those ruling ideas which decide our ethical behaviour and have such important influence on our practical life" (16). But the issues which intrigue Jung most are those dominant in Christianity: Christ as a symbolic figure, the apocalyptic Christ-Antichrist antagonism, the doctrines of redemption and of the *privatio boni*. These are the ruling ideas that preoccupy Jung, and which he believes are involved in the Job symposium. In addition Jung is concerned with the *complexio oppositorum*, with the inclusion in the God figure of the opposites of good and evil. It was this, Jung affirms, that recalled to his mind the story of Job —"Job who expected help from God against God" (17).

Jung's *Answer to Job* is difficult to summarize. Its argument is elusive. One cannot grasp it in any sustained comprehension. At times it appears to be clearly crystallized and then it becomes opaque and amorphous— like sludge. It is not possible to establish from his exposition whether Jung conceives of Jahveh as a conceptual projection of Job's tortured mind, or as a heaven-dwelling tribal deity. He reifies his symbols, and appears to treat them as historical substantialities. It is not possible to arrive at any clear and final conclusion as to whether Jung treats of Christ as a symbolic figure, or is concerned with the symbolic potency of the figure of Christ. One thing does appear certain—Jung writes as a believing Christian, believing in the sense that he sees in Christianity the fulfillment of the Davidic promises, that of the birth and martyrdom of the Messiah. And yet, though patently believing, Jung is not pristinely orthodox. He scorns and ridicules the Christian affirmation that God so loved mankind that for its redemption He martyred His only begotten son—Jesus: "One should" Jung writes, "keep before one's eyes the strange fact that the God of Goodness is so unforgiving that he can only be appeased by a human sacrifice!" "This," he states, "is an insufferable incongruity which modern man can no longer swallow, for he must be blind if he does not see the glaring light it throws on the divine char-

acter, giving the lie to all talk about love and the *Summum Bonum*"
(18). Nor does Jung subscribe to the fundamental Article of Faith, that
Christ *is* the Redeemer, the Messiah, and the Ultimate. He envisages,
rather, if not the advent of a second Messiah, the sustained and continued
operations in man of the Paraclete, the Holy Ghost of Christian dogma.
Half apologetically, half accusingly, Jung writes: "In the interest of continuity and the Church the uniqueness of the incarnation and of Christ's
work of redemption has to be strongly emphasized, and for the same
reason the continuing indwelling of the Holy Ghost is discouraged and
ignored as much as possible. No further individualistic digressions can be
tolerated" (19). Apologetically he adds: "If everybody had tried to thrust
the intuitions of his own private Holy Ghost upon others for the improvement of the universal doctrine, Christianity would rapidly have perished
in a Babylonian confusion of tongues" (20). But the times have changed,
and now, Jung affirms, "the psychotherapist has more to say on these
matters than the theologian, who has remained caught in his archaic
figurative language" (21). The doctor very often is forced by the problems
of psychoneurosis to look more closely at the religious problem, for "in
the last resort the principles which, spoken or unspoken, determine the
moral decisions upon which our existence depends, for weal or woe" are
embraced "in the positive or negative concept of God." In a footnote
Jung adds: "Psychologically the God concept includes every idea of the
ultimate, of the first or last, of the highest or lowest. The name makes no
difference" (22).

Those who are not at home in the vernacular of theological exposition,
and who confront them in the same frame of mind that they bring to
the consideration of mundane matters, must find Jung's words and ideas
wearisome and arid. They are likely to react as Glover did, with a gesture
of total rejection. It's all archaic and vapid nonsense. But, I would humbly
submit, it isn't. Jung speaks an odd and esoteric language, and frames his
argument in the provincial format of Pauline Christianity, but he is a
seer and his vision reveals deep and great profundities. For all the labors
involved, for all the toil it takes, Jung's *Answer to Job* is deserving of
patient and sober study. In the end, it is a rewarding work, an inspiring
and stimulating contribution to the understanding, if not the solution,
of the problem of Job, the problem of the evil inherent in life. For Jung
goes beyond the simple issue of God's justice, and treats of the *function*
of evil in human existence. He posits that evil is an inseparable part of
good, as death is inseparable from life; that good itself would not be
good, apart from evil. Indeed it is the disjunction of the two—the dark

from the light, the left from the right, the low from the high—that has brought our culture and the human race to the brink of individual and collective disaster and annihilation.

This formulation is easily misconceived, for so much depends upon what is intended and understood by evil. Thus Auschwitz was not evil. It was beyond evil, was a prelude to Armageddon. The evil intended is that inherent in existence, and indwelling in the human psyche. It is that part of being which when reconciled and integrated yields all that is uniquely beautiful and esthetically good in culture and in civilization, and which in its highest transmutation engenders the vision of, and devotion to, the God concept.

It is interesting and noteworthy that when disencumbered of its Christian accents, Jung's dicta on good and evil are very similar to the Hasidic version. "The basic doctrine which fills the Hebrew Bible," wrote Martin Buber, "is that our life is a dialogue between the above and the below" (23). This is more explicitly affirmed in the Kabbalah which so largely inspired and fashioned the teachings of Hasidism. ". . . the togetherness of man with God, with God who 'dwells with them in the midst of their uncleanliness,' purifies and hallows all; . . . man must serve God with the evil impulse too; . . . the redemption overcomes the division between clean and unclean, holy and profane; *all* becomes pure and holy," are articles of Hasidic faith (24). It is written: "The abyss has opened; it is no more allowed to any man to live as if evil did not exist. One cannot serve God by merely avoiding evil; one must grapple with it" (25). But to grapple with does not mean to destroy or to repress. "The sparks of the light of God yearn for release from their deepest exile in that which we call evil" (26).

The Talmud teaches that man must serve God with both impulses (good and evil). "The Shekhina embraces both, the 'good' and the 'evil', but the evil not as an independent substance, but as the 'throne of goodness,' as 'the lowest step of utter good.' " (27).

I must resist the temptation to quote more and to expound further, lest this be turned into an essay on Hasidism. Yet I would counsel those who are interested, to read Martin Buber's illuminating book on *Hasidism* (28). It stands in effulgent contrast to Jung's profound but murky exposition.

Freud, too, can be quoted to show that he was not unaware of the problem of good and evil. But Freud was confessedly no philosopher, and the oceanic feeling so requisite to a full appreciation of these matters was alien to his experience, and probably missing among his otherwise rich and varied endowments. His most pertinent contribution to this subject was his *Civilization and its Discontents* (29), a work which he himself felt was rather "commonplace."

I fear that in this exposition Freud may appear to have fared badly and Jung more favorably. I would submit that I am not biased, nor a pleader. Certainly I must not be taken for a Jungian. If I must subscribe, I would subscribe to Paracelsus' motto *"Alterius non sit qui suis esse potest."*

At this point, coming to the end of my presentation, I want to anticipate and to respond to what I would consider a warranted query, namely: "What bearing has this upon psychiatry, and how can it profit the psychiatrist to fathom 'the lesson of Job,' or to wrestle with the problem of Good and Evil?" The obvious answer might be—it all depends upon the psychiatrist and on his understanding of what psychiatry embraces. But such an answer would be rather glib and uninforming. I'd rather respond to the query in earnest and confessionally, that is, in terms of how *I* became involved in this problem.

It was not any religious preoccupation that brought me into this realm, but rather certain very impressive and challenging experiences in psychiatric practice. Over a stretch of time I encountered a significant number of patients whose psychopathies seemingly derived from the absence of an effective Super-ego in the structure and operations of their psychic organism. They apparently did not and could not differentiate between good and evil in an operational sense. They were not dull, they knew in an informed way what the world at large terms "evil," and what it holds to be "good." They furthermore were as law-observing and as honest as the average person, or perhaps not quite as much, but sufficiently so to keep out of legal difficulties. The good and evil they could not understand or appreciate was that which is involved in interpersonal relations. They were not altruist even in the most elementary sense. They were unhappy souls and knew not the sources of their unhappiness. They belonged to that category of patient currently described as suffering from a character neurosis, a designation which I find adequately descriptive but not illuminating as to etiology or psychodynamics. Their pathology could not be understood or explicated in the framework of Freudian psychodynamics, nor in that of any other school of psychiatric thought or teaching. In working with them I was in time persuaded that they lived life primitively, that is, without any orientation as to the human meaningfulness of the living experience. They had no sense of the evil inherent in life, nor of the need to accept and to reconcile the evil in order to gain the good. They were unwilling and unable to renounce, to give up, to yield, what was *seemingly* good, that is pleasurable and gratifying. They saw no reason for doing so. On the contrary, their reason argued *to the contrary*. Why love your neighbor when it was more reasonable and more gratifying to hate him, and besides, as any one can perceive, the neighbor was more deserving of hate than of love? Furthermore, your neighbor takes you for a sucker if you do show him kindness and affection. But for the patients I have in mind the neighbor was not merely *the* neighbor, it was mankind entire.*

The fact, the resulting effect, that they themselves were not loved, that they were unhappy and ineffective, that they were as outcasts among men, taught them nothing and served only to embitter them. When they entered upon therapy, they did so in the expectation that somehow the therapist would conspire with them to devise means and to structure ways by which the nasty horde of humankind might be brought to its kness.

Confronted with this type of patient, with this order of psychopathy, how is one to deal with it? How is one to help the patient? One thing appeared certain to me—no therapist could help who had not in his own way, for himself, and beyond himself, grappled with the problem of Job, with the issue of the evil indwelling in Life. It is not requisite that he should have solved it, only that he should have grappled with it—as Jacob did with the Angel at *Peniel*.

In grappling with the problem of Job, I have taken my stand 'tween Job, Jung, and Freud. It is by the side of Job. I cannot reconcile myself to, nor accept, the Christian faith in a life hereafter, wherein and whereat all injustices will be righted. This is seemingly Jung's ultimate answer to the problem of Evil.** To this extent I am more proximate to Freud than I am to Jung. And yet I cannot subscribe to Freud's mordant atheism. Freud understood very little of religion. He was compulsively obsessed with the rejection of that infantile consolation which Christianity and the later corrupted Judaism offered to the credulous, the belief in a life hereafter. In the Book of Job there is not one word of the hereafter, and the orthodox addendum pictures the Almighty rewarding Job's piety in the here and now, and not in

---

* Freud expounds this argument with his accustomed forcefulness in his *Civilization and Its Discontents*. But Freud is not on the side of the angels.

** In *God and the Unconscious* by Victor White, the following is quoted from one of Jung's letters: "On empirical grounds I am convinced that the soul is in part outside space and time (i.e., relatively eternal). Similarly the continuation of personal consciousness after death appears to me, on grounds of experience, to be probable" (30).

In view of the fact that Jung wrote the introduction to this book, it may be assumed that the quotation is correct.

the great beyond. But there is vastly more to Christianity than the myths of resurrection and Judgment Day, and more to Judaism than the archaic laws of Kashris. The totality of religion cannot be adjudged an Infantile Illusion. Religious faith is the supreme achievement of the human spirit, infinitely higher and greater than either Art or Science. For without it there would be no humanity, and hence neither Art nor Science.

Religion is not to be encompassed within reason, as Freud and many others have attempted, but it can be intelligized. The dimensions of one man's life experiences are too constrained to encompass the full magnitude of the meaning of life, and his vision too feeble to perceive its outlines in the limitless expanse of time. And yet it lies not beyond the competences of man's understanding to perceive that living man is a time- and space-bound congelation of matter suspended between two eternities, the eternity of the past and that of the future, and serving to bind them together. For his soul's sake he must reconcile and subserve both. In this understanding man can achieve his attestation of the God-head, gaining and bringing his tribute.

REFERENCES

1. JUNG, C. G.: *Answer to Job,* translated from the German by R. F. C. Hull. London, Routledge and Kegan Paul, 1954.
2. FREUD, S.: *Totem and Taboo.* New York, Moffat, Yard and Co., 1918.
3. FREUD, S.: *The Future of an Illusion,* translated by W. D. Robson-Scott. London, L. & V. Woolf, 1928.
4. FREUD, S.: *Moses and Monotheism,* translated from the German by Katherine Jones. London, Hogarth Press and Institute of Psycho-Analysis, 1939.
5. KING, A. R.: *The Problem of Evil: Christian Concepts and the Book of Job.* New York: The Ronald Press, 1952.
6. JASTROW, M.: *The Book of Job: Its Origin, Growth and Interpretation,* together with a new translation based on a revised text. Philadelphia, J. B. Lippincott, 1920.
7. JASTROW, *ibid.,* p. 82.
8. JUNG, *op. cit.,* p. 68.
9. JASTROW, *op. cit.,* Chapter V.
10. JASTROW, *ibid.,* p. 71.
11. FREUD, *The Future of an Illusion, op. cit.*
12. FREUD, *ibid.,* p. 28.
13. FREUD, *ibid.,* p. 71.
14. FREUD, *ibid.,* p. 26.
15. FREUD, *ibid.,* p. 78.
16. JUNG, *op. cit.,* p. 83.
17. JUNG, *ibid.*
18. JUNG, *ibid.,* p. 11.
19. JUNG, *ibid.,* p. 116.
20. JUNG, *ibid.,* p. 117.
21. JUNG, *ibid.,* p. 153.

22. JUNG, *ibid.*
23. BUBER, M.: *At the Turning.* New York, Farrar Strauss and Young, Inc. 1952.
24. BUBER, M.: *Hasidism,* translated by Greta Hort, New York, Philosophical Library, 1948, p. 9.
25. JUNG, *op. cit.,* p. 68.
26. JUNG, *ibid.,* p. 30.
27. JUNG, *ibid.,* p. 52.
28. BUBER, *op. cit.,* p. 9.
29. FREUD, S.: *Civilization and Its Discontents,* translated by Joan Rivière, London, L. & V. Woolf and the Institute of Psycho-Analysis, 1930.
30. WHITE, V.: *God and the Unconscious,* Chicago, Henry Regnery Co., 1953.

Part III:
ON THE SOCIOLOGY OF PSYCHIATRY

20

The American Family in Crisis

OF ALL PEOPLE, those that are concerned with mental health should be, or so it seems to me, the very first to embrace within their concern the community as well as the individual. They should labor under a compelling need to inquire—how healthy is the community, and also, how much and in what way does the community contribute to the breaking down of the individual? They should, in other words, bring social as well as intra-psychic etiology into the picture.

And yet, it isn't the community *per se* that calls for scrutiny, but rather its social integer, the family. According to the famous anthropologist Claude Lévi Strauss, "the family, consisting of a more or less durable union, socially approved, of a man, a woman, and their children, is a universal phenomenon, present in each and every type of society" (1).

Historically and culturally, the family *is* the social integer of society. The family is the reflex of, the begetter and the begotten of the community. In studying the community, we can begin with the family, even though, as we need to note, the community is more than an aggregate of the families it embraces.

It is the family I would consider with you, not the hypothetical or universal family as defined by Lévi Strauss, but rather the American family, which, as I see it, is in a state of crisis. I plead with you not to pick a quarrel with me over the issue, is there such an organism as the American family? I know how this matter is "teased to rags" by the sociologists, who only particularize and never generalize about the family. I can even sympathize with their scruples, and agree that there are really only nascent families, maturing families, upgrading families, and so forth. Yet for my purpose it is safe and sound to postulate the existence of an

281

American family, for what I treat of is not a parochial variant, but an all-pervasive dynamic, which embraces and affects us all. It is a socio-economic, cultural and psychological disorientation to which all of us are subject, and which is most patently affecting the American family.

Our experts on communication advise us that a thing is not a thing until you've named it. I've therefore named it. I've named the crisis of the American family as the Menace of the Matriarchoid Family. The American family is losing, has lost, its patriarchal pattern, and is becoming matriarchoid in character. The term *matriarchoid* is a neologism. I intend it to mean "resembling but essentially different from matriarchy." The term is my own, but I share with a few others an awareness of the crisis that it labels. Several sociologists and psychiatrists have taken note of this change in family pattern. You have, I am sure, come upon the term *momism,* coined, I believe, by Philip Wylie, and first used in his book *A Generation of Vipers.* David Levy, a pioneer in this field, has studied the subject obliquely, dealing mainly with the over-protective mother and her psychological effects upon the family. Sorokin has skirted about this thesis in his embracing diatribes on current society. The Gluecks in their studies on juvenile delinquency have provided us with telling data on the evil consequences of the familial change. Parenthetically I would add that in several of these works Mother has been made the scapegoat, and womankind in general has been made the target of blame. It's Adam's old trick of blaming Eve and I'll have no part in it. As I will undertake to show later, it is woman, even more than man, that has suffered by this change in familial pattern although in truth I do not see how the suffering of the one sex can fail to involve and affect the other.

If you require me to describe or to define the matriarchoid family, I can do so only in negative terms. Its predominant features are the abandonment and denial of the patriarchal patterns, values and mores. The matriarchoid family is in *status nascendi.* What its ultimate features may be we cannot anticipate, but its current pathogenicity is all too clear. I will revert to this later. Here I need to define what I intend by patriarchal patterns, values and mores.

First of all allow me to go on record that I am not a defender of the patriarchal family. My role is that of an expositor not that of a pleader. I do, however, believe that what was originally a descriptive term has been converted of late into a term of opprobrium. The patriarchal family is too commonly envisaged as a marital group, in which the wife and children are tyrannized by the husband and father. No doubt such family groups do exist, but I would rather describe such groups as "male tyrannized," or, as not infrequently happens, as "woman tyrannized" families. Historically, that is, as far as historical data are available (and I must add that the data are scant and the conjectures multiple), the outstanding characteristic of the patriarchal family is not male tyranny, but rather the domestication of the adult male. The patriarchal family gave rise to "husbandry," that is, to the more or less lifelong "enslavement" of the male to the arduous task of providing for the care of his marital partner and the defense and upbringing of his children. This association and commitment of necessity involved governance which in some instances no doubt led to tyranny—for, as Lord Acton observed, all power tends to corrupt.

The extent and degree of masculine authority no doubt varied from age to age, but a complete and abiding arbitrary mastery of man over woman is hardly conceivable, not only for the reasons so pointedly exhibited in Lysistrata, but also because all males are perforce the sons of mothers.

The patriarchal family came into being as a result of the economic progressions of primitive society. "One of the reasons why the patriarchal family is not to be found in lower cultures," wrote Briffault "is that it (the patriarchal family) is founded on property, and that the dominance of the husband in that family and the subordinate position of the wife rests ultimately upon the economic advantage of the former and the economic dependence of the latter." We do not know precisely when the patriarchal family became the norm among European peoples. For our purpose it suffices to appreciate that the patriarchal family has existed for a long time, for a time longer than the span of recorded history. To the economics of this family pattern, to its expanded and planned husbandry, we can trace almost the entirety of our socio-cultural history and heritage.

Both the relationship and the economy of the patriarchal family are contractual in nature and committed in spirit. Planning involves coordination, pledged promises and obligations which are to be fulfilled. Failing of these, both plans and planners face inevitable ruination.

A vast portion of our ethos, and much of our socio-cultural heritage revolves about contracts, pledges and commitments. It is not for naught that one of the earliest sociologists, Jean Jacques Rousseau, titled his classic although naive masterpiece, *The Social Contract*.

This is not, and to my mind, never has been, a man's world. But for many millenia it has been a "patriarchal world." I am not referring solely nor mainly to man's position in the family. I mean rather that our value systems have been patriarchal—that is, reflexive of the pattern and purpose of the patriarchal family. We are likely to describe them as masculine values or virtues—values such as work, order, discipline, insistence on the fulfillment of pledge, promise and contract, and so forth. But they are neither purely masculine nor are they pristinely native to him. They are virtues, or values if you prefer, which have been assessed as such in the operational relationship of the patriarchal family.

It would be an enormous task to trace the many ways in which these patriarchal values are manifest in our traditions, laws, customs, habits and arts. These are so native to us that we must hold them off at a distance, by an effort of deliberate intention, to examine them. Consider, for example, the most obvious instances, those of style and dress, and our sense of the beautiful in the human form, both male and female; the arts graphic and plastic, literature, poetry, the drama, and above all our sacred texts, the Bible and its commentaries, our ecclesiastic history, its numerous rituals and traditions—all these carry the patent imprint of patriarchy.

This I believe to be historically true. But the patriarchal family is rapidly disintegrating, and in that process we are experiencing and witnessing a negation of those patterns, values and mores on which and by which our multi-millenial culture has been structured and buttressed. The effects are witnessed in social misery and what collectively must be termed socio-cultural delinquency. These are the challenges which confront the psychiatrist in the lives of those who turn to him in search of sanity.

Society is sick, and its morbidities are most clearly exhbited in the family. Juvenile delinquency, divorce, alcoholism, drug addition, homosexuality, and frantic promiscuity are widespread. They are not the result of the change in the family pattern; they are rather the concomitants thereof. They issue from the same complex of forces which has so disruptingly affected the family structure. Among these prevailing social morbidities none is more terrifying than the anarchy of youth—wrongly termed juvenile delinquency. I find this term most objectionable, because it misleads and corrupts our understanding of the faults involved. A delinquent is one who has failed in the fulfilment of an obligation or a duty. But this presupposes both knowledge and wilfulness. To prove delinquent I must both know and wilfully fail to meet my obligations. But if I do not know my duties nor my obligations, if I do not know them in the compelling manner of an indwelling conscience or ego ideal, how am I then to be adjudged a delinquent? At most I deserve to be named no worse than an ignorant, uncultivated or asocial fellow. And that's precisely the point. Our young at times do not know their duties and prerogatives at the cognitive or informational level, because they have not been informed (the ignorance of patients is often appalling) or, knowing of them, their knowledge is not supported or activated by the affect charge of an ego ideal. They are without a conscience, super-ego, ideal ego or ego ideal. Freud has taught us that the super-ego represents the introjected or incorporated father image. In the matriarchoid family there is no conscionable father image to introject. I believe that the societal ethos contributes no less to the structure and content of the super-ego than does the father personage. But as I have already observed, our very ethos is growing more matriarchoid—and less patriarchal.

The anarchy of youth is more embracive and meaningful than juvenile delinquency, the latter being a term heavily freighted with legalistic implications. The anarchy of youth is to be witnessed even in the absence of crime or violence.

I cannot here elaborate upon the other instances of social delinquency which I named—divorce, alcoholism, drug addiction, homosexuality, etc. I must rather turn to the question—*What is behind this change?* What is the derivation of this pervasive dynamic that has resulted in such a profound cultural and psychologic disorientation? The answer is rather simple but too frequently misconceived. It is our changed and changing economic and industrial system. What comes to mind with this phrase? Most commonly the marvels of modern technology, the steam engine, the electric dynamo, the telephone, radio, television and so on right down to atomic energy and automation. But it is not these technological marvels that I have in mind when referring to our changed and changing economic and industrial system. I intend something more revolutionary, more fundamental, more fateful. I mean the advent of the modern industrial manufacturing system. I doubt that mankind in its long existence on this earth has ever before experienced so profound an ecological disorientation as that effected in the advent of modern industrialism. Only the mastery of fire and the conquest of the metals in the bronze and iron ages can be conceived to have so profoundly affected the lives of mankind as did the industrial revolution.

We are all aware of and indeed are surrounded by the technological marvels which the industrial revolution has yielded. But in the main we are unmindful, except in a vague and possibly troubling way, of the other yields of the industrial revolution, those involving man as a psychologic, social and spiritual creature. Let me touch upon these "other yields" and detail a few of them. The industrial revolution was vastly more than merely industrial in nature. In effect it produced the most cataclysmic social disorganization man has experienced since Prometheus, by robbing the gods, made man a gift of fire. For one—it distanced man from the earth. For thousands upon thousands of years (the estimate is half a million), man lived in and on, but ever in the most intimate contact with the earth. He lived off, or worked, the soil or the sea, or, if he chanced to be a craftsman, merchant, soldier, minister or king, he was but a pacing distance from those who did. As late as the fifteenth century eleven-twelfths of the population of England were employed in agriculture. Now I will not dwell upon the tutorial effects of such proximal and intimate relation with the earth or on all that it can teach a man of life and living. I want rather to single out one disastrous effect that followed on the separation of man from the earth. He suffered the chronic starvation of malnutrition. That is not the same as the starvation of want or of famine. It is much worse. To this alienation of man from the immediate and native sources of his food may be charged, in a very large measure, the major epidemic diseases of the nineteenth century, diseases such as tuberculosis, typhoid, cholera, scarlet fever, diphtheria and the infant diarrheas, and of such chronic disorders as rickets and chlorosis. The nineteenth century man was not a healthy specimen, and a great deal of his ill health can be traced to his malnutrition.

I have underscored the separation of man from the earth mainly because the fact itself is so little appreciated and because its effects are so little realized. To my mind, however, even more disruptive were the effects of the industrial revolution upon the homestead, the family and the inter-relations of man, woman and child. The homestead, which in its more ideal pattern embraced three co-existing generations, was an institution of far-reaching effects. It was in substance a school for living, wherein the young were indoctrinated by practice and precept in the techniques and wisdoms requisite for making a go of life. It was the repository of a man's enterprise, his security against advancing years and failing strength, his heritage gained and his heritage transmitted. It gave the testament of endurance, of meaningful continuity, to the succeeding generations. True, it exacted the performance of duty and the fulfilment of obligation, but it redeemed the travail of both in the rewards that were attested in the prospering family. Above all, it gave clear meaning, a transparent rationale, to those virtues which the moralists taught—the virtues of honest husbandry and of good will.

The industrial revolution disrupted the homestead, negated the rationale for its being, and created a world inimical to its very existence.

The industrial revolution weakened the structure and dissipated the native functions of the family. Since time immemorial men and women were more bound in union by the mutuality of services rendered to each other and to their progeny than by the warm but evanescent charms of romantic love. The family was not merely a conglomeration of persons but rather a productive organization, a working union. With the industrial revolution, and because of it, most of the productive functions of the family organization were taken over by other organizations. The intrafamilial "mutuality of services" has been reduced almost to the vanishing point.

One of the warrants for union in marriage of men and women was, as it remains, the desire for progeny. But whereas in time past children were an asset, in the real as well as in the affectional sense, they have become more recently, if not entirely a liability, certainly something of a luxury —to be indulged in circumspectly. The child too has suffered a severe dislocation in its intrafamilial relations. During its youth it is now largely a supernumerary. It has no organic, functional role in the current familial scheme of things. This is especially the case with the urban child. Save for its school work the child has little to do, and that little is of a make-work character. Contrast this with the many chores which the child performed in time past, and still performs in some of our rural homes.

Nowhere, however, are the disruptive effects of the industrial revolution more clearly reflected than in the degradation that woman has suffered in her familial position and function. For thousands of years woman was the mainstay of the family. She was wife and mother, nurse and teacher. She spun the yarn and wove the cloth. She tailored. She gardened for the kitchen and the medicine chest. She it was who molded candles, preserved foods against the winter seasons, made soaps, cooked, baked, laundered and tended to the hundreds of functions and details that were so vital to the maintenance and the flourish of the family. She bore sons and daughters, to be of aid to herself and their father, to be their pride, their consolation and their support. Doubtless she worked long hours and hard, but for all this she had her rewards, the greatest among them the secure knowledge that she was needed and wanted, that she was indispensable in the scheme of the living pattern. There was for her, too, the sense of accomplishment, the satisfaction that comes with the fulfilment of the primal urge to create, to dispense of self in the process.

Thus it was for thousands of years. But thus it is no longer. One after another of the woman's functions, of her utilities in the home, have been taken from her—first by the machine and then also by the mercantile, commercial and social agencies. Now she neither spins nor weaves. She has neither greens nor herb garden. She does not bake, though she may yet cook. She has been, as some of our feminist and liberal friends say with such eager enthusiasm, "she has been freed of the yoke of household chores." She is a free woman —free for what? To the man from Mars, for he alone could be considered a true outsider, it would appear that woman, so largely deprived of her ancient prerogatives, is free to seek retribution, and is doing so in a mighty wrath of frenzied aggressions.

The socio-economic changes to which I trace our social disorientation have taken place in our sphere during the last 150 years, and this is but as a moment in the long span of man's habitation on this globe. We then must ask: Can the primal hungers and wants of men and women be readapted to fit this changed and changing world? Can we with impunity deny, gainsay, block out, impede, divert that *élan vital,* that upsurging drive that lifted man out of the primal ooze and that has through the eons of time brought him to the forefront of creation? Can we, without paying a fearful price therefor, meddle with that order of relations between men and women that has in the span of time yielded us love and song, the plastic arts, poetry, the dance, the culture of beauty, of form and color, of adornment, of perfume; that has given us courtesy and grace, manners and spirit; that has fostered home and friendship, and the strong bonds of blood kinship, the *Anlage* of all that is civil and civilizing? Can we? All the available evidence speaks against it: witness the so-called battle of the sexes, hate and love, and momism.

I have referred also to the negation of the ancient wisdoms. I intend by this the decline in prestige and power of those institutions whose primary function it has been to indoctrinate man in the habitudes and practices of altruism. I mean primarily religion and the church, intending by the latter every order of congregation and place of worship, although among the indoctrinating institutions one could and should include also the enlightened professions and the universities.

Few among us today can fully appreciate the role that the church and the synagogue played in the lives of our own ancestors. The place of worship served for more than worship. It was where acquaintances were made and friendships were engendered. It was where romance insinuated its sparkling, bright spirit, to give temporal pertinence to the timeless verities. It was where courtships were often first inspired and ultimately sanctioned. The church was an instrument of charity and of mercy. It succored the orphan and sustained the widow. It cheered the sick and consoled the bereft. It tempered the galling guilt no less than it goaded the slothful conscience. It reconciled the estranged, and fostered justice. It gave refuge to the persecuted, and aid to the abused. It was, in a word, a realm apart, wherein by his own efforts and with the aid of the anointed, man could reconcile the temporal with the timeless, the mortal with the immortal, the particular with the transcending, and thus achieve an effective relationship with both the immortality antecedent to his earthly advent and that beyond his demise. The church helped our ancestors to appreciate, even when they did not understand.

The church was the one place where music was written and rendered, where the staged spectacle taught both the doctrine and the mystery, where the painter adorned the walls with his graphic portrayals of Old and New Testament scenes, where calligraphy was practiced and taught, where the young learned their alpha and beta, and the more advanced embrace the cumulative knowledges and the wisdoms of the ages. Here, in a word, the liberal arts were cradled and nurtured. To its congregation and to the community, the church was club, theater, opera, museum, library, school, welfare agency, nursing service, foundling home, funeral parlor, and much, much more besides.

Man is a creature that lives by values, no less than by bread, and of late too many of his traditional values have been cast into doubt. In the cataclysmic upheavals of two world wars, goodness, love, charity, mercy, truth, humility, brotherliness, have been violated and mocked. There is current a highly organized, energetic and cunningly resourceful propaganda which makes the homely virtues and the religious persuasions and faiths of our fathers appear like a compound of neurotic anxiety, infantile delusion, political-economic naiveté and mean escapism. Many who are caught in the tension field of this propaganda seek refuge in doctrinaire bigotry; hence the resurgence of orthodoxy in morals and religion.

My original proposition was to the effect that an effective resolution of the mental hygiene problem requires not only persons, tools and places but also, and primarily, a healthy community.

I have expounded all this not in the spirit of a Jeremiah. I call neither for repentance nor for a return to the faiths and ways of our forefathers. That is beyond and behind us all—for all eternity. We must rather seek for new ways, for an effective reconciliation of the abiding needs of man with the new ways and needs of our changed and changing world. But seek them we must for they will not come to us of themselves. We must seek them in the light of a clear understanding of the nature of the crisis confronting the American family. It is to this end—the illumination of the nature of the crisis—that I have directed my exposition.

REFERENCES

1. SHAPIRO, HARRY L. *Man, Culture and Society,* New York, Oxford University Press, 1956.
2. BRIFFAULT, ROBERT. *The Mothers,* New York, Macmillan Co., 1931, p. 158.

21

The Rise and Decline of Fatherhood

WITHIN OUR DIVIDED and divisive country there is one affirmation on which we can all agree, and that is that we are in one hell of a fix.

Considerable agreement also exists about the evils of that fix—the disintegration of the family, the generation gap, drug abuse, promiscuity, crime and violence, racial conflict, the whole spectrum of discontent and disruption. But there is wide divergence of opinion as to what has gotten us into this situation. A bedlam of theories is loudly advanced by a host of seers and sages, who are convinced that they know how we got into it and the way out.

The first of these sages is the "Jeremiah person," who bewails the deterioration of the generations and castigates the elders for the faults of the young. He preaches a return to the past and is a stern advocate of law and order.

Next is the starry-eyed visionary who sees in the prevailing turmoil the birth pangs of a new world—a green world, governed by a third order of conscience. He sees no evil where evil is, rationalizing away the rebellion of the young and perceiving in them a praiseworthy prelude to a redeeming future.

Then comes the nihilist who decries both past and future, glooms about the destiny of mankind, and sees in our contemporary difficulties the inevitable consequences of man's historic hypocrisies and vanities. The nihilist has no program for salvation and nothing but contempt for law and order. He advocates the chaos of every man doing his own thing in his own way.

The seer I find most interesting, and also menacing, is the amateur sociologist who elaborates the dynamics of our discontent in terms of the struggle between classes: the conflict between the haves and the have-nots, those who are "in" and those who are "out," those who move laterally and those who move vertically, those in the majority and those in the minority, and so on. I would call these pseudosociologists neo-Marxists if I thought they knew anything about Marxism. But I see little evidence that they do. At best, I see in their position a mixture of some righteous indignation with a large measure of superficial and erroneous thinking on social dynamics. Their sociological potpourri is unhistoric; it represents an uncritical reaction to a challenging situation that urgently demands critical accounting.

Why do I find them menacing? Because their arguments are so seductively simple, and seemingly so rational. Society, they say, is divided into classes; these classes are competitive, antagonistic, and belligerent. And that explains everything! Of course society is divided into classes, and these classes are competitive, antagonistic, belligerent; but it has always been so, since the time of Cain and Abel, and it promises to remain so until all men are cast, like ants, in one identical and unchanging mold. A truly, absolutely classless society is a fantasy that, if realized, would be a disastrous nightmare. Society would stagnate, social progress would be arrested, and culture would be frozen.

All these seers and prophets fall wide of the mark, not so much in their analysis of what is wrong in the current state of affairs, but in their judgment as to what are its causes and its remedies. Collectively, their major defect is that *they are unhistorical.* This is witnessed by their failure to recognize that ours is but the latest in a series of crises which mankind has encountered and resolved during its long existence. Ours may be a more grievous, more complex crisis than any of the preceding ones. But to every man who ever faced a crisis, his own contemporaneous confrontation must always have appeared more menacing than those of the historic past. Thus I can read about, but cannot truly experience, the pall of anxiety, dread, and despair which engulfed much of the Middle Ages. Writing of the 14th century, Huizinga (2) described the spirit of the times: "A general feeling of impending calamity hangs over all. Perpetual danger prevails everywhere." This has a familiar ring, has it not?

In the literature of crisis lamentation, the following is a prize specimen: (1) "The father will not agree with his children, nor the children with their father, nor guest with his host, nor comrade with comrade; nor will brother be dear to brother as aforetimes . . . there will be no favor for the man who keeps his faith, or for the just, or for the good." This was written more than 2700 years ago, by the Greek poet Hesiod.

But although mankind has experienced numerous crises, these have not all been of equal magnitude and gravity. Some were exceptionally complex and menacing, and the present-day crisis is of this nature. Its historic origins, however, are discernible to those who take the trouble to study the technological, economic, and social developments that led up to it. I will discuss these developments later; at this point I want to consider just what characterizes the exceptional crisis, what distinguishes it from the common and frequent variety. In this I am indebted to the work of the Spanish historian and philosopher Ortega y Gasset (4), who defines the exceptional crisis as an *historical crisis,* one that involves and disrupts the social and cultural fabric of society.

During normal change, Ortega states, the basic framework for understanding the world remains the same; only slight modifications occur, smoothly and without a break, from one generation to another. But in an historical crisis, the entire system of convictions about the world collapses. "Man returns to a state of not knowing what to do, for the reason that he returns to a state of actually not knowing what to think about the world." He has no positive beliefs on which to build, only negative ones. He may try to assuage his feeling of being lost by assuming a skeptical frigidity, anguish, desperation masquerading as heroism, or an attitude of vengeance.

This seems to be a fair and fitting description of the mood that affects an appreciable number of people in the Western world. But granting that we are currently in such an historical crisis, the question remains, how did this come about? More pointedly, what was the system of convictions that has collapsed, and how did it collapse, and why?

Answered categorically, the system of values and convictions which has seemingly become invalid is that of the patriarchal family. Its validity is questioned because its structure and operations have been breached—by technological changes and by their derivative economic and social effects.

Origin of Patriarchal Family

The terms *patriarchal, patristic, paternal,* once so honorific, are now terms of equivocal merit at best, and at worst terms of contempt. But historically the patriarchal family was the *fons et origo*—the source and origin—of our culture and civilization, and if at present our civilization is menaced and our culture challenged, it is less because of any mortal flaws in the nature of the patriarchal family than it is because of what has happened to that family.

The patriarchal family is of comparatively recent origin; it came into being with the invention of agriculture, which probably occurred about 11,000 years ago. Its precursor was the matriarchal family. Precisely when matriarchy yielded place and patriarchy became the predominant pattern of the family is undetermined. But we can witness the stark affirmation of patriarchy in the Biblical story of the creation of woman. Here woman is not the prior creature, but is derivative: "The rib which he took from man, Jehovah fashioned into a woman and brought her to man." This account of the creation of Eve appears to be essential to the story of the fall, for without her man would not have been tempted nor sinned against God, and would not have lost Paradise.

The Biblical story of the temptation and fall of man has a counterpart in the Greek myth of Epimetheus and Pandora. Here, too, man (in the person of Prometheus) had offended the gods by stealing fire, and in retaliation the gods fashioned Pandora, the all-gifted one, and placed her among men. She tempted Epimetheus, the brother of Prometheus, and she was all too successful. He opened the casket she brought as a bridal gift (could this be a picturesque and suggestive Freudian fantasy?), and as a result, in the words of Hesiod, "Countless plagues now wander among men; for earth is full of evils and the sea is full," a painful contrast to prior times when "the tribes of men lived on earth, remote and free from toil and heavy sickness."

Both these tales of the creation of woman and the fall of man recount the loss of a mythical life of ease and abundance and the consequent curse of toil and strife placed upon man. They strongly suggest that their essential meaning is the change in man's pattern of living, from that of the nomadic food-gatherer and hunter to that of the relatively settled farmer and animal-breeder.

It is this which most likely precipitated the shift from matriarchy to patriarchy. With the development of agriculture and animal husbandry, the human family acquired the character of a social and economic organism, where previously it had been essentially a biologic union. It was not love, at least not in the sense we understand it, but necessity and the benefits of mutual services that founded the patriarchal-economic family. Man settled down, first in villages and then in cities, where his genius could operate under favorable conditions to invent the plow, the loom, the wheel, and metal-working. With the introduction of the plow, agriculture became man's work, for handling the plow (especially when oxen were used to draw it) required more strength than the average woman possessed.

Patriarchal Accomplishments

These basic inventions lifted man economically above the level of sub-sistence living, and facilitated and encouraged division of labor, specializa-tion, barter, and exchange. Commerce necessitated the keeping of accounts and records. Counting, measuring, writing, and ultimately the alphabet—signs that stood for single sounds—were developed. Man began in earnest to order his encounters with experience, and science, religion, and law were the products of his efforts.

All the evidence available, prehistoric as well as historic, credits the major attainments in civilization and culture—technology, science, reli-gion, law, literature, music, aesthetics, and philosophy—to the efforts of the male.

Deterioration of Patriarchal Family

Though living conditions for most individuals in the economically de-veloped countries have improved immensely, the deterioration of the patriarchal family and the cultural environment has continued unabated. In effect, the deteriorative process is now irreversible. The patriarchal family suited and served a given economic-technological period, one which has been of long duration but which is now, in the Western world, ap-proaching its end.

The tragic accompaniment to this end of an era is that as yet we have nothing to take its place. The disintegration of the patriarchal family has also involved a weakening of the institutions which supported its ethos. Religion and law, morals and discipline, are openly flouted and aggres-sively challenged. The traditional masculine virtues—work, order, dis-cipline, the fulfillment of pledge and promise, judicious husbandry neither niggardly nor wasteful—have become trivial in our times.

This is the global picture; it is reflected in the microcosm of the fam-ily, which is now also in a condition of historical crisis. The traditional ethos, during its long development, had undergone numerous and radical changes, but in none of them was the institution of fatherhood challenged. The individual father might be rejected or discredited, but not the office and the role of the Father. Indeed, in the past the rebel himself was more than likely to justify his rebellion by an appeal to the ideal of fatherhood, claiming that his father was not a good father, or that he himself aspired to be a better one.

The father's loss of power has disrupted the means and process of ethos transmission. When this process breaks down, as it has on a limited scale in the past because of wars, revolutions, or natural disasters, the consequence is that the affected group tends to become lawless. That, of course, is not the same as becoming criminal, though some of the lawlessness is likely to fringe on the criminal. The young are likely to be the most lawless, for they are on the receiving end of the broken communication exchange; little or nothing comes through to them, save only perhaps what is to them incomprehensible noise. Interestingly, our particular term for lawlessness in the young, "delinquency," has as its core meaning not willful criminality but failure or neglect, perhaps due to ignorance or lack of conviction.

Sheldon Glueck was probably the first to emphasize clearly the negative influence of the weak or absent father, especially when combined with the domineering and castrating mother, in the development of a delinquent child. But the delinquent is not created; he is engendered. The absent father does not teach his son criminality. He fails, most often now he is made unable, to pass values on effectively to his children. The result is a protean psychopathology, that of paternal deprivation.

This deprivation is built into contemporary society. Our modes of living deprecate and nullify the role of the father. The agitation some years ago about "momism" and the "generation of vipers," which pictured the mother as a conspirator bent on castrating both husband and son was grossly misdirected. Her role has grown only because that of the father has so greatly diminished. The functions of ethos indoctrination have been taken over by the agencies that have so largely displaced the father—schools, television, comic strips, glossy magazines, the morbid realism of ultramodern fiction and advertising. They have served us badly. The results are reflected in growing delinquency, both juvenile and adult, and in the far more numerous mass of asocial, ineffectual persons, whose serious paternal deprivation has left them handicapped in the process of self-fulfillment because of their inadequate superego formation.

Youth has rejected our patriarchal ethos. I do not protest against this, for though the ethos had great merits and served the conditions of past generations well, many of its elements are unsuited to present-day life and most certainly to the emergent world, product of the technological revolution confronting us all.

Current Protest

The spectrum of current protest is broad, ranging through long hair, general dirtiness, identical patched dungarees for all, talismans, charms, mystic symbols and cryptic gestures, to the more serious and socially disruptive riotous actions in schools and colleges and in the political arena. Three major challenges emerge, and these intimately affect the structure and function of the family. One is the relationship between men and women within and outside of marriage. The second involves sexual relations and has gained the title of the Sexual Revolution. The third, still poorly defined, concerns the relations of parents in particular, and older persons in general, to all who have not yet grown to full adult status.

Without question, woman in the patriarchal family was, and had to be, subordinate to man. The family was founded on property, and the dominance of the husband rested ultimately in his economic power over his wife. But these economic relationships are no longer operational, either in kind or in degree, in the present-day family. One third of our working population is female, and the proportion is increasing. Women are pressing for equality, and it is widely recognized that they are not only entitled to this, but have the means to gain it.

The word *equality* is problematic; taken in its ultimate sense, not only are men and women not equal, but no two men or two women anywhere in the world are equal. More often it is used to mean denial of an all-inclusive superiority attributable to any aggregate class of human beings. A white man is not superior to a black man, a European to an Asian, nor a man to a woman. Superiority among human beings can only be partial, fractional, particular.

As I see it, the family of the future will be one in which the issues of equality will have been submerged in the achievement of a free collaboration allowing the exercise of each member's unique gifts and competences. This is not mere fantasizing or wish fulfillment, though I do earnestly hope for such a development. The prediction is based on possibility because, free from its ancient economic bind, the family will be able to be founded on love, on mutual respect, and on good will.

Not very long ago, the only way in which nearly every adult woman could gain her living was to marry a man willing to support her in return for her domestic contributions. Once so involved, she was bound to stick it out, no matter what. Today women have more and better options, the most significant being that they can earn their own living, if they so choose, and remain free of economic dependence on father or husband. But a woman who is gainfully employed and economically independent is not necessarily independent of men in other respects. I rather foresee the emergence of a greater interdependence, a more free interrelationship between men and women, one initiated, cultivated, and maintained by choice, rather than by compelling economic and social forces.

Women's Rights

The second major challenge is that of the sexual revolution, especially as it relates to women (3): "freedom to dress so as to enjoy unhampered movement; freedom to move outside the family and escape familial or communal taboos and ostracism for deviant behavior; the right and possibility not to have one's procreative functions dominate all one's life; the right to divorce without social stigma."

These freedoms, stated here in a general way, clearly refer to certain easily-recognized exactions and taboos imposed on women in the patriarchal family: premarital virginity, fidelity in marriage, "fatherless motherhood," and what have been termed perverted sexual practices. Here, too, it can be argued that some of these demands were warranted in that family system because they contributed to its security and stability. And under the present social and economic conditions their practical implications are, perhaps, not so significant as they formely were. The arguments for the sexual revolution may have merit, but the troubling question is how much merit and in which issues. One of the defects of its credo is that it affirms the desired freedom without mentioning any of the derivative responsibilities. And it treats of sex as if it were a "right apart," like the right to hold a job, or vote, or wear pants, and not as what it is—the matrix of human interaction, the pervasive power that binds together the sexes and the generations.

However, I am persuaded that much good will come of the sexual revolution, though like all revolutions it has been disfigured by excesses and hampered by Utopian aspirations that do not consider the basic needs and limitations of human beings. In the end, I think, the current revolution in sexual mores will yield less exploitive, more honest, and more rewarding relations between men and women, and thus it will foster better families.

And finally, what of children in relation to parents, and parents in relation to children? Bear in mind that by children we mean all the young, including the preadult. In prior times we tried to mold them in our own image, perhaps hoping to improve on our own past but retaining the basic form in which we ourselves were cast. For it was our own world that we expected to pass on to our children, and we assumed that we understood the nature and requirements of that world. We looked on our children as our inheritors, and it was certainly our moral and practical obligation to make sure that our children would be able not only to take over and care for the patrimony we left them, but also to advance it.

But now the flow of life through succeeding generations has become discontinuous. We of the older generation cannot, except in a few respects, "prepare our children for the world that will be their own." We do not know that world, and it certainly will not be much like our own. We therefore must, by obligation, let the young make their own adaptations to life, grope their own way to the mastery of their own existence. But that does not mean that we must abandon all efforts to offer them guidance and understanding, for certain human values remain valid whatever the prevailing economic, technological, or social conditions may be. Truth is one, honesty is another, kindness a third. We must differentiate here between moralisms and morality; the former are temporal injunctions, while the latter are timeless and abiding human values. We have all too often, in the past, confounded the one with the other, urging them both alike upon the young and thus discrediting both.

Youth, in its protest and rejection, has tended to throw out not only the dirty water and the baby, but also the tub. Not all the components of the patriarchal ethos are transient, valid today but not valid on the morrow. Some of its components are beyond the reach of time and circumstances; in human terms, they are eternal. Such are truth, authenticity, charity, love, work and creativity. No matter what his economic or political state, without these virtues man is not man.

I believe we of the older generation have failed our youth in not insisting, against all odds and opposition, on the validity of these virtues. We need to stand firm on these elements of our own faith, to cultivate a historic perspective and to regain our lost courage. By doing this we might, with the young participating, forge an ethos suited to the new order of living now so painfully emerging.

REFERENCES

1. HESIOD. *Works and Days.* Trans. Hugh. G. Evelyn-White. The Loeb Classical Library. Cambridge, Harvard University Press, 1943.
2. HUIZINGA, JOHAN. *The Warning of the Middle Ages.* London, Edward Arnold, 1924.
3. LERNER, GERDA. Women's rights and American feminism. *The American Scholar 40* (Spring, 1971), 235-248.
4. ORTEGA Y GASSET, JOSE. *Man and Crisis.* Trans. Mildred Adams. New York, W. W. Norton, 1958.
5. POLANYI, KARL. *Origins of Our Times.* London, V. Gollancz, 1945.

22

Our One-Generation Culture

THE THESIS I wish to submit is as precious as it is simple. And yet, though *both* precious *and* simple, it seldom finds a place on the agenda of the councils on gerontology. In essence it is this: Among the dimensions of being, meaning is one of the most significant.

Commonly we are concerned with but two dimensions—the dimension of duration, which we call longevity, and the dimension of physical integrity, which we gauge under the plus and minus signs of health and disease. But, I submit, there is a third dimension which overrides both the others, and which can be expressed in the colloquialism—Life, what for? This is the dimension of meaning.

It is my deepest conviction that unless we take into account this element of meaning, neither longevity nor physical integrity can ultimately prove a social asset. On the contrary, of and by themselves, they threaten to engulf us in a quagmire of futile endurance, burdensome alike to the aged who endure and to the young who must endure their endurance.

Already there is a good deal of evidence to support this dire prophecy. One such is the lugubrious statistic of suicide. It was Pliny the Elder who said, "Against the outrage of life I have the refuge of death." Seemingly there are many among our aged who are impelled to seek and to find this refuge. Life proving intolerable, outrageous in extreme, they find surcease in death. Scanning the tables one finds that it is not the young, the passionate and the impetuous who most commonly destroy themselves, but rather the older ones. The suicide rates increase consistently and significantly from the fifth through the eighth decades of life. It was 12.3 per 100,000 population in the age group 35 to 44, and 27,9 for the age group 75 to 84 for the year 1955.

More telling is the differential between the rates for men and women. The ratio is one female to three males in the earlier age group, and one to 6.5 in the older age group. The quest for meaningfulness evidently bears down more heavily upon the male than on the female. In women it may be in their very femaleness.

Suicide is a datum hard to grasp and difficult to interpret. One is always prompted to implicate the suicide's psyche, to postulate that suicide is always an act of madness. I'll not press this issue, but only ask, "Why should man or woman, mature in years and seasoned in experience, and surely many among the older suicides are such, elect to put an end to their lives?" Is it too much to suppose that in some instances, and I'd guess in many instances, the individual found life to be meaningless, and meaningless life to be intolerable?

Clearly, however, not all who find life meaningless destroy themselves outright. Some, it would seem, do it in a leisurely fashion, finding refuge not in death but in senility. This, too, is a datum hard to grasp and difficult to interpret. Experience in England and in the Scandinavian countries has shown that the person adjudged senile in the complex setting of an industrial city can at times become a well adjusted geron in the less demanding environment of a village or farm, not only because, the environment is less taxing but because he can more readily find some answer to the question "Life, what for?" in small usefulness and in the affect relations which rural life affords and urban life denies.

Senility cannot in every instance be established on the basis of cerebral sclerosis and behavioral criteria. It is a very disquieting fact that our population seems to be deteriorating more rapidly than it is aging. From 1936 to 1951 admissions to state mental hospitals of persons 65 years and over with disease of the senium increased 99.9 percent (1). In Connecticut between 1950 and 1954 the number of people 60 years and over in the general population increased by 14 percent, while the number of admissions to the state mental hospitals from the same group increased by 39 percent (Kolb).

These statistics, however, cannot be taken at their face value. As Lawrence Kolb observes: "The increased use of mental hospitals by the aged is not altogether due to the higher incidence of mental disease among them . . . it is widely felt and feared that many feeble old people are being sent to mental hospitals for sociologic rather than for mental health reasons." It is sociologic rather than organic senility that afflicts this group. We can interpret the sociological in terms of the dimension of meaning.

However, the dimension of meaning must be defined; and the meaning of meaning must not be taken for granted. What can and does make the life of an individual meaningful? Gerontologists, of course, are not unaware of this problem. They know that merely to stay alive, and to be tolerably healthy, is not quite enough. A man needs also to be occupied. What an odd and yet most expressive phrase this is. To be occupied! An apartment is occupied; so is a seat in the theatre or on the train. A man can be occupied with his thoughts, his plans, his dreams. Palpably then, occupied means "to be filled" or to be "taken up." Man needs occupation. He needs to be "taken up" with something. He himself is a vacuity unless he is "devoted to," "concerned with," or "taken up by" something worth his while; and "while" refers to his life, to his endurance. Seemingly then, it is his occupation that gives meaningfulness to his life.

There is much to support this proposition. Consider how many familial names derive from occupational functions: the Smiths, Weavers, Coopers, Farmers, Shepards, Carpenters, Taylors, and so on. In the social system apparently a man *is* what he does. His identifying signature is his occupation.

With this awareness, gerontologists have been preoccupied with "jobs for the aged." They look upon retirement not as an occupational terminus but as a junction station for a switch in occupation. This, I am sure you will agree, is very much to the good. A man *should* be occupied as long as he lives and is capable of working.

But one cannot pursue this argument without awareness that something is wrong with it. If work is really that significant, men would love it, and loving it would crave it. But men notoriously do *not* love work, and that is not always the fault of the job. Many men look forward to retirement, which to them means a time when they won't have to "put up" with all the unpleasantness of their job and work. True, once retired they may dream of their old bondage and wish they were in harness again, but even this does not attest to their love of work. It may be rather that between work and retirement, they find work less galling.

We have a something akin to this in what psychiatrists call the weekend neurosis. Those who suffer this neurosis appear to do fairly well during the work week, but wilt as personalities during the work-free weekends. But it isn't because they so love their work that they miss it on weekends. It is rather that they do not know what to do with themselves when they are not working. That is phrasing it in colloquial terms. The basic fact is that weekend living confronts them with a variety of interpersonal affect relations which they cannot effect with satisfaction and which they do not encounter in the same kind or degree at work.

It appears, then, that occupation cannot be entirely subsumed under the heading of work. Or to phrase it otherwise, work is a part, but not the whole, of occupation. To apply this directly to gerontology, work will help the aged but does not provide them a full measure of that third dimension of being which we have defined as the meaningfulness of life. Something else is wanting. That something is of the order of consanguineous relatedness and of altruism.

Because of the somewhat scholastic overtones of my exposition, I have been wondering what a man of the sixteenth, seventeenth, or even of the eighteenth century would think of all this. I suspect he'd understand little of the argument. He would be aware that we are troubled about something, but he wouldn't quite grasp what it was. All this talk of the meaning of life, of work, of retirement, would sound strange to his ears. Yes, he'd be likely to observe, one can retire to monastery, but not from work. And as for the meaning of life, that is simple; life is for the good of man and the greater glory of God.

He would be right to find our preoccupations odd. They were largely unknown to his age and period. They are derivatives of the Industrial Revolution and of the new economic system. In his time, age was what Rabbi Ben Ezra said of it—the best that was yet to be—the last for which the first was made. For then a man, rich or poor, worked and lived with his kin, and, in the measure of his circumstances, lived for the good of man and the greater glory of God. The good of man and the greater glory of God were implemented, realized, eventuated, in the embracive family, which provided consanguineous relatedness and the initial as well as the most immediate evocation to altruism.

Of all the multiform effects of the Industrial Revolution and the new economic system, none perhaps has proved more of a challenge to the meaningfulness of life than the disruption of that familial pattern upon which our culture and our ethos were founded and which, by the best available evidence, had endured for more than twelve thousand years. This was the pattern achieved when man abandoned the nomadic life of the hunter and food gatherer and learned to cultivate the land; when, in other words, he became an agriculturalist.

The initial home was, in effect, a homestead in which three coexisting generations lived and labored in a meaningful and rewarding union. This homestead, with its familial pattern, was an institution of far-reaching effects. It was a school for living, wherein the young were indoctrinated by practice and precept in the techniques and wisdoms requisite to effective living. It was the repository of a man's enterprise, his security against advancing years and failing strength, his heritage gained, and his heritage transmitted. It gave the testament of endurance, of meaningful continuity, to the succeeding generations. Above all, in the prospering family, it gave clear meaning and a transparent rationale to those virtues which the moralists taught, the virtues of honest husbandry and of good will. Herein lies the meaning of "for the good of man and the greater glory of God." But the Industrial Revolution disrupted the homestead, negated its rationale, and created a world inimical to its very existence.

Ours is not a three but only a one-generation culture. We live not for long, nor in any measure of closeness, either with our parents or with our children. Little wonder then that we are described as a Lonely Crowd, and are spoken of as Outsiders. The Nobel Prize for literature was awarded to Albert Camus, and he was cited as the author who most clearly spoke for our generation. I am willing to recognize him as such. Camus is an Existentialist, and existentialism is the brave affirmation of despair. It is a quest for the meaningfulness of life in the absence of meaning. It proffers the desperate counsel to abandon the search for meaning and to find in existence itself both its means and its end.

All this may seem like a far cry, too distant and too remote from our immediate preoccupation—gerontology. But, I confess, it is a far cry I wish to sound. Gerontology is not a science apart. Neither in its biological, nor in its economic, nor in its social phases is it a discipline unrelated to the rest of the spectrum of existence.

It is said that to live long you must choose the proper grandparents. That applies to every phase of being. But one's grandparents do not suffice to assure effective existence. The cultural milieu, the societal matrix, the prevailing ethos, also exercise their determining influences. And ours are of an inimical character.

Would it strike you as all-too-far fetched were I to relate the problem of juvenile delinquency to that of geriatrics? But it isn't. In a substantial measure they both derive from the disruption of our familial pattern. Bluntly stated, I cannot conceive the resolution of either unless we reconstitute the family—bringing the parents back to their children, and the children back to their parents.

It is not a Canute-like objective that I set before you. I have no nostalgic or romantic hankering for the good old days. They weren't that good, and they are gone forever. But there *is* a limit beyond which we cannot and may not abandon the patterns of cultural relatedness without courting immediate disaster and ultimate annihilation. To this extent I concur with the dire warnings of Toynbee, though I do not entirely subscribe to his patterns of salvation.

I do not know how salvation is to be effected. I cannot offer you a design for redemption. I do, however, believe that we have allowed technology to take over the governance of our lives. We have not subjugated our ways of living to the ends of life, but have rather yielded our ancient values to the prevailing means. I cannot believe that a people skilled and clever enough to fathom the mystery of the atom, enterprising and ingenious enough to invade the firmament with its satellites and space ships, cannot resolve even these issues if it will grasp and confront them.

Crucial to these issues is the fact that all the immediate considerations revolving about the care and physical well-being of our aging population, whether they concern medical services, pensions, work, or custodial provisions, will not suffice unless we also facilitate attainment of a third dimension of being, that of meaningfulness. And the meaningfulness of life is attained primarily through consanguineous relatedness, and its evocation to altruism. I intend the integrated family, bound in love and service.

REFERENCE

1. KOLB, LAWRENCE: Mental hospitalization of the aged. Is it overdone? *Am. Journal of Psychiatry*, Feb. 19, 1956.

23

The Addictive Personality

DRUG ADDICTION is a plague of epidemic magnitude. Everywhere anxious voices cry out, "Beware, Be Warned!" "Our present problem," the distinguished psychiatrist, Dana Farnsworth, has said, "is more serious than anything that we, or any other country, has encountered. We have more people involved on a larger scale and with vastly more drugs than ever before, and we have an intricate mixture of issues generated in part because we have become a society more dependent on drugs, even on legal ones, than any preceding society."

Perry Talkington warns us "Our psychiatric hospitals are being flooded with adolescents. The number of first admissions of patients 24 years old and younger almost doubled between 1962 and 1969. Drug abuse has replaced mental retardation as the third most frequent diagnosis for males between the ages of 15 and 24."

The severity of the epidemic, in terms of the numbers affected, is difficult to establish with precision. The Federal Bureau of Narcotics and Drugs estimates 650,000 addicts for the nation, of which number 300,000 are said to be in New York City alone. The Addiction Services Agencies of New York City estimate that the city harbors 150,000 hardcore addicts, plus from 200,000 to 400,000 others. In 1969, according to the Chief Medical Examiner of New York City, heroin utilization and its complications were the leading causes of death for persons between 15 and 35 years of age—greater than the deaths due to accidents, homicides, cancer and suicides.

The most disturbing feature of these data is that they are exponentially on the increase. There were four times as many heroin-related deaths in the decade of 1960 to 1969 as there were in the preceding decade 1950 to

1959. These more than suggest that the treatment of addiction, notably of heroin addiction, has effected few "cures." Various investigators have found a relapse rate for addicts discharged from hospitals after having undergone treatment ranging from between 90 to 95%. Of course, this does not establish that treatment *per se* is of no value. Insulin, as we all know, does not cure diabetes. But it does highlight the fact that the prevailing methods of treatment, punitive with drugs, notably methadone, are not enough. They do not "cure," and, of course, do not help to prevent addiction.

Three components enter into the addiction complex. These are the addictive agents—the drugs, the predisposing conditions and the addictive personality. Of the three components, we know most about the addictive agents and least about the addictive personality. Yet it is clearly manifest that the crucial factor in addiction must be the personality of the person who is prone to addiction. The addictive agents are protean in nature, multiform in substance and ubiquitous in distribution.

The predisposing conditions are anything but uniform. They range from those of abject misery to those of sumptuous luxury. The evident constant in the addiction complex is the character of the addict, his addictive personality. But then, what precisely is the character of the addictive personality? How is it defined? How recognized? Can this perception be utilized in the treatment of the addict? Could it serve as a basis for the prevention of addiction? As noted, we know a great deal about the addictive agents. The law has concentrated on the control of their availability and distribution. Treatment has for its main objective the elimination of the addict's dependence upon the addictive agent. And public education has focused on the hazards of addiction. However, as I said before, little attention has been devoted to the factor *primus inter omnes* (first among the rest) of the addictive personality. But there are some who vehemently deny that there is any such psychological entity as an addictive personality. We must, therefore, come to grips with this issue before we can further pursue our theme.

The difficulty in this "issue" derives, I believe, from the impreciseness of the word "personality." It is, in effect, a vague term. Personality derives from the root term "persona," which in Latin means "a mask," such as, in ancient times, was worn by an actor playing a role. We use the term "personality" in quite the same sense today to express just how *we see* an individual, how he appears to us. We say so-and-so has a pleasant or an appealing, or, to the contrary, an ugly and repugnant personality. In the main, then, personality is a something *in the other person,* his mask of presenting features, to which we react subjectively. It is not really an objective evaluation of the individual we make in terms of good or bad, but rather an expression of our own likes and dislikes. It is not uncommon to hear it said of a man that he has a fine character, but a poor personality.

Now this brings us to the term "character," frequently used as a synonym for personality, which it is not. Character refers to a quality of being quite different from that of personality. Personality relates to appearance, character to operation, to behavior. We speak of character as good or bad, weak or strong, decisive or otherwise. Hence, what, we must ask, is the basis for such a judgment? This question is intensely relevant to the problem of addiction, and it merits deep exploration. We have noted that personality relates to appearance, and character to operation, to behavior. Character is dynamic, and in human experience, the dynamic instance is initiated by the making of a choice between two or more options. Man, more than any other living creature, must perforce make choices, must elect not only between alternates of good and bad, but also at times between bad and worse, and between good and better. From this it follows that the so-called good character must be such because the individual more or less consistently makes the better choices from among the available ones. Of course, this in turn leads to the derivative question, namely, what distinguishes the good from the inferior—from the bad choice? Or to paraphrase this, wherein lies the goodness of the good choice? Now this is a tantalizing question—one that has made many a holiday for such moral sophists as Szasz and Laing for example. But, in effect, the question can be dealt with in a very simple and direct way, not speculatively or metaphysically, but empirically, and I would like to say, biosociologically. Thus, *that* choice is good which favors the advancement and self-realization of the electing individual, and also of those with whom he is intimately coexistent. This definition could be extended to embrace more of the realm in which the individual exists, to include, for example, the community, the state, society in general, etc. For this occasion, however, I prefer the simpler definition, so let me affirm that by self-realization I intend nothing more, though in itself it is already a good deal of accomplishment, nothing more than normal growth, development and normal life experience, including the competence to earn a living, to marry, to raise a family and to meet the exigencies of aging. At this point of the exposition I have in the past asked myself the question, which I suspect you, too, are likely to ponder, namely: Why speak of addictive personality when in effect we are concerned not with personality, but with character? The answer to this question is in part trivial and in part very much in earnest. The trivial part is usage. The addictive character is less euphemistic than the addictive personality, and in psychiatric nosography, as well as in psychiatric literature, the term "personality" is encountered much more frequently than is "character." Also, quite frequently, these terms are not differentiated from one another or are used in an associative bind to imply that character molds personality, which affirmation, of course, is only partially true.

Now the earnest part of the answer I offer is that "it wouldn't matter." Those who deny the validity and the concept of the addictive personality would likewise deny the validity of the addictive character. And they do this because of a simple misconception. They see in both of these terms the implication of genetic predestination, as if individuals so described were simply and inescapably doomed to become addicts. In fact, however, these designations—addictive personality and addictive character—carry no such implications. On the contrary, when understood in depth, the phrase addictive personality, and, even more pointedly, the phrase addictive character argue that addicts are not born such—they *become* addicts. The issue of how much loaded genetics enters into the creation of the addictive personality, if any at all, is a sticky problem. For certain, there is no evidence whatsoever to even suggest, let alone prove, that there are any genes which specifically foreordain an individual to become an addict. But genetic factors, insofar as they may influence an individual's physical, mental and emotional endowments, can, and probably do, enter into the complex of determinants which in one case make for, and in another case fortify against, addiction. But even so, it is inconceivable that a genetic factor could be the single, primary, determinant agent in addiction.

To sum it up then, there are no born addicts. There are only some individuals who become addicts and others, far more numerous, who do not become addicts.

We have thus far discussed addicts and addiction as if we had already agreed on the precise meaning of these terms. But, of course, we haven't. In a general way, I suppose, when we speak of one as being an addict, there is in the back of our minds the awareness and persuasion that such a person is perversely dependent upon the use of some substance deleterious to his health and disruptive of his individual and social operation.

In addition, we may think that the use of such substance is prohibited by law.

In the broader sense of the term "addiction" we must perceive several distinctive components. Two such are habituation and dependence. Habituation is a psychological state. Dependence is a physiological condition. Then, too, there is the component of legality, what the law will forbid or permit an individual to use. But not every habituation and not every dependence, or dependence-evoking substance, are legally taboo. The smoking of tobacco is a good example, and the drinking of alcoholic beverages is another. Furthermore, addiction can be perceived in many phases of life; some of them are not usually recognized as addictive and, indeed, are socially sanctioned, even though they may prove deleterious to individual and group living. Examples of such are the addiction to work, to the amassment of much wealth, prestige or power. In moderation, that is when commensurate with other essential operations in living, these are commendable pursuits. They acquire the character of an addiction when they are pursued to an extent which cripples individual and social living. This analysis of the several components that enter into the concept and reality of addiction throws a clear light on the relationship between the addictive agent and the addictive personality. The addictive agent, as we have noted, is protean, of many shapes, forms and substances. Nominally, everyone is exposed to addictive agents in one form or another. The addictive agent carries the potential for addiction, but only the addictive personality, or preferably the addictive character, exposed to an addictive agent, becomes an addict. The potential of the addictive agent is activated by the addictive character's need and desire to escape from confronting realities with which he believes he cannot, or, in effect, really cannot deal effectively.

The nonaddictive character, confronting a challenging reality not manifestly overwhelming (as someone in a concentration camp, for example), will gird to meet it, compromise with the challenge when necessary, and when unavoidable will accept and adjust to defeat. He will not run away from the challenge, nor from defeat; but the addictive character is prone to avoid challenge. He is an escapist. Life confronts him with many challenges throughout his life, and the world also affords him many means and routes of escape if and when he is so inclined. Now whence comes such inclination to run away? I will deal with that question a bit later.

Lest I be charged with being some sort of social Darwinian, some privileged "tough" who despises the so-called "weak in spirit," let me make it clear that I do not look upon addiction to alcohol or to drugs, soft or hard, as degeneracy, nor on the addict as a degenerate. I do not brand, nor do I condemn. Basically I am compassionate. But even more, I am eager to highlight what in my opinion is the crucial factor in addiction, the recognition of which should serve to make treatment of addiction a bit more effective and also make the prevention of addiction possible. I am keenly aware that some challenging realities are beyond the resources and competences of most men to meet and overcome. Weekly, I travel by train between Bridgeport, Connecticut and Grand Central, New York and pass by Harlem, that hellhole of poverty and degradation. I would not know how, in any decency, I could stand in judgment over any of its numerous and swarming inhabitants; and yet, miracle of miracles, even in Harlem, there are many, so very many, who do meet and successfully overcome their confronting and bitterly adverse realities. Poverty and adversity do contribute to the creation of the addictive character. Escapism is more likely among the deprived, but the addictive personality is encountered at all levels of society and at all levels of economic status, among the educated, as well as among those without learning.

Now let us come closer to the actualities of the addictive personality, to observe his characterological features clearly, and to describe them in fine detail.

I have described the addictive personality as that of an escapist, as of one who, unable to master confronting realities, runs away. Israel Zwerling, a psychiatrist of broad experience and keen clinical acumen, found that the addictive personality (he dealt mostly with alcoholics) presented a quite constant constellation of traits. To him, they seemed to be schizoid people, fearful and withdrawn. They were depressed, and gave a history of frequent suicide attempts, as well as of numerous self-inflicted injuries. He found them to be basically dependent, taking and grasping in their relations. They frequently exhibited both overt and unconscious rage. Their sexuality was immature.

Dr. Howard Zucker describes his addictive patients as "showing marked social anxiety, usually generalized." They had the tendency to form intense relationships with a remarkable lack of ego-boundary. They exhibited exaggerated and lifelong dependency needs. Psychoanalytically, the addictive personality can be defined as a severely regressed, pregenital character with primitive defenses, obvious oral and anal traits, severe depressive elements and pregenital sexuality. This conglomerate of characterological and behavioral symptoms can, I believe, be subsumed under the rubric of developmental inadequacy with resultant bizarre and aggravating defenses. I name the complex simply *Escapism*. It is a fugue from adult life from adult responsibilities.

John and Elaine Cumming have also dealt with this complex. They named it "the inadequacy syndrome." "This term," Elaine wrote, "refers to those characteristics which can be thought of as the result of a general failure to adapt because of ego-poverty. Ego-poverty means a lack of inner resources for solving crises and even solving day-to-day problems." How, we may ask, is such ego-poverty engendered? Paul Agnew, writing under the title "Cultural Deprivation and Mental Illness," offers the following explanation. Ego-poverty results from inadequate enculturation. "The cause," he wrote, "is failure of the individual to internalize the cultural content, value systems, ethos, ideal patterns of behavior and culturally approved goals and aspirations, because these were not transmitted to them." This statement needs a bit of sharpening. The failure is not that of the impoverished individual, but of those who failed to enculturate him. It is to be assumed that enculturation was potentially possible. Otherwise, the problem would be of an entirely different nature. To paraphrase the foregoing in terms of arguments relative to my own presentation, it can be said that the escapist runs away because he was not taught nor trained how "to stay with it." And the escapist is and must remain ego-impoverished because ego-capital derives from the effective dealing with life's presenting evocations, confrontations and challenges. Herein lies the sense and wisdom of the common saying, "Nothing succeeds like success." The escapist does not succeed.

The concept of the inadequacy syndrome as a resultant of failure in enculturation provides us with ideological orientation in the problem of the genesis of the addictive personality and suggests a methodology for treatment and the prevention of addiction. To quote Paul Agnew again "Treatment of inadequate enculturation," he wrote, "would consist of developing means of transmitting the culture to persons already old enough to be considered as having been deprived of adequate enculturation. Treatment would be a teaching-learning process in the comprehensive sense. It would be involved in the active transmission of values, ideals, patterns, role responsibilities and other elements of the prevailing culture." "For prevention," he wrote, "means would have to be developed for breaking into the cycle of generations and seeing to it that culture is adequately transmitted to individuals who otherwise would experience inadequate enculturation. This would have to be an endeavor of the community through its publicly supported professional agencies specifically created and organized for this purpose."

Enculturation is a suggestive rather than an explicit term. We can understand its indicated results, but it does not instruct us as to how these results are to be achieved. We need to ask, "How does one enculturate a person?" The answer appears to me to be: by disciplined instruction, discipline being the dynamic component of the operation. It is no mere coincidence that learned professions are termed disciplines, as the discipline of law or that of medicine.

Discipline is a term misunderstood nowadays. It is a term misunderstood and eschewed. To many, the term has the twang of compulsion, if not of tyranny. Not discipline, but permissiveness is the order of the day. It appears that we have taken in earnest Rousseau's fiction of the noble savage. Mankind surely was savage, but never noble. And most certainly, whatever of nobleness of spirit, or of manner, man had developed down the ages came to him by way of a discipline which bridled his unreasoned impulses and his savage passions, and taught him to share his existence with the rest of the living world, and thus, also to meet his life's obligations. May it not be then that the enormous problem of alcohol and drug addiction is in essence a problem of missed discipline? And hence characterological in nature? And if such indeed is the nature of the problem, is it not clear that such also should be (in part) the nature of its solution?

At present, the effort to contain (there is no pretense at overcoming) the so-called epidemic of addiction has two components, diverse in nature but frequently used in combination. One is punitive and the other medical. Neither the one nor the other, nor both in combination, has proved effective to any significant measure in curbing addiction. This does not argue that such efforts should be relinquished or abandoned, though for certain, the punitive phase could be much refined and humanized. It does argue that the present punitive and medical means are in themselves not effective in reducing the incidence of drug addiction. There is no point in my citing statistics in support of this affirmation. The evidence is all about. Thus, a ghoulish item appearing in a recent issue of the *New York Post,* November 3, 1972, reports that the deaths in New York City during a ten-month period in the current year numbered 1176 drug addicts. The number, so stated the Medical Examiner's office, is expected to go even higher when a backlog of almost 1000 autopsies still awaiting final laboratory reports is completed. The average age of these victims of addiction was about 25. The youngest was 15 years of age. But the significant point is that one-third of these were on methadone. Clearly, something more than methadone and the police is called for in the struggle against the spreading epidemic of addiction. That something, I submit, is the perception of the problem of addiction in a new gestalt, not primarily as illegal, nor yet primarily as a medical problem, but rather as one characterological in nature. And thus, the remedy for the cure of malignant addiction would be seen to lie in the correction of the character deficiences that afflict the addicted personality.

Here I must anticipate the despairing query: "Is it really ever possible to correct character difficulties and deficiencies—to reform a personality?" On the basis of what history clearly shows, and on the derivatives of my own 50 years of psychiatric experience, I would unhesitatingly say, "Yes, it *is* possible, provided that the effort is sufficiently intensive, adequately prolonged, and the subject still young, to wit, under 30."

Plato based his paideia on like convictions. The teachings and the practices of all religious bodies are directed toward such ends and are based upon such persuasions. Otherwise there would be no redemption for the sinner and no reform for the evil ones. But such historic references, I am afraid, may prove antipathetic to some. They suggest, as I said before, regimentation, constraint, exaction. In effect, they do. Plato's Republic, if established, would be very much like a Communist polity. And the exactions of the churches, at least some of them, were and remain galling indeed. But then, is it possible for mankind to live a civilized life without discipline? Man is defined as a creature with a culture, and culture implies discipline. Innately, discipline need not be harsh or cruel. It can be, in its end results, an elected commitment arrived at by indoctrination and persuasion. To be a disciple does not mean to be enslaved. It means to be dedicated.

What I propose is this—that those not adequately encultured, that is, the addicted and the addiction-prone persons, should be engaged in a teaching-learning process which would enable them to internalize the culture content, value system, ethos, ideal patterns of behavior and culturally approved goals and aspirations which, because of varying reasons and conditions, were not transmitted to them. Such a proposal, I know, must seem staggering in magnitude and in complexity. It also evokes among some of the cynics the memory of such past attempts which it is said always failed. But what I envisage has not been attempted on the scale and with the intensity I deem necessary. It is forecast faintly and in small dimensions in such laudable efforts as Synanon, Phoenix House, Daytop and other like efforts. But what is requisite is of much more heroic dimensions in spirit, vision and effort. Dare I say that I see in the addiction epidemic a moral crisis and that it calls for a moral remedy?

The moral crisis manifest in the individual derives from the world he lives in. If he is not properly enculturated it is because the culturally approved goals and aspirations have not been transmitted to him. The exceptions are few and irrelevant.

What precisely the moral remedy to our moral crisis is to be, I have hinted at, but cannot spell out in detail. I take refuge and some consolation in the sage saying that the correct asking of a question already provides half the answer.

24

Community Psychiatry — Its Social and Historic Derivations

THE BANNER of the crusade launched by the late President Kennedy against mental illness and mental retardation carried the envoy, "Psychiatry must be returned to the mainstream of medicine." The tone is imperious, like the Elder Cato's *Delenda est Carthago*. But unlike Cato's injunction it is a bit cryptic. One is moved to ask, "Just what does this mean? Is not psychiatry now 'in the mainstream of medicine?' And if psychiatry is not in the mainstream, what channeled it off, and how is it to be brought back?"

Dwelling on this injunction to "bring psychiatry back into the mainstream of medicine," one grows to appreciate that it *is* indeed pregnant with meaning. One perceives, in time, that it expresses in a sophisticated way the essential and strategic requisites for the effective realization of community psychiatry.

Psychiatry must be brought back into the mainstream of medicine! But to understand the 'why and how' of this injunction, we need to turn to history. There we find that psychiatry was indeed an integral part of medicine in times past, as far back in time as medicine was practised by man. Psychiatry was the mainstay of the primitive medicine man and of the shaman. "Nowhere is the reliance on psychotherapy in general and suggestion in particular more obvious than in the medical lore of primitive society," wrote Erwin H. Ackerknecht (1). If, by a long leap in time, we pass from primitive medicine to the medicine of Ancient Greece, we find that Hippocrates was well instructed and widely experienced in psychiatry, and that this psychiatry was an integral part of his medicine. Asclepiades of Bithynia (142 B.C.), called by the moderns the "Father of Psychiatry," was a competent physician who treated the mentally ill by means of diet, baths, massage, emetics and bloodletting. He advocated a pleasant environment, social activities, pleasant companions and music in the treatment not only of the mentally ill, but of all patients.

To the names of Hippocrates and Asclepiades can be added those of Galen (A.D. 130-200), Caellus Aurelianus (A.D. 400) and Soranus, each a distinguished physician and well informed in psychiatry (2).

It is not my intention to survey ancient medicine and to list those other physicians whose knowledge and understanding of mental illness is noteworthy. For the points I wish to make are well enough reflected in those illustrious physicians I have mentioned, to wit, that the ancient physician well appreciated mental illnesses, that he treated them with a fair degree of effectiveness, and that the treatment of mental illness was then not a "practice of psychiatry," but an integral part of the practice of medicine. None of the ancient physicians was in effect a psychiatrist, nor would he consider himself as such, not even Asclepiades of Bithynia, the "Father of Psychiatry."

We see then that psychiatry was from its very beginning in the mainstream of medicine. It remained so until the Eighth Century, A.D. when it was, so to say, diverted. Thereafter psychiatry pursued a separate course, for the Ancient World, the Græco-Roman realm, was conquered by the Arabs in the seventh century. "The fall of the Roman Empire of the West," wrote Castiglioni (3), "marks a period of arrest in the history of (Western) civilization. Rigidified in a system of formulas and dominated by mysticism, medicine was forced to exist in a state of scholastic dogmatism, in which it is difficult to find any animating ideas."

The Mohammedan conquest of the Græco-Roman realm had a blighting effect upon Europe's cultural life, and Europe did not begin to recover until near to the end of the eleventh century. During this interim of 300 years, the pursuit and the practice of medicine deteriorated greatly, and psychiatry fell into the hands of "the exorcizing priest and the priestly witch hunter" (4). The psyche was no longer the realm and concern of the physician. As the *soul*, it became the domain of the priest and the religious inquisitor. "The whole field of mental disease," writes Gregory Zilboorg, "was torn away from medicine. Medical psychology as a legitimate branch of the healing art practically ceased to exist. It was recaptured by the priest and incorporated into his theurgic system. Seven hundred years of effort seemed for a long while to have spent themselves in vain. The ardent voice heard in Hippocrates' discourse on the 'Sacred Disease' was lost in the wilderness; it was silent for nearly twelve centuries" (5).

Zilboorg's poetic allusion to the "ardent voice heard in Hippocrates' discourse on the 'Sacred Disease'" must not escape us. It is in that discourse that Hippocrates is said to have taken his place among those who did *not* attribute disease to the ill will of the gods—but rather, to natural causes. Hippocrates scorned superstition and the quackery that dissimulated its cupidity by ascribing disease to the Godhead. "Being at a loss," wrote Hippocrates, "and having no treatment which would help, they concealed and sheltered themselves behind superstition and called this illness sacred, in order that their utter ignorance might not be manifest" (6). "It is not in my opinion," wrote Hippocrates, "any more divine or more sacred than any other disease, but has a natural cause" (p. 139). And as to the gods, according to Hippocrates, "A man's body is not defiled by a god . . . a god is more likely to purify and sanctify it than he is to cause it defilement" (7).

The profound sanity of Hippocrates' teachings was, however, overwhelmed by the madness of a new era in which church and clergy excluded psychiatry from medicine, and gave it over to demonology.

It is an easy but rather fatuous sport to make much of the Church's demonology, to accent the scourge, the faggot and the stake. But we who have witnessed the carnage of two World Wars, the brutalities of the execrable Hitler, and the horror of the Bomb are ill suited to point a scornful finger at the errors and madness of the ancients. I dwell on the demonology of the Church because it marks the separation of psychiatry from medicine and because it served as prelude to the advent of the mental hospital.

But there is more to be considered before this progression becomes clear. Thus we need to appreciate that when we speak of the Ancient World, of Græco-Roman culture, and of Græco-Roman medicine, we refer to but a very small area of Europe, to a narrow band of land figuratively encircling *mare nostrum,* the Mediterranean Sea. In historic times this was an area peopled with a cluster of nations that had been for thousands of years under the tutelage of great minds, of named and unnamed philosophers, scientists, poets, artists, and moralists. These peoples had by dint of much labour ascended from the semi-brutish levels of primitive man to the higher levels of cultural attainment. To this day we marvel at the ingenuity of those men who created the alphabet, invented the wheel, learned to sail the seas, fashioned the lyre and the flute, speculated so sublimely on Nature and man's place within it, wrote poetry and drama, fashioned marble and bronze so that they became animate with the voice of eternal beauty.

That was the Ancient World that *was,* that was, as we have already noted, disrupted in the seventh century by the invasion of Islam. "Islam," in the words of the historian Henri Pirenne, "was thrown across the path of history with the elemental force of a cosmic cataclysm. Its sudden thrust had destroyed ancient Europe" (8). When, some 400 years later, Europe experienced the stirrings of a revival, it was sensed not in the Mediterranean perimeter, but rather in the northern lands of Europe. "The centre of gravity," to further quote Pirenne, "heretofore on the shore of the Mediterranean, was shifted to the north. As a result, the Frankish Empire, which had so far been playing a minor role in the history of Europe, was to become the arbiter of Europe's destinies" (9). "Without Islam, the Frankish Empire would probably never have existed and Charlemagne, without Mahomet, would be inconceivable." From whatever standpoint it is studied, the advent of the Frankish Empire marks a distinct break with the civilization of antiquity.

To understand then why psychiatry was taken over by church and priest, why in later years it was relegated to the *Narrenturm* and *Irrenanstalt,* and why indeed some of the earliest hospitals for the insane were founded in the Germanic cities, we must first understand what in the main happened in the lives of the northern peoples, those embraced in the Frankish Empire, who later became the arbiters of Europe's destinies. These peoples were different, much unlike the Mediterranean hosts whose civilizing experiences, gained in a long travail of social coexistence, these northerners had yet to face and suffer. Europe had to pass through its medieval era.

It was an era of great madness: one of widespread *furor,* violence, cruelty, anxiety, sadness and depression. It was an era racked by famines, wars and pestilences. It was a time of cruel and bitter strife among the princes of the lands, among workers and masters. "A present-day reader," writes Huizinga, "studying the history of the Middle Ages based on official documents will never sufficiently realize the extreme excitability of the medieval soul" (10). "A general feeling of impending calamity hangs over all. Perpetual danger prevails everywhere. Bad government, exactions, the cupidity and violence of the great, . . . brigandage, scarcity, misery and pestilence—to this is contemporary history nearly reduced in the eyes of the people. No other epoch has laid so much stress . . . on the thought of death" (11). "Until far into the sixteenth century, tombs are adorned with hideous images of a naked corpse with clenched hands and rigid feet, gaping mouth, and bowels crawling with worms" (12). "Is it surprising then," Huizinga adds, "that the people could see their fate and that of the world only as an endless succession of evils?" "The background of all life in the world seems black. Everywhere the flames of hatred arise and injustice reigns. Satan covers a gloomy earth with his sombre wings" (13).

In this atmosphere rationality was suffocated and demonology thrived. "The fear of sorcery and the blind fury of persecution continued to darken the mental atmosphere of the age." The times were full of strife and sorrow, and hence of great madnesses. The Black Death, raging between 1347-1350, had carried off, it is estimated, a third of the population of Europe, and utterly demoralized those surviving. "The effects of the Black Death," wrote Hecker (14), "had not yet subsided and the graves of millions of its victims were scarcely closed, when a strange delusion arose in Germany which took possession of the minds of men and . . . hurried away body and soul into the magic circle of hellish superstition." This was the dancing mania that affected the whole of Germany and spread to the neighbouring countries. Italy had its counterpart in Tarantism. In Hungary there arose the mad Brotherhood of the Flagellants, called also the Brethren of the Cross. Gross and pitiless were the persecutions of the Jews, which, to quote Hecker, "were (now) committed in most countries, with even greater exasperation than in the twelfth century, during the First Crusades" (15). An ancient madness named Lycanthropy, known in Greece and described by Aetius, Oribasius, Paulus, and Avicenna, now reappeared. In this madness men were said "to run howling about graves and fields in the night, and (would) not be persuaded but that they were wolves, or some such beasts."

The temper of the people of Europe was such that they were open to every credulity, superstition, fear and madness. "Men's minds were morbidly sensitive," writes Hecker, "and as it happens with individuals whose senses are suffering under anxiety, become more irritable, so trifles are magnified into objects of great alarm, and slight shocks, which would scarcely affect the spirits when in health, give rise in them to severe diseases, so with this nation, at times so alive to emotions, and at that periods so sorely pressed with the horrors of death" (16).

The frenzy and the madness of this mood is perhaps nowhere better mirrored than in the paintings of Hieronymus Bosch (1460-1516), Matthias Grünewald, and Pieter Brueghel, the Elder (1525-1569). Though these artists painted their fabulous paintings in the dawning years of the Renaissance, the hyperrealism (the term is Huizinga's [17], of their bewildering, satirical mordant *exposé* of life as it was, appears like the lingering memory of a desperate nightmare. And no doubt it was, for as

Huizinga observes in his essay titled *The Problem of the Renaissance* (18), "The Renaissance is only a very superficial phenomenon; the true essential cultural transition flowed out of the Middle Ages." And the flow was rich also in promise and attainment. Like Bosch and Brueghel, I have indited the desperate side of the Middle Ages. But these ages also had their bright, their redeeming side. I have accented the griefs and the travails of Europe's northern peoples as they advanced from the initial state of primitive hordes and marauding bands, to form, in the faith of the one God, large nations, strong principalities and kingdoms, in order to highlight the historic rationale for the diversion of psychiatry away from medicine, to the church and priest.

In the Middle Ages there was a great work to be done, and it was in the main a moral work. The picture, therefore, must not be distorted. The church for all its errors, crudities and persecutions did a noble work in humanizing, educating and disciplining the savage and illiterate hordes of Europe. If the church was but a poor custodian of the wisdom of Hippocrates, yet custodian it was—and at Monte Cassino in Italy, at Oxford, Cambridge and Winchester in England, at Tours in France, and at Fulda and St. Gall in Germany, it was monastic medicine that kept alive the memory and works of Hippocrates, of Galen, of Dioscorides, and of Caellus Aurelianus, the latter pre-eminent for his psychiatric knowledge.

"Literary medicine," wrote Castiglioni, "took refuge in the churches and cloisters; and the medical learning of the period, as was also the case with philosophy, had its protection and development almost exclusively in the monastery" (19). The church, too, was the founder of the hospice, the forerunner of the hospital, which, as we have indicated, in time took over the care of the mentally ill.

The Monastic Orders not only were the custodians of ancient learning and educators in their own right, but some among them concerned themselves with man's plight this side of heaven. Among these the Cistercian Order, founded by Robert, Abbot of Molesine, in 1098, was the most preeminent. "The Cistercians came to be more widespread, more influential than any order; their fame was based not only on their zeal for purity and simplicity, but also on their skill at organization" (20).

The Cistercians are of immense historic relevance to our central concern, Community Psychiatry, for in the pattern of "This is the house Jack built," they were contributory to the great agricultural revolution wherein large portions of wooded Europe were deforested, bogs reclaimed, swamps and littoral areas redeemed, thus greatly extending the land available for agricultural use. They likewise improved agricultural and husbandry practices. The ultimate effect was more food, enabling more persons to survive, this resulting in a remarkable increment of population. To carry the story further, it is from this increment in population that the town and village laborers derived and these, with the advent of the Industrial Revolution, were converted into the proletariat. Their descendants, the children of the emergent Age of Affluence, now press for the services of Communal Psychiatry. And, therein lies the full promise of the return of psychiatry to the mainstream of medicine.

To revert to the agricultural revolution in which the Cistercians played so significant a part, we need to appreciate the significance of food production in the history of mankind, and of its effects on population.

During the thousand years that followed on the dissolution of the Roman Empire, population dwindled. "It is impossible," wrote Pirenne, "to estimate, with any approach to accuracy, the density of population, as no reliable data are available. All that we can say is that in the Carolingian Epoch (that is, in the ninth century) the population was very small, undoubtedly smaller than in any previous epoch. . . . And it seems to have remained stationary until the beginning of the eleventh century, for the natural excess of births did no more than fill the gaps made by famine, war, and the disturbances and catastrophes of every kind that descended upon the West from the middle of the ninth century" (21).

Of the afflictions suffered by the people, none was worse than famine. Charles Creighton, in his *History of Epidemics in Britain,* wrote, "The history of the English epidemics, previous to the Black Death, is almost wholly a history of famine sicknesses; and the list of such famines with attendant sickness, without mentioning the years of mere scarcity, is a considerable one (22). Famine was endemic in all of Europe, sometimes in one region and sometimes in another (23). In France, between 970 and 1100, there were no fewer than sixty famine years. England suffered terrible deaths in 1086 and in 1125. And then came the agrarian revolution.

About the year 1000, there began a period of land reclamation which was to continue intensively to the end of the twelfth century, and with an abated intensity up to our own days. "At no period," wrote Boissonnade, "has the conquest of agricultural land been carried on with so much discipline and ardour" (24). Thousands of pioneers came to prepare the way for the work of plough and hoe by burning away brushwood, thickets, and parasitic vegetation, clearing forests with the axe, and uprooting trunks with the pick. As a result the face of Europe changed.

"Germany in particular was transformed. In its immense forests, through some of which an eleventh century missionary could ride for five days on end in complete solitude, pioneers made clearings . . . established great farms all along the side of the roads or on the edge of the woods" (25). In England the woods were attacked with such vigour that nothing was left of the ancient forest which once covered the soil of Britain, save a few rare remnants. In the Low Countries, France, Spain and Italy, the forest fell before the axe of the pioneer, and with this a pitiless war was waged against wild beasts.

The plough followed in the wake of axe and pick. "Side by side with the labour of hoe and spade, the use of the iron ploughshare allowed the earth to be ploughed deeply, sometimes seven or eight times on end" (26). Improved ploughing and manuring of the land, the superior cultivation of cereals, and of vegetables, yielded better harvests and a larger food resource for both animals and humans, and in consequence by the end of the thirteenth century the population of the six states of the West contained together perhaps 60,000,000 souls, twice as many as they had numbered before the fifth century (27). (It is of interest to note that from the fourteenth until the sixteenth centuries there was no radical change in the magintude of Europe's population.)

Much of this increased population was in effect 'surplus,' that is, a population that could not be absorbed by the agrarian economy that made possible its survival. It was this population, harnessed by the initiative of the newly emergent *entrepreneur* class, that in time made possible the capitalist economy with its *bourgeoisie* and its proletariat.

The increase of the population naturally favoured industrial concentration. Numbers of the poor poured into the towns . . . where trade grew proportionately with the development of commerce, and guaranteed them their daily bread. Their condition there, however, seems to have been very miserable (28).

The working group emergent at the end of the Middle Ages was historically unique. It was 'the proletariat,' the group that possessed nothing but its labor power "to sell on the labor market for a living." The rise of this 'propertyless' class, the proletariat, is accounted for in the rise of capitalism, not as a result of expropriation—i.e., because they were deprived of their rightful ownership of the tools for their work—but rather, in the seeming paradox, because it became possible for this added population to survive. Prof. F. A. Hayek expounds this seeming paradox as follows:

"For the greater part of history, for most men the possession of the tools for their work was an essential condition for survival or at least for being able to rear a family. The number of those who could maintain themselves by working for others, although they did not themselves possess the necessary equipment, was limited to a small proportion of the population. The amount of arable land and of tools handed down from one generation to the next limited the total number who could survive. To be left without them meant in most instances death by starvation or at least the impossibility of procreation. It was only when the larger gains from the employment of machinery provided both the means and the opportunity for their investment that what in the past had been a recurring surplus of population, doomed to early death, was in an increasing measure given the possibility of survival. Numbers (i.e., population) which had been practically stationary for many centuries began to increase rapidly. The proletariat which capitalism can be said to have 'created' was thus not a proportion of the population which would have existed without it and which it had degraded to a lower level; it was an additional population which was enabled to grow up by the new opportunities for employment which capitalism provided" (29).

This 'additional population' added up to a massive increment. Thus, to cite but one country, the population of England in 1600 is estimated to have numbered 4,460,000; a century later in 1700 it was 5,653,000, and in 1801 it was 8,331,000. In 200 years, between 1600 and 1800, England's population almost doubled. Sir Robert Peel in 1806 saw in the industrial revolution the mainspring of "an additional race of man" which he credited to the greater "comforts of the population and early marriages."

On this score Sir Robert was an enthusiast. In fact there was both want and misery, and a great deal of it. This has been amply detailed by the Hammonds in their classic works on *The Village and The Town Labourers* (30).

The misery of the proletariat inspired a great deal of humanitarian concern, which materialized in social legislation and in the development of the sanitation movement. Society became acutely aware of disease and death, for both were startlingly manifest in the industrial cosmopolis: in Boston, London, Birmingham *et al*. The '*Zivilisationsseuche*' as the Germans termed them, the 'plagues of civilization,' the diseases of malnutrition, of overcrowding, of insanitation, of overwork—cholera, tuberculosis, typhus, typhoid, the infant diarrheas, rickets, the pneumonias, scarlet fever, diphtheria—all these were rampant, most intensively among the working class, but also among the middle class.

Thus with the development of industrialism, the rise of the proletariat, the concentration of great numbers of human beings in industrial centres, much disease was engendered, and to phrase it tersely, the greater need for medical service of superior competence became manifest and urgent.

The 'market' for medical service was greatly extended. Its consumers clearly were divisible into two groups. The middle class which constituted the bulk of 'private practice,' and the poorer class, which was served in clinics, dispensaries, in 'contract practice,' and as charity patients.

The extension of the 'market' for medical services, is tellingly mirrored in the remarkable increase during the eighteenth and nineteenth centuries of hospitals, medical schools, and medical personnel. This increase was not only numerical but also qualitative. "For 200 years after the Reformation," wrote Sir Arthur Thomson (31), "England was virtually without hospitals of any kind." "England then was a rural and semifeudal country; the sick were scattered in villages, and it was not until the end of the eighteenth century that the picture was completely and quickly changed by the Industrial Revolution."

"Sickness, widely spread in an agricultural community with village workshops, might escape notice, but the misery of the sick poor congregated in makeshift towns without sanitation was intensified and compelled attention." "It is not surprising, therefore, that the eighteenth century witnessed the foundation of a large number of charitable institutions in the shape of voluntary hospitals." Among these hospitals, now founded in all parts of Europe, were some devoted to the care of the insane, and the mentally ill became the responsibility of the public rather than, as before, of the church.

But psychiatry cannot be said to have been rehabilitated even at the end of the eighteenth century. For psychiatry had been subjected to a schism which, dating from the time of Paracelsus, had riven brain and psyche apart, making the one the domain of the anatomist and physiologist, and the other that of the psychologist and philosopher. Psychiatry did not come into its own until the latter half of the nineteenth century when, as Nolan D. C. Lewis has phrased it, "The first systematic reaction against a mechanistic and static attitude in psychologic medicine developed in France, where interest in purely mental phenomena was *not* considered as a regression into medieval superstition" (32). Lewis here refers to the work of Bernheim (1840-1919), of Liebault (1823-1904)), of Jean Charcot (1825-1893) and of Sigmund Freud (1856-1939), who in their separate ways founded what now is known as dynamic psychology, psychoanalysis, and psychotherapy.

The history of these developments is, I am certain, too well known to you to warrant dwelling upon them, but what is all too little appreciated is the fact that it was dynamic psychiatry that "brought psychiatry out of the hospital and back into the community." This phrasing is a little more pat than apt, for dynamic psychiatry also penetrated into the mental hospital and influenced its therapeutic practices. This much is certain: were it not for the development of dynamic psychiatry, communal psychiatry, as we now envisage it, would be impossible. For it must be acknowledged, as it seldom is, that dynamic psychiatry has enabled us to understand and to treat vast numbers of the mentally and emotionally ill, who in times past were not suited for hospitalization, and for whom the so-called alienist or neuropsychiatrist had little meaningful to offer.

William Alanson White, in his autobiographical recitation, *Forty Years of Psychiatry* (33), attests to this, as likewise, does Clarence Oberndorf in his *A History of Psychoanalysis in America* (34). In the chapter entitled "Psychiatry at the Turn of the Century," Oberndorf tells of the psychiatric practices he encountered at the New York City Psychopathic Pavilion at Bellevue Hospital. "Through these low-ceilinged, dark, overcrowded wards," Oberndorf wrote, "patients suffering at the same time from medical conditions and psychopathy passed to form a series of never-ending, kaleidoscopic, dramatic, unforgettable pictures of human misery" (35). "Psychically determined somatic conditions were treated with foul-smelling, punitively invested placebos, such as asafetida and valerian, and by some surprise manipulations such as a sharp slap or plunging a hysterical patient into an ice-cold bath" (36). Sometimes the Paquelin cautery was used. A woman obsessed with the thought that she was suffering from a growth in her abdomen, and who on thorough examination revealed no growth, was subjected to a phantom operation. A superficial incision was made while the women was under ether. She was later told that the growth had been removed. Oberndorf, laconically, observes, "But, as might have been expected, the symptoms did not change."

This was in 1910. Since then psychiatric hospitals and the practice of psychiatry, both in and outside the mental hospital, have changed greatly for the better.

Psychiatric treatment, the need for which was once considered a misfortune and a disgrace, is to-day sought and accepted by many. The 'open door' has increased rather than reduced mental hospital admissions. There is indeed a greater demand for psychiatric services than it is currently possible to provide. The demand is mounting and it is likely to increase with time, rather than diminish.

Whence comes this demand for psychiatric service? What is the force behind the movement for communal psychiatry? The answers are not difficult to find. They derive from the same sources, from the same socio-economic and cultural factors that have enlarged the market, that is, the demand for medical services in every other department of medicine. Psychiatry has been broached rather late in the order of medical specialties, most likely for the very reason that it has been outside the mainstream of medicine. It has not been, except since very recently, and at that not in every hospital, a department on a par, say with surgery, opthalmology, obstetrics, gynecology *et al*.

The market and the demand for medical services have increased. This is reflected in a variety of statistical data. Thus, between 1909 and 1955, general hospital beds in the United States increased by about 200 per cent. During the same period the population increased by about 80 per cent. There was also experienced a marked increase in the utilization of the beds and a shortening in the average length of patient stay in the hospital. This held for both general and special hospitals. In 1933 the admission rate to general and special hospitals per thousand population was 56. In 1951 the rate more than doubled; it was 136. The total days in hospital per thousand population was 859 in 1931, and 1,269 in 1961. In this period the average length of stay was reduced from 15.3 days in 1931, to 9.3 days in 1961. Clearly many more persons per thousand population were making use of available medical services in 1961 than they did thirty years before. Clear, too, is the fact supported by other statistical data that the population in the relatively lower economic brackets now use physicians' services about as much as do those in the higher economic brackets. The average annual visits per person is roughly 4.5 for the lower economic groups and 5.0 for those with an income of 7.5 thousands of dollars and over. Thirty years ago the respective visits were 2.7 for the low income group and 4.2 for the high income group.

By now it should be clear that during the past thirty years (the period is arbitrary) we not only have witnessed an extension of the market for medical services, but we also have been and are now more extensively facing a new order of medical consumer. This is a most important realization. Modern medicine was historically a derivation of the socio-economic developments initiated and fostered by the *entrepreneur* class. Specifically, it was engendered by the growth of cities, by the development of modern commerce and industry, by the rise and extension of the middle class, of the professional and functionary groups, and of the proletariat.

It was in the larger cities, the principal commercial and government centres, that the great universities were first founded. In certain of these

—namely, Salerno, Bologna, Padua, Montpelier, and Salamanca—there developed great schools of medicine. Here too, there were established notable hospitals. Here gathered the new class of *entrepreneurs,* the *bourgeoisie,* the town and city dwellers, the merchants, crafts masters, apprentices, and common workers. And with them also were the growing masses of civil and clerical functionaries, the forerunners of the modern bureaucrats. It is in these centres, proximate to the universities and hospitals, inspired and animated by the new learning emerging therefrom, and responsive to the needs and demands of the more numerous and wealthy new class of citizen (the *bourgeoisie*), that the modern patterns of medical practice had their origin. Here the cardinal elements of free choice, fee for service, and the confidential relations of patient and doctor were crystallized and soon acquired the sanction of established principles. Heretofore, the practice of medicine was, at least in tradition, a consecration, a devotion to the service of man, wherein the compensation received was not a reward for that which was given, but only an incident in the business of living. Medicine, losing none of its idealist heritage, did in effect take on the ideational and practice patterns of the emergent and dominant middle class, the class which directed the rise and attainments of modern Europe.

To-day medicine, as society itself, is confronting a new class, *entrepreneurs of another order,* and far more numerous than even was the middle class. I call them *proletbourgs,* for they are in effect derivative from the proletariat of past times now grown akin to the *bourgeoisie.* They are a product of our mounting and spreading affluence. Also, they are better informed, more articulate, and financially more competent than were their ancestors. They know what medicine has to offer and they rightly believe that they are entitled to its benefits.

It is this new order of medical consumer who today crowd our hospitals and tax our medical personnel and resources, wanting to be treated for and relieved of those illnesses and physical disabilities, the like of which their elders years past would have carried and suffered their whole life. It is the psychiatric needs of this new order of medical consumer that has animated the movement for communal psychiatry.

These patients constitute a new class of medical consumer, different from those we have known before. They are unlike the traditional poor and the familiar prosperous. They are not the historic middle class. Psychiatrically they present us, in the main and in the majority of instances, with disabilities that are non-organic, that are character-faulty, neurotic, situational. Not infrequently their complaints revolve about common problems of common existence, problems which they experience with uncommon intensity and which, lacking adequate comprehension, ego strength, frustration tolerance, in a word, inner and outer resources, they cannot deal with adequately or effectively. Not infrequently these patients are also boxed in by constricting material, social, and cultural circumstances within which they can manœuvre but little. With such patients one is in most instances restricted to the practice of that order of therapy which is descriptively to be termed restitutional. In these instances, there is seldom available the opportunity or the inner and material resources requisite for deeper therapy aiming to help the patient to reconstitute his personality. The avowed philosophy of this order of treatment has been well defined in a statement issued on behalf of the New York Joint Board of the Amalgamated Clothing Workers of America—the statement dealing with a plan for Mental Health Rehabilitation for a Union Population. "A mental health program," the statement read, "will have to be geared to improving social functioning as an immediate target, rather than being considered only as a consequence of a treatment regime. Though treatment and rehabilitation (my preferred term is restitution) efforts are in many ways indistinguishable, they can be conceptually differentiated. Rehabilitation is geared to influencing performance in social roles. On the other hand, the objective of treatment is to improve the patient's psychological state. A rehabilitation approach, while aware of the patient's underlying pathology, directs its primary attention to the functional roles of the individual." And there, it may be added, it usually rests.

That despite, restitutional therapy is not to be conceived of as a Grade B therapy or as the therapy we commonly practice, only watered down a bit.

By definition, restitutional therapy is a therapy with limited objectives. Its therapeutic goal is to help restitute the patient to his previous operational self. But it is a grave mistake to think of restitutional therapy as simple and easy. On the contrary, restitutional psychotherapy involves the exercise of uncommon skills, of timely and discreet initiatives, and the judicious venturing of more calculated risks than is common in our ordinary institutional or private psychotherapeutic practice. Restitutive psychotherapy must perforce be an active therapy and also one that involves the therapist in the immediacies of his patient's world and existence. This pattern of active, time and occasion-bound therapy perceptibly differs from what most of us now practice. It is a pattern of practice not easy to master. It is one which thus far has only been partially explored.

Communal psychiatry will most assuredly develop into an extensive service engaging the participation of numerous psychiatrists and of a large professional personnel drawn from the other disciplines.

Those whom, for want of a better name, we designate as the ancillary professions must perforce play a large role in communal psychiatry, and the psychiatrist, if he is not to lose out, will need to know how to work with, and at times direct and orchestrate the activities of these, his co-workers. He will also need to know a great deal more than he now does about the family, about sociology, economics, group dynamics and culture.

Communal psychiatry is an historic emergence that is responsive to current needs. It is not the ultimate in psychiatric service. If past experience is to be trusted, communal psychiatry will solve some of our present service problems and also bring to the fore a great many new ones. Contrary to the persuasions of some, the overall patient load will not decrease with the extension of communal psychiatry. On the contrary, it is more likely to increase. Because of better nutrition and the declining prevalence of infectious diseases, viral as well as microbial, we may have many fewer young seniles and brain-damaged individuals. But for a long time to come, I am persuaded, the numbers of psychiatric patients will continue to increase. This, plus the likely recognition of the full extent to which psychological illness is involved and in fact 'masks' as organic and functional disease, will ultimately impress upon us the need to take a more sophisticated look at the prevention of mental illness. I say sophisticated, for the mention of prevention immediately exacts from some psychiatric quarters the oh so pure-science retort, "We know next to nothing about prevention." But that is an unhistoric snobism. We may not know the specific cause or causes of schizophrenia but we do know a great deal about the psychophysiological needs of the developing child, and we know too what psycho-emotional input is requisite to the maintenance of an effective adult ego. Prevention is to be approached from the physiological as well as the pathological.

A critical scanning of medical history will show that the greater contributions to the attainment and maintenance of good health, as well as to disease resistance, derived from the application of the knowledge and understanding of normal physiological needs and requisites to the regimen of man. The pertinent realization on this score is that it is not the physician nor the psychiatrist who determines or molds the regimen of man or his ecology. And it does not entirely lie in the power of the individual to do so. The basic fact is that in the largest measure it is the community which shapes man's setting, his regimen, and ecology. And by community, I intend not only the individual's immediate physical and social milieu, but the larger community as well, the one that embodies and propagates the prevailing ethos. It is and will be increasingly incumbent on the profession and the discipline of psychiatry to foster a psychologically salubrious regimen and ecology—for every child, youth, man and woman. This does not mean that the psychiatrist will be called upon to be everything for every man. Indeed, the psychiatrist is not to be educator, criminologist, legislator friest and politician. But to each of these he may, and increasingly is likely to, contribute a something or much, learned from his unique professional studies and experiences, that must prove useful. This is a deliberate understatement, for who is in a better position to perceive and to appreciate the extent to which the community, the human aggregate, contributes to the engenderment of disease, both physical and psychological?

Communal psychiatry will require close contact between the psychiatrist and the educator, the law practitioner, the law enforcement agents, the ministry, labor and industry. The contacts should in time extend further, to include say, the communication and entertainment services, and advertising. But that perhaps is looking too far ahead.

One final observation it to be made, and that in the nature of a caveat. Communal psychiatry must not be allowed to starve out, to throttle, that order of psychiatry which is so aptly described as the "one to one practice," that is, the private practice of psychiatry. For this was and is bound to remain the fountain source of dynamic psychiatry, of the depth insight into the labyrinthian operations of the human psyche.

REFERENCES

1. ACKERKNECHT, E. H.: Ciba Symposia, Vol. 9, No. 1, 1948. p. 826. Yet primitive medicine was by no means exclusively psychotherapeutic. The primitive healers used physical treatments and drugs still highly valued in our own medicine.
2. In the judgment of W. D. C. Lewis, about 1,500 years in advance of his times, "for he placed the patient under the best conditions of light, temperature, food and quiet and insisted that all elements of an exciting nature be excluded. He denounced simple starvation, bleeding, chains, alcohol and excessive drug therapy." (Lewis, D. C. Nolan, *A Short History of Psychiatric Achievement,* W. W. Norton, New York, 1941, p. 53.)
3. CASTIGLIONI, ARTURO: *A History of Medicine,* New York, Alfred Knopf, 1947, p. 258.
4. "Die Psychiatrie fiel in die Hande exorzisierender Priester und priesterlicher Hexenverfolger," Ackerknecht, *op. cit.*
5. ZILBOORG, GREGORY: *A History of Medical Psychology,* New York, W. W. Norton and Co., p. 103.
6. JONES, W. H. S.: *Hippocrates,* Vol. 11, p. 141.
7. *Op. cit.,* p. 149.

8. PIRENNE, HENRI: *Medieval Cities*, New York, Doubleday Anchor Books, Garden City, p. 15.
9. PIRENNE, *op. cit.*, p. 17.
10. HUIZINGA, JOHAN: *The Waning of the Middle Ages*, London, Edward Arnold, Ltd., 1955, p. 11.
11. *Op. cit.*, p. 124.
12. *Op. cit.*, p. 126.
13. *Op. cit.*, p. 21.
14. HECKER: *The Epidemics of the Middle Ages*, London, Sydenham Society, 1840, p. 87.
15. *Op. cit.*, p. 40.
16. *Op. cit.*, p. 115.
17. HUIZINGA, JOHAN: *Men and Ideas*, New York, Meridian Books, Inc., 1959, p. 307.
18. *Op. cit.*, p. 270.
19. CASTIGLIONI, ARTURO: *A History of Medicine*, 2nd Ed., New York, Alfred Knopf, 1947, p. 293.
20. BROOKE, CHRISTOPHER: *Europe in the Middle Ages*, London, Longmans, Green and Co., 1964, p. 295.
21. PIRENNE, HENRI: *A History of Europe*, New York University, 1955, p. 105.
22. CREIGHTON, CHARLES: *History of Epidemics in Britain*, Vol. 1, Cambridge University Press, 1891, p. 15.
23. CURSCHMAN, F.: Hungersnote, Mittelalter, Leipzig, 1900.
24. BOISSONNADE, P.: *Life and Work in Medieval Europe*, London, Routledge and Kegan Paul, Ltd., 1927, p. 229.
25. *Ibid.*, p. 229.
26. *Ibid.*, p. 230.
27. *Ibid.*, pp. 237-38.
28. PIRENNE, HENRI: *Medieval Cities*, New York, Doubleday Anchor Books, 1925, p. 110.
29. *Capitalism and the Historians*, pp. 15, 16, edited with an Introduction by F. A. Hayek. Chicago, The University of Chicago Press, 1937.
30. HAMMOND, J. L., and HAMMOND, BARBARA: *The Village Labourer, the Town Labourer*. Longmans, Green & Co., 1920.
31. History and Development of Teaching Hospitals in England, in *Brit. Med. J.*, p. 749, Sept. 10, 1960.
32. *A Short History of Psychiatric Achievements*, W. W. Norton, 1941, p. 160.
33. *Forty Years of Psychiatry*, Nervous and Mental Disease Monograph Series, New York, 1933.
34. *A History of Psychoanalysis in America*, New York, Grune & Stratton, 1953.
35. *Op. cit.*, p. 64.
36. *Op. cit.*, p. 65.

25

Psychiatry for the Millions

AT THE FIFTH INTERNATIONAL PSYCHOANALYTIC CONGRESS, meeting in Budapest in September, 1918, Freud did not, as was his custom, deliver a lecture but instead read a carefully reasoned paper. The title of his paper was, "Turnings in the Ways of Psychoanalytic Therapy." This was a meaty paper, one that is pivotal to the history of what, using Freud's words, can be properly termed "turnings in the ways of psychoanalytic therapy."

Particularly interesting and significant in this paper is Freud's clairvoyant prophecy of things to come—the challenge that psychoanalysis will face when "the conscience of the community will awake and admonish it that the poor man has just as much right to help for his mind as he now has to the surgeon's means of saving life" (1). What was likely to happen then? "Then," said Freud, "clinics and consultation departments will be built, to which analytically trained physicians will be appointed, so that the men who would otherwise give way to drink, the women who have nearly succumbed under their burden of privations, the children for whom there is no choice but running wild or neurosis may be made by analysis able to resist and able to do something in the world. . . ." Freud however was not happy about these prospects. "For," Freud continued, "the task will then arise for us to adapt our techniques to the new conditions. I have no doubt that the validity of our psychological assumptions will impress the uneducated too, but we shall need to find the simplest and most natural expression for our theoretical doctrines." "It is very probable" he forecast, "that the application of our therapy to numbers will compel us to alloy the pure gold of analysis plentifully with the copper of direct suggestion. . . . But whatever the elements out of

332

which it is compounded, its most effective and most important ingredients will assuredly remain those borrowed from strict and untendentious psychoanalysis" (2).

It is on this lugubrious note that Freud ended his discourse on "the new directions in which it (psychoanalysis) may develop." Here I want to draw your attention to a suggestive peculiarity in Freud's final sentence. Freud did not say simply that the important ingredients would be borrowed from psychoanalysis, but rather, from "strict and untendentious psychoanalysis." Why this caveat? The answer is simple. Freud's paper was polemical rather than expositional. This is reflected in the different titles given to this paper in English translations. The original German title is "Wege der Psychoanalytischen Therapie." In Joan Rivière's translation it is titled "Turnings in the Ways of Psychoanalytic Therapy." The significant term in this title is "turnings." That which turns clearly does not move in a straight line. James Strachey's translation carries the bland title "Lines of Advance in Psychoanalytic Therapy." In a separate notice Strachey points out that the main stress in Freud's paper was "on the 'active' methods chiefly associated (later) with the name of Ferenczi" (3).

In historic retrospection it is clear that Freud's paper signaled the first break in his relations with Ferenczi. While seemingly endorsing Ferenczi's advocacy of "active" therapy, Freud unconditionally and emphatically reaffirmed what he termed the fundamental principles of psychoanalysis. Psychoanalysis, Freud argued, is active enough in pursuing its therapeutic task which consists of two things, namely making conscious the repressed material and, uncovering the resistance (4). Furthermore, Freud reiterated, it is a fundamental principle that "analytic treatment should be carried through as far as is possible under privation—in a state of abstinence" (5). Keeping the patient in a state of privation Freud construed as a form of activity. "As far as his (the patient's) relations with the physician is concerned," wrote Freud, "the patient must have unfulfilled wishes in abundance. It is expedient to deny him precisely those satisfactions which he desires most intensely and expresses most importunately" (6).

Taken in its entirety Freud's address to the Fifth International Psychoanalytic Congress must be construed as a warning to those in attendance, and in particular to Ferenczi, that deviation from what Freud termed the common ground of psychoanalytic assumptions would not be acceptable.

In this connection it is worth noting Jones' astute comment that "more than individual friendships Freud had come to treasure the value of his discoveries and all that ensued from them. It would be a mistake to think that Freud felt any personal dependence on any member of the Committee, even on the one nearest to him, Ferenczi" (7).

It cannot be said, despite the cordial exchange of letters that continued between Freud and Ferenczi following the Budapest meeting, that Ferenczi missed the warning. Ferenczi attempted in various ways to propitiate Freud, to gain his understanding and his support. Some of his endeavors now seem pathetic, almost pusillanimous. But he did not, for compelling reasons, as will be shown later, prevail. Freud was obdurate and in the passage of time grew ever more so.

Ferenczi though deeply affected and very unhappy, still pursued his own thoughts and persuasions. For as Franz Alexander wrote "Ferenczi had a vital interest in therapeutic problems, an incessant urge toward therapeutic experimentation that sprang from his dissatisfactions with the accepted psychoanalytic techniques, and it was this experimental attitude toward therapy that eventually caused his rift with Freud" (8).

It was more than dissatisfaction with the accepted psychoanalytic techniques that caused Ferenczi to confront Freud. He was also dissatisfied with the theoretical pathodynamics of the Freudian system, with what Freud termed the "common ground of psychoanalytic assumptions," specifically with Freud's theories on the etiology and the therapy of the neuroses.

The ultimate break with Freud (even though they remained on seemingly friendly terms) came at the Thirteenth International Psychoanalytic Congress, meeting in Wiesbaden in 1932. It had been generally accepted that at this meeting Ferenczi would be elected President of the International. Freud himself had urged Ferenczi to accept the presidency, suggesting, much to Ferenczi's displeasure, that this would act as a "forcible cure" to take him out of his (Ferenczi's) isolation. Ferenczi however declined the nomination, giving as his reason that he could not in honesty accept office in an organization with whose academic and therapeutic principles he was so much in conflict (9).

Ferenczi died in 1933. He had long been suffering from pernicious anemia.

In her introduction to the third volume of the selected papers of Sandor Ferenczi, Clara Thompson wrote, Ferenczi "was a man without great power ambitions, and was a devoted and loyal friend to Freud. The theoretical disagreements which developed between the two men were a source of great unhappiness. He did not enjoy a fight with his respected teacher and yet he had to be true to his own clinical convictions. He never ceased until his death in trying to win Freud's approval. Nevertheless, their friendship was severely shaken, never to be restored on the same basis, by Ferenczi's last paper, 'Confusion of Tongues between Adults and the Child'. In 'The Principles of Relaxation and Neocatharsis' we see especially clearly his frantic attempt to tie his thinking to Freud's leadership. I believe this conflict greatly limited his production in these last years" (10).

Ferenczi did intensively try to reconcile his own maturing insights with Freud's fundamental psychoanalytic assumptions. But he was foredoomed to failure. The monolithic character of the Freudian construct would not, and could not, tolerate the inclusion of any conditioning or added elaborations. It was crystalline in structure, and anything added could only disrupt it. This being the case Freud was right to resist every attempt to modify the basic assumptions embodied in the Freudian construct.

Ferenczi would have been much the wiser had he cut himself free from his allegiance to Freud and the Freudian construct. But he could not, and that is history!

In these last observations I intend to affirm that the issues between Freud and Ferenczi were not personal. Freud and Ferenczi were basically friendly and congenial. The conflict was in a real sense academic, involving an older man, entrapped in his own brilliant but closed complex of ideas, and a younger man of genius and imagination who saw many things beyond that brillant complex of ideas and set out to explore them. Ferenczi could accept Freud's ideas but Freud could not accept Ferenczi's.

The difficulty was not simply due to a lack of goodwill on Freud's part. Given his scientific *gestalt*, Ferenczi's ideas could not but appear, as indeed they were, alien and hence not includable.

What was Freud's scientific *gestalt*? Bluntly stated, it was that of the late nineteenth century medicine, that is positivist, materialist, and specificist. In that gestalt every disorder, psychological as well as somatic, was assumed to be due to a specific cause, and the cure or remedy of the disorder, was to be achieved by the removal, counteracting, or overcoming of the specific cause.

In medicine the preeminent apostle of this school of thought, called etiological, was Emil von Behring, the discoverer of diphtheria antitoxin. Until the early decades of the twentieth century this was the predominant school of medical thought and to this day it still has its numerous adherents.

Freud was in many respects, and avowedly, a disciple and an adherent of this school.

Freud posited that every neurosis is initiated in a specific traumatic experience (or experiences) which, not having been effectively counteracted, is (or are) repressed into the unconscious. It is from such repression that the protean symptoms of the neuroses derive. Furthermore, the specific treatment for the neuroses is free association, the sovereign process by which the repressed is "brought" into the conscious. Awareness, insight, and the implementation thereof effect the cure.

Reject any one of these basic postulates and the Freudian construct collapses. Yet this is precisely what Ferenczi did, but only in a singular manner. He challenged not the validity of the postulates upon which the Freudian construct is based but only their universality. He argued that there were neurotics who seemingly had not experienced any specific ingressive, traumatizing assaults. He reported that free association even when long pursued, failed in some instances to reveal any repressed materials and brought no relief. He reported that some neurotics became well without free association, without being subjected to artful frustration, and deliberate privation. He reported that some neurotics became well when he afforded them encouragement, patent interest, and manifest affection.

Ferenczi, to repeat, did not deny that the classical procedures of psychoanalysis are uniquely suited for and effective in the treatment of certain patients and for given conditions—hysterics for example. But he intuited (the term is intended in its precise meaning) and argued that there are procedures other than frustration, privation, and free association that are effective in the treatment of the neuroses.

These affirmations are scattered throughout Ferenczi's writings. They are compactly and definitively stated in the paper titled (in English) "The Principles of Relaxation and Neocatharsis" (11).

At this point it would be well to step away from the close scrutiny of the differences between Freud and Ferenczi and to regard, as well as to speculate on, what was going on in the intellectual sphere of Ferenczi's mind.

Unbeknown to him, for he never expressed or affirmed it, he was breaching the specificist constraints of the Freudian construct. In this he shared in a liberating movement that radically and profoundly changed the basic orientation of all modern medicine. The specificist contentions that every disorder, physical or psychological, has, and must have, its specific nosogenic agent was proved to be wrong. It was shown incontrovertibly that there are many diseases, demographically important, which are not due to the presence in the body of noxious agents, but rather, to the absence of substances and factors (experiences) essential to normal development and effective living. Such disorders were originally termed the minus sign diseases. Now they are designated as deficiency diseases or disorders of deprivation.

Arnold C. Klebs, the noted medical historian and authority on medical incunabula, wrote in 1917 in his "History of Infections" (12) "the microorganisms as the determining factor of infectious diseases, the specificness of the infection and the invariability of microbic species make this the dominant theory of the day in medicine. Its profound influence is felt in private and public life to a degree unparalleled in the annals of human society. So dominant is this doctrine that the question is hardly ever asked: might there not be, apart from the microbe, pathogenic influences of equal if not of greater importance." Replace in the aforegoing the term "microorganism" with the phrase "repression in the etiology of the neuroses" and you have a succinct description of what confronted Ferenczi when confronting Freud.

The concept of minus sign diseases, of diseases due to deprivation, was neither easily developed nor readily accepted. Thus, Christian Eijkman, the director of the Batavian Pathologic Institute, had clearly demonstrated in 1897 that beri-beri was a disease associated with a diet mainly consisting of polished rice, and that beri-beri could both be prevented and cured by the inclusion in the diet of the pericarp of the rice. Yet Sir Patrick Manson, famous for his discoveries on the transmission of malarial infection, in his presidential address to the Epidemiological Society in London in 1905 maintained, despite his acquaintance with Eijman's work, that "the theory which conforms best to all the known facts in respect to the etiology and pathology of beri-beri is to the effect that this disease is purely an intoxication produced by a toxin elaborated by a germ whose nidus is located outside the human body" (13).

Such was Sir Patrick's opinion according to "all the known facts," and on this score, Sir Walter Langdon Brown has aptly observed "if a new idea can be fitted into the authoritarian framework we are too apt to accept it uncritically, whereas if it breaks new ground we are too likely to reject it" (14).

It took many years to convince clinicians that cretinism, goitre, scurvy, chlorosis, pellagra, rickets, and a host of other disorders were due to what was lacking, rather than to some intrusive pathogenic factor. In the realm of psychiatry the concept of deprivation operating as a pathogenic factor emerged but very recently. It has not as yet fully permeated psychiatric thinking, and least of all formal psychoanalytic thought and theory.

But Ferenczi quite clearly intuited this pathogenic dynamic. "I can picture cases of neurosis," Ferenczi wrote, "in fact I have often met with them in which . . ." the "persons have actually remained almost entirely at child level, and for them the usual methods of analytic therapy are not enough. What such neurotics need is really to be adopted and to partake for the first time in their lives of the advantages of a normal nursery. For the first time in their lives to be afforded that of which they were heretofore deprived" (15).

One can cite much from the miscellaneous writings of Ferenczi showing that he had some sense of the pathogenicity of deprivation. But there is no evidence that he did in fact ever clearly formulate his thoughts thereon. What he did know was that there are cases, numerous cases, in which the usual methods of analytic therapy are not enough. Ferenczi's tie to Freud, his intense craving for the latter's approval, was too great. It impeded the full elaboration and the ultimate maturation of his theoretical insights. When Ferenczi did finally "break" with Freud, it was too late. Ferenczi by this time was mortally sick.

In the contemporary histories of psychiatry and psychoanalysis Ferenczi is noted for having initiated, together with Otto Rank, the quest for increased efficiency of therapy. "The search for ways and means to make analytic therapy more efficient and shorter," writes Hans Strupp, "took its start with the work of Ferenczi and Rank (1925) of which the subsequent efforts by Alexander (1956) and French (1946), Alexander and Rado (1956-1962) are logical efforts" (16).

This acclaim of Ferenczi as the initiator of the move for "active-brief-therapy" widely misses the mark of Ferenczi's significance in the history of psychoanalysis and psychiatry.

Ferenczi disavowed the time curtailment of therapy initially advocated by himself and Rank. In his immensely significant and profoundly insightful paper, "Child Analysis in the Analysis of Adults" (1931), Ferenczi wrote "I must confess two things: that my hope of considerable *shortening* the analysis by the help of relaxation and catharsis has, so far, not been fulfilled, and that this method has made the analyst's work considerably more laborious. But what it has done—and I trust will do still more— is to deepen our insight into the workings of the human mind in health and disease and to entitle us to hope that any therapeutic success being based on these deeper foundations will have better prospects of permanence" (17). Ferenczi's hoped for "deepening of our insight into the workings of the human mind" was attained during recent decades in the recognition of the pathogenicity of deprivation, and more elaborately in the development of the discipline of ethology.

David Levy (1931), René Spitz (1946), John Bowlby (1957), pioneered in the study of deprivation, focusing on disturbances in the vitally critical relations and interactions between mother and child, and their deleterious effects upon the physical as well as the psychological growth and development of the child. The discipline of ethology with which the names of Oscar Heinroth, Nickolas Tinbergen, and Conrad Lorenz are associated brought into our awareness not only the mechanism of imprinting but, what in relation to our concern is equally significant, the existence of critical periods for the acquisition of learning and action-patterns.

W. H. Thorpe describes the so-called sensitive periods as follows. "There do exist specific brain mechanisms ready to be activated during and only during a particular period of the life span of the child and if they are not properly activated at the right time, subsequent activation is difficult or impossible, resulting in permanent disabilities in later life" (18). Thorpe also comments on the consequences of learning missed at the time specific for such learning. "The close of the specific learning period for a simple type of task may result not from a waning of the ability to acquire the simpler performance but because the acquisition of more complex abilities, perceptions and skills, and the tendency actively to experiment with and explore the environment, render the subject less willing to restrict his attention to the simple situation and to play the more passive role" (19).

The above citation aptly describes the mechanism and consequent plight of the "dropout" prematurely entangled in adult sexual and social activities and responsibilities.

It is not my intention to further elaborate either on the deprivations studies, nor on the findings and teachings of ethology, though these are indeed fascinating in themselves. I cited them here to substantiate the affirmation that in psychiatry, as in the other divisions of medicine, there is a growing awareness of the pathogenicity of deprivation, substantive and (as in ethology) experiential. It is also noteworthy that the studies on deprivation and of ethology have introduced into medicine the old concept of ontology (though not in the form of the Aristotelian entelechy) and of the more modern concept of existentialism.

To revert to the main thesis of my presentation—the Freudian construct neither includes nor allows for the existence and pathogenicity of deprivation in the etiology and hence in the therapy of the neuroses. *De-*

privation repressed into the unconscious is inconceivable. It cannot, then, be brought into awareness by the technique of free association.

Judd Marmor in his thoughtful and provocative paper titled "Limitations of Free Association" (20) arrives at a number of conclusions proximate to my own. Thus Marmor affirms, in several versions, that if "material has never been repressed the free association method will not bring it into consciousness" (21). Again, "the significant fact that has been overlooked in most psychoanalytic theory is that material of which the patient is unconscious does not necessarily always reside in the patient's 'unconscious.' There are many aspects of a patient and his character structure that he has never repressed because he has never been aware of them even sublimally" (22).

"The conviction" Marmor writes, "has slowly grown upon me in the course of over thirty years of clinical experience, that there are serious limitations to the free associational method that have gone largely unrecognized and which have an important bearing on certain shortcomings of classical psychoanalysis as a therapeutic method" (23).

Like Ferenczi, Marmor reports that he has "encountered people who have undergone prolonged and painstaking analyses and yet have been left with clear-cut residual patterns of narcissism, exploitiveness, social aggression, rigidity, compulsiveness, and other similar characterological attitudes." "The suspicion," Marmor further states, "begins to grow that perhaps there is something in the method itself that in some cases, at least, is failing to get at some of these fundamental personality patterns."

The nature of those cases wherein classical psychoanalysis cannot but fail as a therapeutic method and the distinctive etiology of these cases their origins traceable to many and different orders of deprivation, have been the burden of this presentation.

Here it may be asked, referring to the title of this paper, but what has all this to do with "Psychiatry for the Millons?" Before undertaking to give the answer I want to refer again to a portion of Freud's address before the Fifth International Psychoanalytic Congress meeting in Budapest in 1918. "The necessities of our own existence," Freud said, "limit our work to the well-to-do classes accustomed to choose their own physicians. . . . At present we can do nothing in the crowded ranks of the people, who suffer exceedingly from neurosis" (24).

Classical psychoanalysis is for the wealthy! What is there then for the crowded ranks of the people, for the millions? Freud left the answer to the future. "At some time or other," he opined "the conscience of the community will awake—then the task will arise for us to adapt our technique to the new conditions."

That "some time" is now and the challenge of a fitting technique is upon us.

It will not be amiss here to scan the historic past that has led up to the new conditions, and to reflect on the modified techniques that may prove useful in meeting current psychotherapeutic needs.

Modern medicine is historically a derivation of the socioeconomic developments initiated and fostered by the entrepreneur class. Specifically, it was engendered by the growth of the cities, by the development of modern commerce and industry, by the rise and extension of the middle class, of the professional and functionary groups, and of the proletariat.*

Today medicine, as society itself, is confronting a new class, entrepreneurs of another order, far more numerous than ever was the middle class. I would call them "proletbourgs," for they are in effect derivative from the proletariat of the past now grown akin to the bourgeoisie.

It is this new order of medical consumes which today crowds our hospitals and taxes our medical personnel and resources. It is the psychiatric needs of this new order of medical consumer that has animated the movement for a new order of psychiatric service.

Psychiatrically these individuals present us, in the main and in the majority of instances, with disabilities that are deprivational in origin. Their complaints most frequently revolve about problems in existence, problems which they experience with uncommon intensity and which, lacking requisite comprehension, ego strength, frustration tolerance, they cannot deal with effectively. These patients are also commonly boxed in by constricting material, social, and cultural conditions within which they can manoeuvre but little.

Such patients are clearly not suitable for, nor do they require, formal psychoanalysis. Their pathology is deprivational in derivation, and not due primarily to repression. They can be treated in what may be fittingly termed restitutional therapy. It is a therapy based on Freudian metapsychology, but it differs from formal psychoanalysis in its objectives and techniques.

Freud had forecast that whatever the new therapeutic technique might be whereby the masses will be treated, its most important ingredients will assuredly remain those borrowed from psychoanalysis. In that, Freud was

---

* Vide "Doctor and Patient in Medical History," Iago Galdston, *Journal of Medical Education*, Vol. 37, March, 1962, pp. 222-232.

proved right. But Freud contemplated such prospects with sorrow and regret. He anticipated that the pure gold of analysis will be alloyed with the copper of other theories and practices—and thus suffer debasement. Freud was not a very good metallurgist or he would have known that all pure metals are made stronger and better by being alloyed. But the analogy apart, restitutional therapy does not aim to displace formal psychoanalysis (when it is applicable) nor does it merely borrow important ingredients from psychoanalysis. *Restitutional therapy is an extension of psychoanalysis to the treatment of the psychopathology of deprivation.* Restitutional therapy aims to bare, to correct, to compensate as well as to help the patient to adapt to, the deprivations experienced by the patient. Restitutional therapy aims as well to deal with the secondary, reactive pathologies manifest in the patient, his defenses, overcompensation, and other malign adaptations.

I cannot here elaborate the therapeutic procedures in restitutional therapy. However they are neither complex nor difficult. Once one has mastered the concept of deprivation as a pathogenic experience, the patterns of therapeutic procedure emanate as a logical consequent. It should, however, be recognized that the secondary derivative pathologies can be and indeed are frequently quite challenging, so that restitutional therapy involves the exercise of uncommon skills, of timely and discreet initiatives, and the judicious venturing of more calculated risks than is common in our ordinary institutional or private psychotherapeutic practice.

The outstanding feature in restitutive psychotherapy is that both patient and therapist are primarily concerned with the patient's immediate "trouble," with the difficulties in which the patient is involved. Symptoms, be they intrapsychic, interpersonal, or socioenvironmental, are taken to represent the "real pathology," and not as secondary manifestations of some deeper etiological dynamics. The deeper dynamics may be intuited by the therapist but he does not "dig for them" as he would in classical psychoanalysis. Yet in restitutive therapy the therapist is more of an inquisitor than a passive listener. In his anamnestic dialogue with the patient, the therapist, always respecting the patient's recital *under pressure,* steers the dialogue away from unessential and repetitive items, and directs the patient to deal with relevant matters. What the latter may be the therapist gathers from the cues provided by the patient in his easy and unguarded recitations.

In restitutive psychotherapy the therapist is deliberately and intentionally an active participant. He helps and guides the patient to understand the nature of his difficulties, their derivatives, and how and wherein the difficulties may be resolved or rendered less onerous. The therapist is uncovering, insightful, tutorial, supportive, and confronting.

The psychotherapist practicing restitutive psychiatry needs to possess and to cultivate a capacity for warm empathic relations with his patient. Patients quite often come to us impoverished in ego strength, despairing in their body image, discouraged about their present and the future, disparaging of self—in a word, defeated souls. They need help to regain the semblance of an upright being, and the therapist in his dealings with the patient can inspire hope, engender self-respect, and evoke the recuperative energies latent in every patient. This he can do without violence to truth and reality and without maudlin sentimentality.

Here I must end my comments on the techniques of restitutional psychotherapy to make a comment on the obvious, namely that restitutional therapy can easily be confounded with brief psychotherapy, intensive therapy, supportive psychotherapy, and others of the like.

Restitutional therapy may be brief in duration, or it may be prolonged. It is likely to be intensive, and is certainly supportive. But it differs from all the others in this respect—that none of the others, to the best of my knowledge, recognizes or takes cognizance of deprivation as the etiological factor in the multiform pathologies from which "the millions suffer." Failing in this, they can only grope in the dark and effect what good they do effect in the exercise of an unilluminated pragmatism.

I am moved to avow here that I have no ambition to initiate a new school of therapy. My intentions, I trust, were clearly manifest in my paper. They were to lay bare the limitations inherent in the classical psychoanalytic construct with repression as the unique pathological dynamic and free association as the equally unique therapeutic means; to sketch the history of the recognition of the so-called minus sign diseases, those resulting from substantive and experiential deprivation; to signal deprivation as a major and widespread pathodynamic force in the psychopathology of "the masses," and to sketch a pattern of therapy, founded on Freud's metapsychology, which could provide effective psychiatric service to the millions. And my transcending ambition and hope is to see all this embodied in the education and training of our young psychiatrists.

REFERENCES

1. Freud, S.: Turnings in the ways of psychoanalytic therapy; in *Collected Papers*. London, Hogarth Press (Joan Riviere, trans.), 1949; Vol. 2, p. 401.
2. Freud, S.: Lines of advance in psychoanalytic therapy; in *Collected Papers*. London, Hogarth Press (Strachey, trans.), 1955; Vol. XVII, p. 168.

3. *Ibid.*, p. 158.
4. FREUD, S.: Turnings in the ways of psychoanalytic therapy; in *Collected Papers.* London, Hogarth Press (Joan Riviere, trans.), 1949; Vol. 2, p. 395.
5. *Ibid.*, p. 396.
6. *Ibid.*, p. 398.
7. JONES, E.: *Life and Work of Sigmund Freud,* New York, Basic Books, 1957; Vol. 3, p. 44.
8. ALEXANDER, F., and SELESNICK, S. T.: *The History of Psychiatry,* New York, Harper & Row, 1966, p. 222.
9. JONES, E.: *Life and Work of Sigmund Freud,* New York, Basic Books, 1957; Vol. 3, p. 172.
10. FERENCZI, S.: *Problems and Methods of Psychoanalysis,* New York, Basic Books, 1955; Vol. III, p. 3.
11. *Ibid.*, pp. 108-125.
12. KLEBS, A. C.: History of infections; *Annals of Medical History,* April, 1917; Vol. 1, No. 1, p. 159.
13. GALDSTON, I.: *Progress in Medicine,* New York, Knopf, A, 1940, p. 126.
14. *Ibid.*, p. 151.
15. FERENCZI, S.: *Problems and Methods of Psychoanalysis,* New York, Basic Books, 1955; Vol. III, p. 124.
16. STRUPP, H. H.: Psychoanalytic therapy of the individual; in *Modern Psychoanalysis,* Marmor, J., editor. New York, Basic Books, 1968, p. 317.
17. FERENCZI, S.: *Problems and Methods of Psychoanalysis,* New York, Basic Books, 1955; Vol. III, p. 141.
18. THORPE, W. H., and LANGWILL, O. L.: Sensitive periods in learning; in *Current Problems in Animal Behaviour,* London, Cambridge U. P., 1961, p. 200.
19. *Ibid.*, p. 200.
20. MARMOR, J.: Limitations of free association, *Archives Gen. Psychiatry,* Feb., 1970; Vol. 22, pp. 160-165.
21. *Ibid.*, p. 161.
22. *Ibid.*, p. 161.
23. *Ibid.*, p. 160.
24. FREUD, S.: Turnings in the ways of psychoanalytic therapy; in *Collected Papers;* London, Hogarth Press (Joan Riviere, trans.), 1949; Vol. 2, p. 401.

Part IV:
EXISTENTIALISM

26

Existentialism and Psychiatry

IT IS DIFFICULT to define precisely what existentialism is, not because existentialism is lacking in definable components, but because it is endowed with so many.

Existentialism has many substantive manifestations, in art, literature, philosophy, etc. But in and of itself existentialism is not "demonstrable." It is a dynamism, a social, cultural and intellectual movement. As such, it can best be understood in its historic derivation.

Existentialism is primarily and essentially European but it needs must concern us deeply. Our interest in existentialism is not a pure exercise in intellectualism, but a wise attempt to anticipate what is bound to confront us in the not too remote future.

Europe and we are an ocean apart, but we are culturally contiguous. Between Europe and ourselves there is a time lag of some twenty years or so, in the emergence of historic and cultural issues and problems. It is therefore a safe assumption that what is culturally crucial to Europe today will be crucial to us one generation hence. Existentialism agitates Europe today. It will stir us on the morrow. Even now one can perceive its prodromal signs in our midst.

What is existentialism? First and foremost it is a movement of protest. It is a challenge to, and a denial of, things past, of the philosophical, the theological, the psychological, the aesthetic, the moral, and, I need add, the scientific theories, dogmas, and assumptions of the past. It is, in the phrase of Nietzsche, an attempt to transvalue values—by initially denying the validity of existing values.

Existentialism is revolutionary and culturally discontinuous. Existentialism does not offer to modify classical thought—it denies its validity.

347

In contrast to classical philosophy which tries to make life conform to thought, existentialism seeks to make thought conform to life. Existentialism reduces life from that which we would like it to be to what it is.

The existentialist movement constitutes an unprecedented reorientation of human thought in that it denies existence to everything of which we are not immediately and indubitably aware (1).

Existentialism is a challenge of colossal dimension and of transcending importance. Existentialism has engaged the interest, and has enlisted the intellectual, aesthetic, and creative energies of some of the most competent and earnest of men: poets, philosophers, playwrights, painters, novelists, theologians, psychologists, and psychiatrists.

Existentialism has its antagonists as well as its protagonists, and both are in earnest. Norberto Bobbio, Professor of Legal Philosophy at the University of Padua, and Editor of the *Revista de Filosofia*, wrote a series of essays on existentialism, titling them *The Philosophy of Decadentism.* "Existentialism," he wrote, "is a mode of philosophizing which in a strange and wonderful way accords with the philosophical vocation and, I would say, the philosophic vogue of our time. As such, we harbor it with an easy conscience or defiantly, with pride or repugnance, and we harbored it as an aspiration or as a temptation even before it was revealed to us in specific terms" (2).

Bobbio recognizes that existentialism is a philosophy of crisis. He fails however to identify the true derivation of that crisis. He ascribes it to the disordered exuberance and unrestrained vitality that follow on the weakening of authority. By authority he intends "the supreme principles which inspire every manifestation of spiritual life both in the theoretical and in the practical spheres" (3). It were profitless to argue Bobbio's criticism of existentialism. However, we can accept his notations on "crisis" and "the weakening of authority."

Existentialism *is* a philosophy of crisis, and this being the case we needs must ask what is the derivation, and the nature of this crisis. Also, since the weakening of authority is both antecedent and consequent to crisis, we need to inquire what authority has been weakened.*

As the starting point I would take the years that witnessed the rise of the Modern Age and the birth of Modern Science—that is, the last decades of the sixteenth and the early years of the seventeenth century. These are the years of Galileo (1564-1642) and of Descartes (1596-1660). This was

---

* Those who would study these matters more deeply will find Ortega y Gasset's *Man and Crisis*, W. W. Norton & Co., N. Y. and Luis Diez del Corral's *The Rape of Europe*, Macmillan Co., 1959, most helpful and illuminating.

the *new* era, emergent from Mediaevalism, and the Renaissance. This was the Age when mankind, aided and abetted by its scientists and determinist philosophers, took in earnest the exhorting counsel of Francis Bacon, to wrest from nature the secrets of its ways, so that man might master both nature and his own destiny.

No age had ever been ushered in so brilliantly, and with so much hope and expectation. No age had been welcomed with so much enthusiasm by those who were called, and who considered themselves to be "the enlightened."

It was not long, however, before both the hopes and the expectations of that nascent era were dimmed by frustrating reality. Life became not better, but worse. The common man suffered not only physical hardships and deprivations, but what was even worse, moral degradation and a deep, inextricable confusion as to life's meanings and values. Emergent science implemented the industrial revolution, with its nasty slums, its disenfranchised proletariat, its ugly factories, and its gross inhumanities.

The Modern Age had hardly reached its adolescence when it was literally macerated by the bloody and disruptive French Revolution. Inspired as it was by so much of the heroic and the humane, this revolution, as revolutions are likely to, soon "got out of hand," monstrously consuming countless thousands of humans, including most of its own initiators. The French Revolution was even more disruptive than bloody. The French Revolution left in its heritage the miseries of Nationalism and of the Citizens' Army. The French Revolution made way for the man on horseback, for Napoleon, the ambitious and unscrupulous usurper. His breed has become all-too-well known to us in the passing decades. Titled as they are—Duce, Gauleiter, Caudillo, Fuehrer, or Comintern Secretary— they have taken it upon themselves to "carve out" the destinies of Europe in the patterns of their ambitions. They have brought misery and death to countless millions, and have sown dissension, suspicion, hatred, and blood feuds among the peoples. Yet they, the ambitious and the unscrupulous usurpers of power, are not the primal evil. They are secondary and consequent evils. The primal evil is of another and deeper nature.

The crisis of our age, as has been observed, is of a moral, of a spiritual nature. Ortega has phrased it well in affirming that "crisis occurs when the system of convictions belonging to a previous generation gives way to a vital state in which man remains without these convictions and, therefore, without a world" (5). It is the loss of convictions that engenders our world crisis, a crisis which is moral in nature, and hence more menacing.

The modern crisis was long in the making but precipitous in its emergence. It came to the fore with the First World War, and has become enlarged and intensified ever since. How well, and with what keen prescience, Viscount Grey summed up the tragic outbreak of the World War of 1914: "The lamps are going out all over Europe; we shall not see them lit again in our lifetime."

For more than three score years, that is, from the middle of the nineteenth century until 1914, Europe lived in the persuasion that it had attained basic stability and had mastered the means for a continuing melioration of mankind's lot. The means were obvious and simple, interrelated and mutually reinforcing. They were: education, industry, and democracy. They were means, but also innately good and rewarding in themselves. It was good to be educated; industry yielded the products essential to a good life; democracy extended the prerogatives and the responsibilities of government and enhanced the dignity of the individual.

These persuasions were bolstered by the moralisms and "sage saws" native and dear to the Victorians. There is, it was argued, a logic, a rationality, a basic sense to life. If one played the game according to the rules, worked hard, stayed sober, saved his money, was decent, and otherwise did his duty by God, country and family, one was bound to prosper, and the world too, accordingly. The great number of Europeans believed all this in earnest.

But then came the World War with its Armageddon aftermath. The conceits, the persuasions, and the faiths of the world were now discredited by gaunt reality. Experience proved them hollow, false, corrupted, and corrupting, thus giving warrant for Sartre's later affirmation, "Human life begins on the far side of despair" (*The Flies*).

The newer generations of sensitive, inquisitive, thoughtful men, contemplating the ruin about them, denied the household gods of their fathers. But, they sought no new gods! They turned to other ways and other sources for the meaning of human life and of human experience. Their search and their labors came to fruition in existentialism.

As I have noted, the crisis was long in the making. There were, in effect, existentialists before existentialism came into being. There were some early "prophets of doom," a clutch of Cassandras, who foresaw and foretold the oncoming tragedies. They were a varied lot, including theologians, philosophers, poets, novelists, and artists. Kierkegaard was among them, and Nietzsche, Baudelaire, and Kafka. These early existentialists were the "odd men" of their era.

The global crash of 1914 heralded the emergence of the Crisis of our Age, and to this Crisis we can credit the materialization of Existentialism.

Existentialism is, as we have already noted, a movement of protest, and a philosophy of despair. These are its initial and elemental qualities. But existentialism is more than formalized protest and despair. It is creative far more than it is polemical.

Existentialism is not nihilism. It is, on the contrary, an energic, creative impulsion. It has animated and inspired the graphic arts, poetry, drama, and every form of prose literature. It has productively agitated and illumined the philosophers, the psychologists, and the theologians.

That is precisely why it is so difficult to "define" existentialism, save in terms of its historic derivations. For the problem is: whose existentialism is prototypical—Sartre's, Camus', Kafka's, Nietzsche's Kierkegaard's, Jaspers', Heidegger's, Tillich's, or Martin Buber's? Existentialism, however, is not a babel of tongues, not a rat's nest of confusion that carries a delusionally unifying label. The accents differ—but the tongue is common. It is that of existentialism.

The key factor in the comprehension of existentialism is existence. This affirmation seems tautological. All existing things—exist! But that is not the sense in which existentialism speaks of existence. For the existentialist, existence is not, like endurance, a derivative state. Existence is dynamic, creative, emergent, mercurial—a flux of "being, becoming, and being." This affirmation is not novel nor entirely new. The Greek philosopher Heraclitus propounded a comparable version of living experience. Nothing remains what it is, everything passes into its opposite, all comes out of all; all is all. But where the Greek theory was formulated primarily to *describe* the flux of experience, the existentialist intends his version of existence initially as a protest against the philosophical and moralistic systems which have arisen in time and which hedge existence with a host of logical formulations and moral injunctions. Secondarily, but in an even larger intent, existentialism affirms the sovereign creativity and "rationality" of pristine existence, of existence unencumbered by preconceptions as to what existence *ought* to be. The rationality of existence, the existentialist insists, is innate in existence and emerges in the existence of being and becoming. All of this is reflected in the existentialist affirmation that "Truth is not formulated but lived." "Classical philosophy considers existence a secondary phenomenon, an appearance behind which it should be possible to discover a rational order, invisible on the surface" (5). But the existentialist reverses the order and the emphasis: existence is primary and authentic—thought and theory are secondary and derivative. The world and life do make sense, but not in the way orthodox philosophy, and doctrinaire moralities suppose they do. Certain it is that historically, and most notably during the past century, the orthodox philosophies and the doctrinaire moralities have been shown to have only the most tenuous relevance to experienced reality.

The emphasis here, be it noted, is on the *orthodox* philosophies, and the *doctrinaire* moralities. Existentialism does not deny the possibility of philosophy, or morality. But the existentialist affirms that to be authentic, philosophy and morality will need to be not *antecedent* and *a priori* to experience, but derivative from existence.

There is a good deal that is seemingly paradoxical and contradictory in the existentialist contentions as represented in the aforegoing. If existence is neither to be envisaged nor governed by any antecedently formulated theories or preconcepts, but is conceived as purely self-emergent and auto-directive, then can existence in effect add up to anything more than a spiraling anarchy that must inevitably end in dissolution? Reading Sartre, one can perceive in the destinies of his principal characters just such spiraling anarchy that ends in dissolution.

"Sartre's man," wrote Norberto Bobbio, "is the sheer antithesis of the Christian God, who creates the world out of nothingness; he (Sartre) creates nothingness out of the world" (6). But that is Sartre's existentialism, predominantly protest in character. Other existentialists, notably the philosophers, psychologists, and the theologians, have gone beyond the protest phase and have concerned themselves with the ontological aspects of existence. Ontology investigates the nature, essential properties and relations of being as such.

The term ontology is commonplace in existentialist vernacular. Sartre's *L'Etre et le Néant* carries the subtitle *Essai d'ontologie phénoménologique*. Existentialism itself is not infrequently referred to as an ontological philosophy. However, ontology in existential expositions most commonly refers to the operational modality of existence: to the *becoming* phase of existential being.

Confessedly, the ontological is the least well developed and the least well defined component of existentialism. Yet it is crucial to, indeed the very complement of, existentialism. For it is its ontological perimeter, framing the miscellany of existential critique, psychology, and philosophy, that renders the existentialist entirety meaningful and comprehensible.

In existential psychology, as expounded by Heidegger, being is of two orders, *being* with the small "*b*," and Being that is written and understood with the capital "B." The initial *being*, that of the small "*b*," emerges out of nothingness, and sequentially yields to nothingness, which, in turn, yields *being* of the small *"b."* The whole experimental process adds up, in the ·perspective of extended existence, to Being with the capital "B." This cyclical process involving the sequential flow of nothingness into being and being into nothingness *is* the ontological dimension of existence.

All this is confessedly an uncommon formulation, and difficult, at first, to comprehend. It will help to understand that by nothingness the existentialist intends not insubstantiality but an irrelevant state, that is one that is not pertinent to any immediacy: like "yesterday's snow."

Existential psychology strongly emphasizes the certainty and the authenticity of the experienced moment, in the here and the now. This existential moment is forged into being out of the antecedent nothingness. The existential moment in turn will yield to nothingness, from which the succeeding authentic existential moment will emerge.

This formulation displaces and discredits the Cartesian *cogito ergo sum* —I think, therefore I am—and affirms instead "I am what I am," or "I am as I am," or "I am because I am." This, in effect, is a paraphrase of Jahve's answer to Moses. When Moses, in the presence of the Burning Bush asked God (Jahve) what is his name, God answered Moses: "I am that I am."

There is something appealing in the affirmation of the authenticity of "being in the here and the now." It is so patently real, so immediate and so undeniable. And yet it is also so very inadequate. For the here and the now brings with it the echo of the "there and then" of the "here and the now *that was,*" and that now is melted into the nothingness of the past, that no longer has an immediacy, save in the residual pattern of individual antecedent, and collective history. The "here and the now" is authentic and immediate, but it is also impermanent, fugitive, and evanescent.

Contemplated in the larger perspective, the existential moment is seen as the link between past and future. The existential moment of the *here* and the *now* is bounden to, and gives issue to the *there* and *thereafter.* In this sense then, the existential moment is ontological. But it affirms only the ontology of the operational modality of existence. It is initial but not amply definitive. It relates to process, not to end result.

It must be said that if existentialism did no more than propound the *operational* ontology of existence, it would already have done a great deal; for modern science has shied away from ontology: ontology smacks too much of vitalism.

The philosophic and the theological existentialist—among the latter we may count Paul Tillich, Martin Buber, Jacques Maritain, and Nicholas Berdyaev*—are not, however, content to rest with an operational ontology of existence, one that is merely concerned with the *process* of being; they reach beyond, to the ontology of the total experience of being, of being with the capital "B." Existence, they argue, cannot be the ultimate rationale of existence. All human experience controverts that postulate. There is, they insist, a perceptible pattern to human life, a pattern which emerges from the immediacies of sequential existence. This pattern is not accidental to existence, but rather attests to the significance of extended existence pattern indwelling, but not manifest, in the singular existential moment. This pattern is the ontology of Being, with the capital "B."

The philosophic and theological existentialists are not thus attempting to sneak in, under the cloak of existentialism, the old and familiar ontology of predetermination. They most earnestly subscribe to the existentialist faith that "the visage of the world was not preordained, that man is free to mold one that suits him, and to abandon it as soon as it ceases to suit him" (7).

It is here that we come aplomb of the relevance of existentialism to psychiatry. The metaphysics of existentialism and its psychological *aperçus* may interest the psychiatrist as a man of this age, himself involved in its cultural crisis. The ontological concepts of existentialism, however, deeply relate to the *métier* of the psychiatrist, and involve his professional operations.

Let me state the arguments bluntly. All problems that properly fall within the psychiatrist's ambient are ultimately existential in character, and ontological in nature. The psychiatrist is called on to treat the individual who is experiencing an existential thwart, whose being and existence encounter frustration and negation, who cannot, in other words, get on with the flux of his existence, and is thus hampered in effecting his unique ontologic fulfilment. To continue in this metaphoric mood, it may be said that classical psychiatry, including psychoanalysis, is primarily and almost exclusively concerned with "what blocks or diverts the individual." Existential psychiatry, on the other hand, is concerned with what blocks the individual from getting *on to where.***

The extension of concern from "what blocks the individual" to "what blocks him from getting where" is of crucial significance. Failure to

---

* Will Herberg, *Four Existentialist Theologians*, Doubleday & Co., N. Y. 1958.

** I must hasten to add that I cannot really conceive of an existential psychiatry, *sui generi*, though I can appreciate how much psychiatry stands to gain by the incorporation of existential insight.

comprehend this is responsible for the frequency of that cynical comment: "His analysis was successful, but he himself is no better." The "where" of the psychiatric problem is not to be determined by an *priori* judgment, nor in accordance with some pattern or schedule of normalcy. It can be grasped only by an intimate study of the existential history of the individual, and this is more than his anamnesis, or the produce of his free association. Reference to free association raises the question of the relation of psychoanalysis to existential psychiatry.

Freud was no existentialist, though he had a profound regard for Nietzsche's psychological insights. But Freud was something of an existentialist, at least in his recognition of the extent to which modern man is alienated from his primal self, from that which is Nature in Man. Freud regarded both nature and culture as twin millstones that grind the marrow of man's being and render his life bitter and a trial. But that despite, Freud was a 19th Century man, and shared in that Century's faith in the ultimate competence of Science to render man free, prosperous, and happy.

That was Freud's belief, his faith, and many shared it with him; but with time and experience, some grew disillusioned. Freud and psychoanalysis, they found, were not enough, not adequate, to illuminate the psychological problems of modern man. Freud's orientation to man as a being, his formulations on etiology, pathology, and therapy in psychic illness, were remote to the living, unique, individual. They were abstractions, or extractions, stereotypic, projective formulations based on the concept of a generic man.

This is perhaps best reflected in Freud's doctrine on the passivity, remoteness, non-participating role of the analyst in Freud's unique therapeutic procedure—that of "free association," and also most tellingly in the many "universals" which he enunciated, such as the Oedipus conflict, the castration fear, the pan-psychism of sexuality.

It was against this dismemberment of man, the remoteness thereby engendered, the falsity of absolute universals, the resultant alienation, the non-participating, non-committed role of the psychotherapist and of psychotherapy, that some among Freud's followers, Ferenczi, Sullivan, Horney, Frieda Fromm-Reichmann, protested.

Among the so-called existential psychiatrists there are many who, if not avowed psychoanalysts, are well informed on, and basically appreciative of, Freud's historic stature and his epochal contributions to psychiatry. Existential psychiatry is not avowedly anti-Freudian nor anti-analysis, but only critical of its limitations. The existentialist emphasis is on the uniqueness of the individual and of his existence, his being. Their protest is against viewing man, the patient, as a stereotypical individual, involved in a psychopathy, to be dealt with "stereotypically." What does this mean? Some insight into its meaning can be gained from Binswanger's concept of man as confronting a triple world in which he lives, and to which he must relate. This triple world Binswanger describes as the *Umwelt* (the world around), *the Mitwelt* (the with-world), and the *Eigenwelt* (the own world).

In existential formulation these three "modes of world" are always interrelated, and always condition each other. Man lives in the *Umwelt*, *Mitwelt*, and *Eigenwelt* simultaneously. It is Binswanger's contention, shared by many of the existential psychiatrists, that classical psychoanalysis is preoccupied primarily, if not exclusively, with the *Umwelt*. In Freudian terms the *Umwelt* would be the reality with which the patient is required to deal "realistically."

Existential psychiatry accents the need of the individual to relate effectively to each of the components of his tri-modal world. The existential psychiatrist maintains that excessive preoccupation with any one of the world modalities, to the exclusion of the other two, is both a product and an attestation of disease.

Perhaps the most important, though rather recondite, element of this formulation is the following: the *Eigenwelt* is not simply a derivative or product of the *Umwelt* and the *Mitwelt*, but rather exercises a shaping influence on the *Umwelt* and *Mitwelt*, which then reflexly operates on the *Eigenwelt;* or to paraphrase this at a simpler level, individuality is not a derivative product of nature and nurture, but itself contributes to the interplay of nature and nurture, and is thus a catalytic morphogenic factor.

This is the accent identified in existential psychiatry as the "ontology of existence." It is here that we can perceive the distinctive orientation of *existential analysis*. In existential analysis the "analyst" seeks to understand, not judgment-wise, but in simple comprehension, how the individual is dealing with his tri-modal existence in his tri-modal world. The "phenomena of his operations," what we might in psychiatry call his psychodynamic pattern, and in the case of the ill person, his psychopathology, thus represent a meaningful understandable operation. Pathology is thus perceived as a mode of relational operation. The existential analyst does not condone or condemn but merely understands.

Binswanger has described the existential analysis of a case under the title "The Case of Ellen West." It makes most interesting and, I must confess, rather disturbing reading. It is strictly a "phenomenological portrait." There is nothing in "The Case of Ellen West" that can warm the heart of the psychiatrist. These is nothing in it of the familiar depth psychoanalysis. We find nowhere any evidence of participation or intercession by the therapist. This case recitation reflects, in truth, a contemplation of the slow ingression and the ultimate triumph of death (10).

Yet the case recitation, chilling in its overall perspective, is instructive in its own, peculiar way. There is a good deal in it that the analytically oriented psychiatrist can absorb and utilize in the deeper and larger comprehension of his patients.

I have underscored the fact that existential analysis, at least insofar as it is represented in Binswanger, offers little illumination on what the existential analyst *does* or, to paraphrase it, what the *technique* of the existential analyst is, and how it differs from the techniques of other psychiatric practices.

Rollo May, in his book *Existence*, emphatically affirms that existential analysis offers no novel therapeutic techniques. "The fundamental contribution of existential therapy," he writes, "is its understanding of man as *being*. It does not deny the validity of dynamism and the study of specific behavior patterns in their rightful places. But it holds that drives or dynamisms, by whatever name one calls them, can be understood only in context of the structure of the existence of the person we are dealing with. The distinctive character of existential analysis is, thus, that it is concerned with *ontology*, the science of being, and with *Dasein*, the existence of this particular being sitting opposite the psychotherapist" (8).

Referring to Binswanger's *Daseinsanalyse*, that is, existential analysis, Rollo May states: "What Binswanger termed Daseinsanalyse (Existential Analysis) represents a synthesis of psychoanalysis, phenomenology, the existentialist concepts modified by original new insights. It is a reconstruction of the inner world of experience of psychiatric patients with the help of a conceptual framework inspired by Heidegger's studies on the structure of human existence" (9).

There is in all this a great profundity and a something which is deeply appealing. And yet, to those who have wrestled with the problems of existence, Existentialism appears incomplete and hence inadequate.

Existentialism conceives of man as a sort of monadic being, floating in a realm of total indifference. It fails to take into consideration *man as a creature with an existential history*. It fails to recognize man as a *social* and hence a cultural being. The individual *emerging* out of nothingness into existence is inevitably confronted by a variety of alternatives. He is confronted with the necessity of selecting one from among the many alternatives. *That* choice is influenced by antecedent existence and by anticipatory evocatives.

To paraphrase this: man realizes his existence in the interplay of the dynamics of his past with those of his future.

I must end with one pertinent observation. Taking a closer view of existentialism one finds that what originally seemed strange and alien begins to sound somewhat familiar. We discover, like Molière's *Bourgeois Gentilhomme,* that we have been, at least in some measure, thinking and acting existentially. Such indeed is the case, yet I submit that it is not quite enough. It is not enough merely to "appreciate Existentialism by non-intention." The existentialist movement, existentialist philosophy, existentialist analysis, confront us as a deep challenge which we need to comprehend clearly and definitely.

REFERENCES

1. KNIGHT, EVERETT, W.: *Literature Considered as Philosophy,* New York, Macmillan Co., 1958, pp. x-xv.
2. BOBBIO, NORBERTO: The Philosophy of Decadentisms: *A Study of Existentialism,* transl. by David More, Oxford, Basil Blackwell, 1948, p. 2.
3. BOBBIO, NORBERTO, *ibid.,* p. 2.
4. ORTEGA Y GASSET, JOSÉ: *Man and Crisis,* New York, W. W. Norton & Co., 1958, p. 86.
5. KNIGHT, EVERETT W., Op. cit., p. x.
6. BOBBIO, NORBERTO, Op. cit., p. 56.
7. KNIGHT, EVERETT W., *Op. cit.,* p. xiii.
8. MAY, ROLLO: *Existence,* New York, Basic Books, Inc., 1958, p. 37.
9. MAY, ROLLO, *ibid.,* p .120.
10. BINSWANGER, LUDWIG: Der Fall Ellen West, *Schwectzer Archiv für Neurologie und Psychiatrie,* LIII (1944), pp. 255-277; LIV, pp. 69-117; LV, pp. 16-40. English translation in Rollo May, Ernest Angel and H. F. Ellenberger, eds., *Existence,* New York, Basic Books, 1958, pp. 237-364.

27

An Existential Clinical Exposition
of the Ontogenic Thrust

EXISTENTIAL PSYCHIATRY though distinctive does not involve any special techniques. Its singularity lies in its biopsychological orientation, captioned as *ontological.*

Existential psychiatry is both protago- and antagonistic. Its impulsion is to break down conceptual barriers, to complement and enlarge and thereby to deepen understanding of the dynamics of becoming and of being.

The language of existential psychiatry is novel and difficult to comprehend. It is difficult to concretize its terminology and to relate it to the already known. Existential terminology is seemingly more suggestive than informing. Yet it needs to be affirmed that he who earnestly desires to understand existential psychiatry must be both enterprising and patient. He must be willing and ready to tolerate the use of old terms for the conveyance of new meanings, in order to acquire new concepts and deeper understanding.

However, despite, its difficult terminology, existential psychiatry is not really difficult to comprehend. Requisite is a reference framework and this can best be gained in a review of the historic growth of modern psychiatry. Here, perforce, the review offered must be very brief, indeed almost skeletal.

Modern psychiatry was in its initial stages predominantly organic. The etiology and the treatment of mental illness were envisaged in terms of the physical constitution of the patient and of its variances from the so-called "normal state and function." This solid persuasion, dominant for more than a century, was breached by Freud.

Freud's epochal contribution to psychiatric knowledge and understanding is designated as the science of the intrapsychic. Freud's psychoanalysis did not invalidate the role of the "organic" in the genesis of mental illness, but only circumscribed it. Freud brilliantly demonstrated that much illness, physical (psychosomatic) as well as psychological, derives from the the psychic internality of man which, without the participation of any noxious physical factors, can yet be pathogenic.

Herein lies what in essence is Freud's greatest achievement. He liberated psychiatry from its enslaving bondage to the physical and the organic, thereby rendering it free to explore the other factors which operate in man's realm to either foster or disrupt his mental and emotional, that is, his psychological being. For this, all schools of depth psychology, including the existential (though it is in effect no school), owe Freud a debt and tribute. He was a pioneer of heroic stature.

Time and experience however, revealed that Freud's theoretical formulations on intrapsychic dynamics, though illuminating in many ways and respects, are not adequate to fully account for the engenderment of the non-organic psychiatric illness, nor do they provide the basis for a comprehensive therapeutic activity. It became evident that not everything that eventuates in the psyche can be accounted for in terms of the interplay of Id, Ego, and Superego. Other factors are participant. A host of dynamisms impinge upon the unitary psyche: personages, for example, in the immediate family and in the extended group.

It becomes clear that the unitary psyche exists in a complex world. It is exposed to and influenced by economic, social and cultural factors. These profoundly affect the psyche, and when of an untoward nature can prove psycho-pathogenic. This extended comprehension of what "shapes the psyche" can be epitomized in the affirmation that there is a *psychological ecology* as real and potent for good or ill as the better understood material ecology of the physical world.

The foregoing is a resume in brief of the productive labors of a splendid host of men and women pioneering in the realms of psychiatry. It were an impossible task to name "the host entire." But though unnamed, they collectively have structured the vision of a psychological ecology, the qualities and dimensions of which profoundly affect the psyche.

The temptation to enlarge upon this vision of a psychological ecology, to treat in this relation of the most recent developments in the studies of ethology, sensory deprivation, sensory overload, et al., is very enticing but must be resisted.

Perceptible in this review of the history of modern psychiatry is the enlarging appreciation of the many factors, intrapsychic, interpersonal, familial, social, economic, cultural, which bear upon and influence the growth, development and operations of the psyche. Perceptible also is the *construct* of the many factors *operating on man*, and, in the ecological sense, his *reacting to their operations*. This construct is dynamic, but it is not ontological, and hence not existential. For, in addition to action and reaction there is a third force in operation—that of the ontogenic momentum or ontogenic thrust. Man (though the process is not limited to man but is shared in varying degrees by all living bodies) does not merely *react* thermodynamically. His reactions are conditioned by an ontological vector. Man is innerly committed to an architectonic pattern to be achieved in the continued process of "being, becoming, being"—that is, the process of living a life.

Man harbors an inner momentum directed toward fulfillment. Existential man moves from being to becoming to being in a long line of successions, until the full architectonic pattern has been experienced and attained. Then death crowns and ends it, even as conception and birth initiated it.

The picture is that of an ideal fulfillment, rarely given to any man. And because it is so rare, because the ontogenic thrust is so frequently blocked, and its momentum diverted, the ontological looms so significant in the pathogenic complex, that is, it looms significant to the informed and perceptive intelligence.

Ontology is at present largely a neglected science. It was once cultivated intensively and with enthusiasm. In the minds of many it is associated with vitalism, which is considered mystical and unscientific (1). It is true, of course, that ontology does cut athwart simon pure materialism and the mechanistic psychologies. But ontogeny cannot be disputed or denied phenomenologically. It incontrovertibly *is*. It is manifest and operational not only in its classical instance, embryology, but also in and throughout the post-uterine existence of the individual. It is "that which gives pattern to existence." Otherwise existence would be, as it indeed is in certain states of psychopathic regression (schizophrenia), amorphous and with but one dimension—duration.

The ontologic thrust initiated at conception is the *kybernetes,* the helmsman, of existence chartered toward fulfillment. But to continue the metaphor—the sailing is usually rough, and the route beset with many hazards.

In this perspective then, the psychological hurt, and also to a somewhat lesser degree the physical hurt, is to be gauged and understood not only in respect to its immediate nature and degree but also in respect to its effect on the existential, ontological momentum of the individual. The magnitude of the psychological hurt does not always have a direct and proportionate relation to the severity of its effects on the ontogenic process.

Most significant is the comprehension of the multiple and different ways in which the ontologic thrust, when thwarted and deflected, is made manifest in the existence, behavior and symptomatology of the individual. The greater part of manifest psychopathology is not to be understood in terms only of its etiology, that is, in terms of the individual's antecedent *determinant* experiences. The effects of these experiences are most frequently modified or compounded by the energies of the ontological drive. The resulting manifest symptom-complex is, in consequence, difficult to disentangle. It is difficult to determine what is primarily pathological, and what in effect derives from the effort to acutalize under untoward circumstances a thwarted existential-ontological goal. Much that appears to be manifestly pathological may, when so examined, be recognized as prophylactic and hence therapeutically useful and productive (2).

It should now be clearly evident that existential psychotherapy is centrally concerned with the patient's ontological experiences, conditions and prospects. Its therapeutic goals and commitments are to uncover the impediments that block and/or divert the ontogenic progressions of the individual; to help him, insofar as that may be possible, to remove the impedimenta and, in certain instances, to reconcile the primal ontogenic thrust with the given limiting circumstances in order to facilitate a compromised but effective self-realization.

Existential psychotherapy is not principally preoccupied with psychopathology, nor does it accept the premise that the correction or elimination of pathology must perforce yield "health," that is, an "integrated individual, one who clearly perceives and relates to reality." Existential psychotherapy, not unmindful of psychopathology, is more affirmingly concerned with psychophysiology and with developmental-ontological dynamics. It regards living as an adventure in ontological self-realization, and the adventure, though patterned on a prototypical core, is unique with and for each individual. The existential psychotherapist is oriented to the prototypical core, but is mindful and respectful of the unique components of the individual adventure in self-realization, this including at times the individual's singular pathologies.

Adolf Meyer did not, to the best of my knowledge, ever concern himself with existentialism or with existential psychotherapy, nor did he interest himself in ontology. But there is much in his concept of ergasial-psychology that is congenial to existential psychotherapy. There is also much that is congenial in Binswanger's tripartite formulation of *Umwelt, Mitwelt* and *Eigenwelt*. The latter, that is *Eigenwelt,* is the ontological component, the catalytic morphogenic factor which exercises a shaping influence on *Umwelt* and the *Mitwelt* and in this exercise is itself reflexly affected.

The *Eigenwelt,* is not, however, to be understood as referring merely to the individual's subjective and private world through the integument of which he experiences the impingements of the *Mitwelt* and the *Umwelt*. The *Eigenwelt* is all that and, in addition, the experienced dynamic of the innate architectonic moving to realization through "being-becoming-being."

The *Eigenwelt* is ontogenic and self-shaping. Its prototypical pattern is not one of simple progression but of qualitative change and alteration. For man lives *as he develops* not on one but on four planes or categories of being. These are: the biological, the social, the aesthetic, and the moral. In the aforegoing, note is to be taken of the phrase "as he develops," for man does not at once enter into these four planes of being. Some do not attain to much "existence" on the aesthetic or moral plane. All, however, share in the biological and the social. The warrant for taking note of "the four categories of being" is that they are components of the ontogenic thrust, and thwart in the attainment of these "categories of being" is likely to prove pathogenic.

Clearly then the existential psychotherapist must be at ease with the modalities of existential-ontological thought, even as the modern physicist must be at ease with mathematical thought (3). He also needs to know the prototypical (common pattern) core of the ontogenic process. He must be competent to recognize in the patient's history and symptomatology the evidences of ontogenic existential thwart, and to define the particular nature of the thwart. He needs to know and be experienced in helping the patient to free himself of his encumberments, and thus to make possible his freer and fuller self-realization. He must know how to be *prosthetic* in the face of limiting possibilities.

If then there are any unique techniques in existential psychotherapy they are *gnostic* techniques, modalities of comprehension and of relating to given data of existential-ontological experience.

The existential psychiatrist must, in a word, be cognizant of the ontogenic thrust and all it involves.

THREE IN AN EXISTENTIAL BIND—A CASE HISTORY

This presentation is supplemental to The Ontogenic Thrust. It is the clinical correlate of that exposition. It is a case report on three patients whose interlocking deviant behavior can, I believe, be understood *best, if not only,* in an existential, ontological perspective. I will accent the latter and be sparing in the etiological psychodynamics that may account for the *origins* or derivations of their behavior. I intend, in a word, to accent the existential, ontological meaning of their behavior, and to show how very useful it is to grasp such meaning.

The three in the Existential Bind are: a professional man, in the latter half of the sixth decade of life; his wife, ten years his junior, to whom he has been married in a childless marriage for twenty-five years; and a younger woman, age thirty-plus. Behind the scenes there is another woman, in her late forties, married, the mother of several children, who had been the man's mistress for a score of years.

The "plot of the story" is this: Several years ago the man in the case became enamored of the younger woman, and she reciprocated his affection. He then decided, after much inner struggle and turmoil, to divorce his wife and to marry the younger woman. He had great compassion for his wife, made careful arrangements and generous provisions for her, but though she protested, he did divorce her. Threafter, he married the younger woman. The old mistress was likewise "generously" discarded.

No children were planned for in this new marriage. Nevertheless, pregnancy did ensue. Shortly after the marriage took place, and before the new wife became pregnant, the man in the case "discovered" that he was living with a stranger in an intolerable bond. He initiated steps for a reconciliation with his wife, with whom in effect he never broke off relations. He also began to set the stage for a divorce from his second wife, subsequent to the birth of their expected child. Remarriage with his first wife is "to follow."

As indicated, the persons involved in this bind are well educated, cultivated, and paradoxical though it may sound, responsible people. Yet their behavior is, to say the least, "out of the common," and seems irrational. And yet, it is *most* meaningful, existentially and ontologically.

To grasp this these added data are requisite. The relationship between the man and his first wife was that of Mother and Son. She was the admiring, indulgent, understanding, jealous and suffering woman. She knew of his philanderings for he "carelessly" left about notes, letters, mementos, bearing on his amours. She spied on him consistently and by querying him cornered him into telling lies. Though he had a series of loves he was not promiscuous, but rather dependently involved in each. The longest "affair" lasted for more than a decade. It is noteworthy that his first wife had been married before *he* married her, and that his second wife was also a "divorcee." His long "affair" was with a married woman.

Why then the radical wrench in his life? And what of the roles of his first and second wives?

His behavior I ascribe to what I would term the Helena complex, the dream most men harbor: meeting the perfect woman, the idealized mother, in the wife (*vide,* Goethe's *Mutter Holle*). Most men shed this dream in the third decade of their life. But the patient in this case had not lived a normal life. He was now in the sixth decade of his life, and ere it was too, too late he grasped at the dream, and woke up in a nightmare. The woman was young, vital, fertile. He could relate to her not as to Mother, but as to the *ideal mother in the wife*. And by engendering his Eupheron he could affirm his manhood.

But then, as he discovered, he was in the sixth and not in the third decade of his life. The eventuation of his ontogenic thrust was dyschronous and pathological.

As for the second wife, patently she gained self-fulfillment in the begetting of the child. Her previous marriage had been childless. She is a sophisticated woman and it is not likely that the pregnancy was either accidental or unintentional. Also, she knew that the prospects for an enduring marriage were slim. She verbalized as much.

What of the first wife? Unwittingly, that is, at the unconscious level, she aided and abetted this Greek drama. By the interplay of the forces unleashed thereby, she broke through her dollhouse existence and gained some belated maturity. She cannot regain any portion of her missed experiences. But she can carry on "from here" in ways that are ontologically more proximate to the pristine architectonic pattern. This woman retains and may regain her man, now somewhat more matured. It is within the realm of possibility that the "second wife" will be adopted as if she were a daughter-in-law, and her offspring a grandchild.

These three beings in an Existential bind did not resolve their respective problems in an *ideal way*. But existentially, ontologically, the problems being given, their efforts at resolution are understandable.

I may add that each of the actors (I conjecture about one, since I had only two in therapy) knew, as actors know, the parts they were playing and the plot's ending. But carry on they did, for they had to.

For me the appreciation of the existential nature of the case made it comprehendable, and also made possible the anticipation of its denouement.

REFERENCES

1. GALDSTON, IAGO: Physiology and the recurrent problem of vitalism; in Brooks and Cranefield, *The Historical Development of Physiological Thought,* New York, The Hafner Publishing Co., 1959, pp. 291-308.
2. GALDSTON, IAGO: Prophylactic psychopathology—the rationality of the irrational in psychodynamics, *The Psychoanalytic Review,* Vol. XI, No. 4, pp. 304-318, Oct. 1953.
3. HARTMANN, NICOLAI: *New Ways of Ontology,* Chicago, Henry Regnery Co., 1953.

28

An Existential Analysis of the Case of Miss L.

MISS L. IS AN ATTRACTIVE young woman in her early twenties. She has that order of handsomeness that is indwelling and that, barring disaster, will endure until the end of her years. She is energetic and generally in good health. She is free of psychosomatic disorders. Her intelligence is manifestly of a high order. She has been, and is, a good student, though her scholarly interests are undisciplined. She presents the picture of an energetic and well endowed person.

She is the youngest of three siblings, each of whom is attractive and intelligent. However, the entire family, that is, father, mother and sisters, is enmeshed in a reticulum of neurotic interactions.

Were this an exposition on family psychodynamics, it would indeed be interesting to sketch the pathogenic relations of the members of this family and to detail the disorders engendered in the different individuals. The family presents a wide variety of disorders and an interesting array of defenses.

However, our concern is not with the family dynamics but rather with the case of Miss L. The intention is to portray and analyze her existential confrontation of her singular existential problem.

Phrased in psychoanalytic terms, Miss L.'s basic problem is "an unresolved Oedipal complex," thus blocking her attainment of mature love and heterosexual fulfillment. In an existential paraphrase, she is to be described as experiencing a serious thwart in the fulfillment of her innate ontological thrust toward maturity.

From the viewpoint of the pathology involved, there is little that is distinctive about the case. Unresolved Oedipal fixations are very common. What *is* distinctive is the history of the patient's efforts to resolve her

367

block. This embraces a series of unpremeditated, yet manifestly relevant existential maneuvers. Viewed singly, that is, without regard to the patient's underlying existential problem (the ontological block) these maneuvers bear the stamp of pathological acting out. The so-called normal and well-adjusted person does not indulge in such maneuvers, hence they may be said to be abnormal and pathological. But viewed in their existential context these maneuvers are as logical, meaningful and purposeful as the contortions executed by the man who, having slipped, tries to regain his balance.

Miss L. passed her childhood and youth in the poorer sections of a cosmopolitan city. She did well in school, but socially was unsophisticated and somewhat restricted. Her home was modest, plain and "uncultivated." A primary concern of the parents was that their daughter should "grow up and marry." Accordingly, when a likely young man did appear on the scene and showed interest in the patient, who was then in her late teens, and asked to marry her, the parents encouraged the match.

The patient was seemingly compliant but, in depth, markedly resistant. Thus the marriage ceremony fixed for a given date was, on her insistence, deferred to a later date, much to the embarrassment of both the families involved. Before the second date arrived, she made a gesture of suicide.

As already noted, overtly she was not averse to marriage. She favored the prospective bridegroom, though she did find him a bit prosaic. She did marry, but the marriage did not last. Within two years, the husband divorced her. Her marriage was unfulfilling in every respect. She neither gave nor gained companionship. She was sexually unavailable to her husband a great deal of the time. In her everyday relations with her husband she was generally freftul and rebellious. Clearly, marriage galled her. It was not the man to whom she was married that made life difficult for her. It was the relatedness of marriage, the "life in common," that she found unbearable. She did everything possible to disrupt the marriage, without knowing why, even while she was troubled by her incomprehensible behavior. Yet, when her husband, who initially was much enamored of her, unilaterally initiated divorce proceedings, she was surprised and distressed. Despite this, she made no effort to retain him, nor did she, when later he showed reawakened interst in her, try to win him back.

Following on the divorce, she neither mourned her "lost husband" nor did she otherwise manifest any reactive regression. It was as if her marriage had been an encapsulated experience, interesting but essentially alien. Separation caused distress but left no wounds.

One marked change in the pattern of her behavior did follow on her divorce. As an adolescent and young woman, Miss L. had been rather reserved in her erotic play and restricted in her sexual activities. Though she grew up in a so-called fast neighborhood where most of the youngsters indulged in what is called heavy necking and not a few among them precociously indulged in sexual intercourse, Mss L., without being a prude, kept her erotic excursions within modest bounds. This, be it noted, was not due to any strong moral inhibitions. It was rather the result of the investment of a great deal of her libido in the non-sexual components of her being and existence. Thus she was intensively and consistently preoccupied with a host of intellectual problems, and esthetically involved in a broad spectrum of subtle moods and fancies.

This intellectual and esthetic preoccupation is not to be construed as a sublimation of her erotic drive. It was, in effect, a simple displacement of libido. In existential terms it may be described as a draining away of some quantity of the energies of her ontological thrust from the erotic channels into those of the intellectual and the esthetic.

As noted before, Miss L. passively resisted her husband's sexual approaches, and when intercourse was "inescapable" she proved neither gratifying nor gratified. Following on her divorce, in marked contrast to her previous behavior, Miss L. became sexually adventurous, receptive and aggressive. There ensued a series of affairs carried out with a variety of men of different races and creeds, and from different stations in life. Some of these affairs were very casual, others were more enduring. None of them proved significant or meaningful. None of the men could bind her in an enduring relationship, they were seemingly units in an extended experience. However, these affairs were not a commonplace promiscuity. They had some distinctive qualities and features. Each of the men with whom she had "an affair" initially interested Miss L. She brought to each relationship a measure of warmth and committedness, but as the relationship waned, she was prone to become hostile, aggressive and castrating. In some instances, this range of mood and relation would be transcoursed in a single day.

The period of erotic adventuresomeness lasted for close to two years and yielded to another order of adventure, one of a more intensive nature. Miss L. attracted and developed a love relationship with a man, whom we will name John, 15 years her senior in age, and her senior by much more in life's experience. John had been married and was divorced. He was the father of several children.

Miss L.'s relations with John have been enduring, but very stormy.

They are characterized by intense affection, bitter quarrels, and numerous misunderstandings. There is a repeated coming together in love and a parting in anger and despair. The relationship is further complicated by the attitude of Miss L.'s parents, who intensely disapprove of it. They disapprove of John as a person, and are grieved at the thought that Miss L. might consent to marry him.

Scanning the situation, it would appear that the lines of tension are clearly drawn between Miss L., her man John, and her parents. Miss L. is seemingly the central figure, and subjected to pulls in opposite directions. Figuratively, if not torn apart by the pull of the opposite forces, she is at least immobilized.

In effect, however, she is neither torn apart nor is she immobilized. Her emotions are intense and varied, but she effectively carries on both her daily activities, that is, her work and study, and also a host of complex relations and interactions which promise to yield a solution to her existential problem.

Events have taken an interesting turn. The parents, to whom John has been an anathema, had a seeming change of heart. They solicited Miss L. to have John visit them at their home. (They had never met him.) This initiative was not the result of an authentic reconciliation nor yet part of a clever scheme. It was the consequence of what I can only describe as existential counterpressures. The parents pressure Miss L. Her involvement with John is a thwart to their own self-fulfillment, which lies in great part in their daughter's marriage to a man who will be congenial to them and with whom they might effectively realize and live out their ultimate being. Miss L., on the other hand, will not yield. She will not give up John, nor will she give up her parents.

Seemingly, she could leave kith and kin and go with the man of her choice. But here precisely lies the crux of the matter. John is not the man of her choice, but only the man that meets her immediate existential needs. The parents have thus been compelled by the force of the existential counter-pressures to yield, to abandon, in gesture at least, their opposition to John. This, in effect, was not only a capitulation but also an overt acknowledgment of Miss L.'s right to a man of her own choice. The parents too, be it noted, could have abandoned their daughter. But they didn't, and the seeming change of heart has behind it an existential reason. For that which in appearance is the embrace of a bitter fate is in effect likely to yield a resolution of the existential thwart experienced both by Miss L. and by her parents. What it will effect for John, I am not in a position to tell.

This prognostic view of "things to come" is founded on a long-range interpretation of Miss L.'s existential maneuvers, that is, on the assessment of the intention and meaningfulness of her efforts to resolve the thwart to her ontological self-realization. It is also based on what has eventuated since the parents have capitulated.

Miss L. now views John more realistically, more objectively, more critically, quite as he is, and as his being currently relates to hers, and as it is likely to in the future. She sees him as an Oedipal *ersatz*.

In one of her dreams, John was with her. I quote from the dream: "Suddenly he was facing me, very close, and saying, 'But don't you think I have taken over those functions of your father, became like a father substitute?' These words, Miss L. continues, "echo like needles into me. He kind of has the quality of screaming in his voice. He is saying something like what K.'s mother (the mother of her divorced husband) said about my meeting K. so early at college, making it easier for me to adjust to the situation with my family. I keep denying. He thinks this is something good, but I know (somehow) that it is horrible and I am ashamed." There follow several other episodes and the dream comes to an end, thus: (This, too, is quoted verbatim.) "We are again in an apartment, in the living room, having an awful fight. He is yelling at me ferociously. I run into the bathroom hysterically and lock the door. . . . I think I am trying to brush my teeth. I am crying and he is pounding on the door. Suddenly, he breaks the door down, and it is not John. It is my father, naked, and he is saying he will kill me if I don't do something. I am screaming and he is about to hit me with his body, when I wake up."

Here we leave Miss L. to further work out her life in time to come, and venture an existential analysis of so much of her life as we now know.

The diagnosis of her existential block, and her ontological thwart, as that of an unresolved Oedipal fixation is, I believe, fully warranted. There is much in the familial history to support this diagnosis. I will detail only a few of the more significant family factors. The parents are ill-matched in respect to education, cultural values, background and much else. The mother is the dominant of the pair, and is the superior in education. She never fully accepted her husband as mate or companion. She aggressively rejected and disparaged the father in the presence of the children. She was also very critical of and hostile to her children, inflicting cruel punishments on them, especially on the older ones. She led her children to believe that the father was to be avoided and that he was sexually menacing. The end result was that the children were bound to and dependent on the mother but had no real love for her. As they grew up, they retained some of the engendered reservation toward their father but found him to be a more responsive person than the mother. The father, on the other hand, disparaged and rejected by the mother, invested much of his libido in his growing daughters. In consequence, the mother grew ever more jealous of and quarrelsome with both her husband and her daughters.

This, in marked brevity, is the familial background of Miss L. and, to my mind, adequately accounts for and supports the given diagnosis.

In the light of this, how are we to view her history? Essentially, not as acting out, but rather as a living through. This difference, that is, the difference between "acting out" and "living through," is of crucial significance. Living through is an existential dynamic. It is an experiential process to which insight is secondary. It is, *when it is,* first lived and then understood. The emergence of the experienced event has its own logic, its unique rationale, best perceptible after its occurence. It can at times be anticipated when the given individual and his past are viewed and understood in an ontological, existential perspective.

Viewed thus, what is, in one respect, pathological, neurotic, self-destructive—her suicide attempt, her precocious and ineffective marriage, her divorce, promiscuity, and her stormy and abrasive liaison with John—all this can existentially be seen as an effort to catch up with life, to amend for deprivations, to correct experiences, to attain, in other words, her rightful position in her ontological *schema*. In this respect then, her pathology is pathologic in substance, but not in essence or effect. It is as I have designated it elsewhere—prophylactic psychopathology.

This seemingly paradoxical comprehension is, I submit, of crucial importance. It distinguishes existential, ontological psychiatry, and points up its unique orientation. This orientation is in my judgment the quintessence of the "technique" of existential psychiatry. It is this I intended when I wrote, "Existential psychiatry is an embodiment of distinctive knowledge and comprehension, rather than the protagonist of novel therapeutic techniques."

We need to pursue these matters deeper. In the main, patients come to doctors with their complaints. Physicians then investigate the patient's complaints in terms of the presenting symptoms and the underlying pathology. Where they can, physicians proceed to relieve the symptoms and to correct the pathology. This, in essence, is the practice pattern of what is known in medical history as the Aetiological School. Today this School is as predominant in psychiatry as it is in clinical medicine. How otherwise is one to account for the so very widespread use of treatment modalities to "repress symptoms" and to extirpate disease"—the chemical, electrical, surgical treatments? The Aetiological School of medical thought and practice cannot encompas and will not tolerate the thought that "disease" has place and meaning in existence, that what, in their criteria of the *normal,* seems and *is* pathological, may existentially be of the essence of the living process; that life in the process of effective existence may require and may utilize what is termed disease—to attain to its ontological ultimates.

All this reduces itself to very practical issues. In the presence of patent pathology, what is the position of the physician, in our case, of the psychiatrist, to be? How does he relate to and deal with the presenting symptoms and with the underlying pathology?

This inquiry, taken in its full embrace, is too large and too complex to be dealt with here. Disease is an intricate concept. There are many orders of disease, and while they have a common connotation, they differ radically in nature and essence. We need here to concern ourselves with a more restricted, that is, partial, version of the problem; specifically, with the Case of Miss L.

How are we to understand and to relate to *her* symptoms, her pathology? I said before, existentially, and as a living through rather than as an acting out, hers was and is an existential disorder. In that purview, her existential maneuvers can be understood thus. In her precocious marriage she extricated herself from the family reticulum. But she was not yet able to engage in an effective, heterosexual co-existence. She thus effected the dissolution of the marriage union. But she retained the gain of her emergence from her family. The period of promiscuity that followed can be understood as a complex effort to gain in erotization, missed out in part during her pre-adolescent and adolescent years, and also, as an attempt to break through her Oedipal bond. Her numerous affairs interposed between her and the binding-father-figure a host of radically different men. This experience made it possible for her to confront her incestuous bind and to "live it through" in her liaison with John. In and through John, seeing him in the bosom of her family, she is *existentially* perceiving that ontological attainment cannot be realized through the father, but "through the contemporaneous lover-husband." Her latest dreams are of the husband who divorced her. She had not dreamt of him before.

One final point, and this one treated all too briefly, since space allows for no more: What is the existential psychiatrist's role in all this? Is he an onlooker, a spectator, viewing the unrolling of a life? Perceptibly he is not an intercessor. He does not repress symptoms, nor attempt to extirpate the disease. What then is his role? What does the existentially oriented psychiatrist do? Like an analyst, he "uncovers." He maintains and promotes an anamnestic dialogue with the patient. He encourages the patient to bring his past into awareness and comprehension. The patient thus learns in time and by effort to understand, existentially and ontologically, the retardations (deprivations and plethoras) he has experienced, the thwarts and blocks he is suffering, and also, this being important to the integrity of his self-image, the *meaning* of his efforts, past and present, to attain to his rightful position in his ontological schema (in common parlance—"to be his age"). He is ontologically and existentially demystified, detoxicated.

Most important is the effect of the therapist's "co-existence" with the patient. The therapist himself needs to have confronted and resolved his own existential being—"being" meaning not a substantive entity, but "process." He must himself represent to the patient a witness of the *attainable* (not ideal) and a living attestation of "the process."

Much of this is evidenced by the Existential Therapist in his manifest relatedness toward the symptomatology and the pathology presented by the patient.

Part V:
SOME HISTORICAL AND PHILOSOPHICAL JOTTINGS

29

The Psychiatry of Paracelsus

In his *Paracelsica* Carl Jung says of Paracelsus:

> Man kann ihm nicht gerecht werden; man kann ihm immer nur unter- oder überschätzen, und darum ist man mit der eigenen Bemühung, wenigstens einen Teil seines Wesens genügend zu erfassen, stets unzufrieden.[1]

However, despite Jung's perspicacious and somewhat despairing comment, it is very timely to scrutinize the psychiatry of Paracelsus. This not solely because we have entered upon the Atomic Age and thus have realized in an egregious fashion the dream of the alchemist, but also because the atomic bomb has in a rude and compelling manner obliged the scientist to take cognizance of the meaning of life. For in the main, and with but very few exceptions, the scientist has been loath to deal with meanings, and most of all with the meaning of life. With an almost arrogant pride the proverbial scientist proclaimed himself an agnostic in all such matters. His was the realm of the "how." The "why" he left to the philosophers and ethicists.

This disassociative process by which the knowledge of matter was divorced from that of meaning began at the time of Paracelsus. He was among the last of that small number of learned men who attempted to amalgamate the ancient and modern learnings. As he was unsuccessful in his own time, so with the passage of time, he lost meaning for the

---

[1] "One cannot do him justice: one can only under- or over-value him, and for that reason one is always dissatisfied with one's own efforts to fathom at least a part of his being." (C. G. Jung, *Paracelsica. Zwei Vorlesunger über den Arzt und Philosophen Theophrastus,* Zürich und Leipzig, 1942, p. 9.)

successive generations of men who clung with increasing desperation to the mensurable data of science, and to whom all that was *unsichtbar* (imperceptible) was mysticism, and hence anathema. On the occasion of the four hundredth anniversary of his death, the Royal Society of Medicine heard this pronouncement on the personality, doctrines, and influence of Paracelsus:

> It cannot be said that the abusive rantings of Paracelsus contributed to the general progress of science and medicine that began in the sixteenth century, principally as to the outcome of the diffusion of accurate knowledge by means of printed books. For he was a rude, circuitous obscurantist, not a harbinger of light, knowledge and progress.[2]

A more sympathetic appreciation is that of Charles Singer, who, though he finds Paracelsus violent, dramatic and repellent, is still willing to allow that his "iconoclasm doubtless did something to deter men from the worship of the old idols."[3] With genial tolerance Singer takes note of the "general agreement among the learned and nebulous band of Paracelsists that their hero did indeed foreshadow the 'new instauration.' "[4] The learned and nebulous band of Paracelsists, however, deems this the lesser of the credits due their hero. Far more significant is his appreciation of the deficiencies, of the pits, and traps that beset the new learning. Paracelsus could not have been either the patron or the disciple of Bacon, though as befits the case, Bacon found something to praise in Paracelsus. Paracelsus was more than suspicious of the persuasion that real knowledge comes through the dismemberment of the whole into its constituent parts. Centuries before the term *holism*[5] was coined to connote to the learned the quality of the whole derived from wholeness, and which is greater than that derived from the sum of its parts, and long before *Gestalt* was

---

[2] H. P. Bayon, "Paracelsus: Personality, Doctrines and His Alleged Influence in the Reform of Medicine," *Proceedings Royal Soc. Med.,* 1942, vol. 35, part I, Session 1941-42, Nov.-Apr., pp. 69-76.

[3] Charles Singer, *From Magic to Science,* London, 1928, p. 105.

[4] *Ibid.*

[5] "It is quite obvious for any impartial student that Paracelsus was remote from the attitude, methods and outlook of the modern scientist, i.e., the investigator of causality in the modern sense. Van Helmont definitely followed the ideal of the modern scientist, with no little success. Nevertheless, Van Helmont realized the paramount importance of entities which are not accessible to causal analysis, especially in Biology, and subscribed, true to Paracelsus' tradition, to 'Wholism,' 'Thinking in Analogies' and Symbolism." (Walter Pagel, *The Religious and Philosophical Aspects of van Helmont's Science and Medicine,* Baltimore, 1944, p. 2 [Supplements to the Bull. Hist. Med., 2]).

applied to denote a psychological concept and to label a school of thought, Paracelsus espoused both thoughts in his criticisms of *der todten Anatomie*. "In der todten Anatomie werdet ihr weder Natur noch Wesen erkennen," wrote Paracelsus. "In the anatomy of the dead you will discern neither nature nor being. Basically it is of no value (that is, in understanding what goes on inside the living body). Essence, uniqueness, quality *(Eigenschaft)*, being and strength, that which is the highest in anatomy, is dead. This has not been dealt with as yet for it is common practice to disregard the best. But it is the living body that teaches the anatomist (the physician) health and disease, not the dead one: he requires therefore a living anatomy."[6]

This persuasion, this conviction that only the living scene in all its multiform parts and in its innumerable interrelations and interreactions, can provide some measure of understanding to those who are concerned with well-being and illness, in body and in mind, characterizes and distinguishes the whole of Paracelsus' thinking. This is in essence his preoccupation with the macrocosm and microcosm to be understood. It is this insight that makes his psychiatry so very modern in spirit and viewpoint. "Er ist nicht veraltet, sondern wächst mit der weiterlaufenden Zeit."[7] For if modern psychiatry is distinguished in any respect, it is in its integrative character, in its willingness and competence to perceive man in relation to the whole world about him. The spokesmen of modern psychiatry do not employ the terms macrocosm and microcosm, but the essence of what is involved and implied in these terms is reflected in both their criticisms and avowals. Adolf Meyer, speaking to the theme "The Contributions of Psychiatry to the Understanding of Life Problems," said, "The human organism can never exist without its setting in the world. All we are and do is of the world and in the world. The great mistake of an overambitious science has been the desire to study man altogether as a mere sum of parts, if possible, of atoms, or now of electrons, and as a machine, detached, by itself, because at least some points in the simpler sciences could be studied to the best advantage with this method of the so-called elementalist. It was a long time before willingness to see the

---

6 "In der todten Anatomie werdet ihr weder Natur noch Wesen erkennen. Nutzt inwendig war nichts. Essentia, Eigenschaft, Wesen und Kraft, so ist das höchst der Anatomie; ist abgestorben. Die ist bisher noch nicht tractirt worden; denn es ist gemeiner Brauch, da Beste wegzulassen. Aber der lebendige Leib ist es, der Gesundheit und Krankheit anatomatiziren lässt, nich der todte; er fordert daher eine lebendige Anatomie." (Paracelsus, *Grosse Chirurgie*, III. pp. 259-261).

7 "He has not become antiquated, but rather has grown with time." (Dr. R. Koch and Prof. Dr. E. Rosenstock, *Paracelsus, Krankheit und Glaube*, Stuttgart, 1923, p. 5).

large groups of facts, in their broad relations as well as in their inner
structure, finally gave us the concept and vision of integration which now
fits man as a live unit and transformer of energy into the world of fact
and makes him frankly a consciously integrated psychobiological individual and member of a social group."[8]

Paracelsus had written "Der Mensch ist eine kleine Welt, ein Auszug
aus der ganzen machina mundi. Im Menschen sind alle Eigenschaften
der Welt in eins."[9]

It is precisely this ample understanding of the little world within the
great world, together with all its vast implication, that renders Paracelsus
outstanding among psychiatric pioneers. With justice Jung sees in Paracelsus "einen Bahnbrecher nicht nur der chemischen Medizin, sondern
auch der empirischen Psychologie und der psychologischen Heilkunde.
Er hat . . . in seiner Art die seelischen Phänomene in Betracht gezogen,
wie wohl keiner der grossen Aerzte vor oder nach ihm."[10]

The most common source of psychological conflict, the most common
cause of psychopathology, is the emotional dissonance between man and
the world he lives in. When the individual and the society in which he
lives are not in psychological harmony, the individual is likely to become
sick.[11] The psychoanalyst will describe this as a conflict between the *Id*
and the *Super-ego,* or as between the primitive drives and the endogenous
as well as the exogenous inhibitions. This formulation is fundamental to
modern psychiatry and is shared by practically all schools. Paracelsus
knew neither the *Id* nor the *Super-ego,* but he did know that those are
sick in spirit in whom that which is *mortal* and that which is *immortal,*
that which is *intelligent* and that which is *unintelligent,* are not compounded in the appropriate proportions and strengths.[12] He saw man as
an amalgam of the divine and the mortal. With superb insight and with

---

8 Dr. Adolf Meyer, "The Contributions of Psychiatry to the Understanding of Life
Problems," in *A Psychiatric Milestone,* New York, 1921, p. 25.

9 "Man is a small world (a microcosm) an extract of the whole *machina mundi.* In
men are embodied all the qualities of the world." (Paracelsus, *Astronomia Magna.)*

10 "A trailblazer not only in medicinal chemistry but also in empirical psychology
and psychotherapy. In his own way he took the phenomena of the soul into consideration, as none of the great physicians had done before him or after him." (C. G. Jung,
op. cit., pp. 177, 128).

11 Dr. E. Jones, *Social Aspects of Psycho-Analysis.* Lectures delivered under the
Auspices of the Sociological Society. London, 1924, p. 6. "The pathological states to
which psycho-analysts have devoted most attention, the various disorders known as
neuroses are themselves not so much diseases in the ordinary sense as forms of individual reaction to social situations, problems and difficulties."

12 J. Huser, *Die Bücher und Schriften des , . . Paracelsi,* 10 vols., Basel, 1589-91,
vol. IX, 1, 2,

comparable vigor Paracelsus expounded his understanding of the human psyche. It is not possible, at least not for me, to translate his words so as to transmit even a modicum of their vigor and beauty. In the original one hears the overtones of his earnestness, of his fullness, of his eagerness. His words mirror a man of strength and conviction; a man too full of the consciousness of what he needs must say, to be halted or gainsaid. "Fleissig ist ein Aufmerkung zu haben auf die Geist der Menschen, dieweil ihr zween seind, die ihm angeboren anliegen."[13] Rendered freely, the author counsels a diligent observation of the spirit (*Geist*) of man,—"the which is composed of two parts, both of which are native to him. For man should live in the spirit of life and be a man, and should not live according to the spirit of Limbus (the primitive-primeval-chaotic) that will make of him an unintelligent creature. For it is indeed true that man is made in the image of God, and so he has a godly spirit in him. But then he is otherwise (*sonst*) an animal and as such has an animal spirit; these two are antagonistic, and yet, however, the one must mollify the other. Therefore, man should not be a beast, but a man; to be a man, he must live in the spirit of life, of human life, and suppress (*hinwegtun*) the animal spirit (*viehischen Geist.*) Therefore it is necessary to recognize both of the spirits, on the basis of which the true spirit of man is distinguished from that of the animals."[14]

In the book *Krankheiten so der Vernunft berauben,* Paracelsus describes and distinguishes between different forms of psychopathy, including also the psychoneuroses. "Viel seind die solch lunatisch Krankheit tragen, deren nicht geacht wird lunatisch zu sein. Denn vielerlei seind Narren, so seind auch vielerlei toub Leut, nich ein Art, nit auf ein Weg, sondern in viel Weg, in viel Art, in viel Gestalt, und Form."[15] "Many are those who are ill who are not thought to be mentally sick (*lunatisch*). For as fools (simpletons, feeble-minded) are of many kinds, so also are there many kinds or crazy people (*toub Leut*) not of one sort, nor in one way, but in many ways, of many sorts, in many patterns and form."

Paracelsus distinguishes clearly between the feeble-minded and the psychopathic (*die Narren und die Touben*). The former, he says, are born simple in mind, whereas the psychopathic are not born psychopathic. The

---

[13] *Ibid.*

[14] "Das seind nun zwei widerwärtige, jedoch aber eins muss dem anderen weichen. Nun soll der Mensch kein Tier sein, sondern ein Mensch: Soll er nun ein Mensch sein, so muss er aus dem Geist der Lebens des Menschenleben, und also hinwegtun den viehischen Geist. Nun ist not die zween Geist zu erkennen, auf dass der recht Geist des Menschen unterscheiden werde von dem tierischen." (*Ibid.*)

[15] *Ibid.*

feeble-minded behave in the wise of an intelligent animal, but the psychopathic in the manner of the irrational *(unsinnige tierische Geist)* animal. To illustrate his meaning, Paracelsus draws upon the analogy of a dog which, while healthy, barks and bites, but does so with the true intelligence of the dog. The feeble-minded may be said to behave in the way of the healthy animal. But the psychopathic behave like a dog deprived of its intelligence, in other words, like a mad dog, for they "bite everyone and rage" *(wütet in alle Tiere).*

Under the caption of *Wahnsinn,* Paracelsus describes mania, of which he recognizes two kinds, that which "springs up" in the healthy body and that which is engendered by other sickness. The periodicity and self-limiting character of the disorder he describes, as well as the tendency of its sufferers to recover spontaneously, make it evident that Paracelsus recognized what we call today manic-depressive psychosis. Paracelsus furthermore includes under the heading *Wahnsinn* four classes of disorders, which he describes as major psychoses,—"die da allzeit bei unsinnigen und unvernünftigen Leben sind."[16] These he names *Lunatici, Insani, Vesani, Melancholici.* It is not possible, the circumstances being unfavorable, to deal in particular with these four classes of disorders. It is, however, important, since Paracelsus is suspect to the uninformed, to underscore the objective and scientific views held by Paracelsus on the origin and causation of the psychiatric disorders which he describes. "Wir erkennen in den Krankheiten, so der Vernunft berauben, durch Experientirung, dass sie aus der Natur entspringen und kommen."[17] "We recognize by experience that the diseases which deprive man of his reason originate and come out of nature (are natural in origin)." In this passage Paracelsus furthermore mocks the priestly clan *(die Götterischen Verweser)* who ascribe such diseases to incorporeal creatures *(uncorporalischen Geschöpfen)* and diabolical spirits. To this belief he will not subscribe, for experience shows that the disorders have their origin in nature.[18]

Nor does Paracelsus prove any less objective and scientific in his approach to psychotherapy. Indeed, he was a psychosomaticist (with apologies for the term)[19] centuries before the concept was reborn and re-

---

[16] *Ibid.,* pp. 45, 62. "Those who are permanently afflicted with an insane and unintelligent way of life."

[17] *Ibid.,* vol. IX, "Das siebente Buch in der Arzenei. *De Morbis Amentium,* das ist von den Krankheiten, die den Menschen der Vernunft berauben." Pp. 38-92.

[18] *Ibid.*

[19] Vide Galdston, I., "Biodynamic Medicine versus Psychosomatic Medicine." *Bull. Menninger Clinic,* 8, 4, July 1944.

christened. Among the general causations of disease he lists as one the *Ens Spirituale,* which can be equated to the psychological factors of disease, somatic as well as psychological. In the section dealing with the effects of the *Ens Spirituale* Paracelsus writes: "Now, then, you should observe and we point out to you that conscience overcomes the guilty one: Similar are the effects of envy and hatred. And we have indicated this to you, so that you should understand, how the *Ens Spirituale* so powerfully reigns over the body, that therefore many sicknesses, and all of the kinds of the sicknesses of men can be brought on; therefore you should apply treatment not as in ordinary diseases, but you should treat the spirit (psyche), for it is the spirit that here lies sick."[20]

Paracelsus dwelt much on the effects of will and imagination on the human body. "You should know," he wrote, "that the effect of the will is of major importance in medicine. For one who does not mean well with himself, and is hateful to himself, it is possible that such a person may be afflicted by the very curse he utters against himself. For cursing derives from the obfuscation (*Verhängung*) of the spirit. And it is also possible that the representations are by curses converted into sickness, into fevers, convulsive seizures, apoplexies, and such like so that they are brought about as indicated above."[21] And with a warning no less timely today than when it was written, Paracelsus continues: "And let this not be a jest to you, you physicians: you know not in the least part the power of the will; for the will is the genetrix of such spirits as the prudent will have no dealings with."[22]

"Great, too, is the power of belief and of faith," wrote Paracelsus, "for belief is of itself capable to make every sort of herb! An invisible nettle, an invisible celandine (balsam), an invisible trioll: and therefore every-

---

[20] "Also wie wir euch anzeigen, sollet ihr merken, dass die Geist den Schuldigen gewältigen: Dergleichen auch die Wirkung verbringen des Neids und Hass. Und haben euch das darumb angezeight, dass ihr verstehen sollet, wie das *Ens Spirituale* so gewaltiglich herrschet über die Leib, dass also viel Krankheiten, und alle Geschlecht der Krankheiten dem Menschen mögen zugefügt werden: Daraufhin nit sollet Arzney brauchen als auf natürlich Krankheiten, sondern ihr sollt den Geist arzneyen, derselbig ist der, der da krank liegt." (J. Huser, *loc. cit.,* vol. I, p. 54).

[21] "Aber ihr sollt wissen in euch, dass die Wirkung des Willens ein grosser Punct ist zu der Arzney. Denn einer der ihm selbst nichts Guts gönnet, und ihm selbst hass ist, ist möglich, dass das, so er ihm selbst flucht, ankommt: Denn fluchen kommt aus Verhängung des Geists. Und ist auch also möglich, dass die Bilder verflucht werden in Krankheiten, zu Febern, Epilepsien, Apoplexien, und dergleichen, so sie gemacht sind, wie oben stehet." (*Ibid.,* vol. I, p. 53.)

[22] "Und lasset euch das kein Scherz sein ihr Aerzte: Ihr wisset die Kraft des Willens nit den mindsten Teil: Denn der Will ist ein Gebärerin solcher Geisten, mit welchen der Vernünftig nichts zu schaffen hat." (*Ibid.,* vol. I, p. 53.)

thing that grows in terrestrial nature the power of belief can likewise bring: therefore the power of belief can likewise create every sickness."[23]

Faith, belief, will, and the passion account in the psychiatry of Paracelsus for many of the ills, and for some of the cures, witnessed in men. Paracelsus is particularly concerned with what we today term the primitive drives, and with the anti-social impulsions. He refers to these components of the human personality as *"das Viehische im Menschen,"*—the brute, beast, or animal in men. To the predominance of these he traces the psychological ills in man. Furthermore, he maintains, in a passage of deep and subtle insight, that "the human intelligence does not become mad, and is not subject to sickness. Hence it is of no profit to search in the human spirit; only in his brute intelligence, therein, reader, peruse. For it is a major achievement to understand the rantings of the lunatic. . . ."[24]

It is only in recent times and largely through the illumination cast upon these matters by Freud and his co-workers that we have come to appreciate the possibility of understanding the "rantings of the lunatic," and indeed it is "a major achievement." So, too, have we learned to understand the "logicalness" of the paranoid and of the other psychopathological reasoning processes. The premises and conjunctions are at fault, but the deductions are keenly logical.

It is appropriate at this point to touch upon Paracelsus' use of the magnet in the treatment of somatic ailments, for this bears not only on the influence of the imagination, but is the derivative starting point of modern psychiatry. The magnet, magnetism, mesmerism, hypnotism, suggestion, psychocatharsis, and psychoanalysis represent a series of stages in the progressive development of modern psychiatric thought and knowledge. The initial impulse to this development came from Paracelsus.

There is no indication that Paracelsus ascribed the influence of the magnet in the treatment of disease to any other quality than the *virtus attractiva macro- et microcosmi*. Imagination, faith, suggestion, did not enter into his account of the powers and operations of the magnet as *specific and separate factors*. Paracelsus was not handicapped by the

---

[23] "Denn der Glaub vermag in ihm selbst alle Geschlecht der Kräuter zu machen, ein unsichtbare Nessel, ein unsichtbar Schölkraut, ein unsichtbar Trioll: Und also ein jedlich Ding das in der irdischen Natur wachst, das vermag auch die Stärk des Glaubens zu bringen: Also vermag auch der Glaub alle Krankheiten zu machen." (*Ibid.*, vol. I ,p. 251.)

[24] "Denn die menschlich Vernunft wird nicht toub, empfächt auch kein Krankheit. Darum ist in derselbigen Menschen Geist nichts zu suchen, allein in seiner tierischen Vernunft, dieselbig, Leser, durchlies. Denn es ist ein grosses, den touben Wüterich zu verstehn, er ist nicht minder denn ein wütender Hund." (*Ibid.*, vol. IX, pp. 1, 2.)

dichotomy of body and soul which has plagued both philosophy and psychiatry since the advent of the Cartesian science.[25] Paracelsus could not have been guilty of such irrationalities as were uttered by the Commission of the French Academy of Science in its report on Mesmerism: *"L'imagination fait tout: le magnétisme nul."* It was quite sufficient for him to state the rationale of magnetic cures in simple and self-evident terms: "For in the last analysis it is thus, that we contain within ourselves as many natural powers as heaven and earth possess. Can the magnet draw the iron to itself even though it appears to be a dead thing: so, too, can the dead person draw the living one to himself. Do the climbing vines reach out to the sun, so too well may man in similar manner have access to the sun. Can the planets draw one according to their wishes, so too can the dead body (i.e. the magnet). These are all invisible works, and yet they are natural.[26]

Paracelsus was fully cognizant of the existence of both folly and superstition, but he would not grant the existence of both natural and unnatural. Had he been confronted with this paradox, Paracelsus would have responded: "the natural embraces all else."[27] With keen insight and as if he were anticipating the criticism of later generations, Paracelsus stated: "No instructed person ever remained misled, him no one has ever seen superstitious. Where is superstition? Indeed, among those that understand nothing. Where is arrogance? But only among those who know nothing. Where is folly? But only among those content in their wisdom and who will seek no further in God's wisdom. And therefore when such an art is expounded and in their thick skulls they cannot fathom it, it must perforce be of the devil and magical."[28]

Paracelsus recognized the existence of the devil but also that far too much was credited to his works. "Ere the world comes to an end, many

---

[25] See Chapter 30, this volume.

[26] "Denn endlich ist dar also, dass wir in uns haben so viel natürlicher Kräfte, als Himmel und Erden vermögen. Kann der Magnet das Eisen an sich ziehen, und scheint do wie ein tot Ding: So kann auch der tote Mensch den lebendigen an sich ziehen. Gehen die Bettler der Sonnen zu, so mag auch wohl ein Mensch dermassen ein Zugang haben. Können die Planeten einen ziehen nach ihrem Gefallen, so kann auch der tot Cörper desselb. Das seind alles unsichtbare Werk, und doch natürlich." (J. Huser, *loc. cit.*, vol. I, pp. 297, 298.)

[27] Goethe's Essay on Nature and its profound effect on Freud.

[28] "Kein wissender Mann ist nie in Verführung blieben, ihn hat auch niemand aberglaubig gesehen. Wo ist der Aberglauben? Doch bei denen die nichts verstohn: Wo is die Hoffart? Als allein bei denen, die in ihren Weisheiten bleiben, und weiter in Gottes Weisheit nit fahren. Und darum so eine Kunst geoffenbart wird, und sie in ihrem dollen Schädel nit mag unergründet werden, so muss sie teufelisch und zauberisch sein." (J. Huser, *loc. cit.*, vol. I, pp. 317, 318.)

arts now ascribed to the work of the devil must become revealed, and it will then be evident, that most of these effects depend upon natural forces."[29]

It is not possible here to deal amply with the so-called demonology of Paracelsus. Yet it would help to understand *his* devil if we equated him to the *death instinct* of Freud. Between the two there is much in common. Both are destructive forces—the one stands opposed to Eros, the other to God. Jung, who among the contemporary psychiatrists is best equipped to fathom and to interpret the demonology of Paracelsus, astutely observes: "For us, the so-called moderns, his Homunculi, Trarames, Durdales, Nymphs, Melusine, etc. are certainly close to the crassest of superstitions, but for his time, not at all. These figures were still alive and effective in those times. They were indeed projections; but even of this he had some appreciation, in that, as is evidenced by many passages, he ascribed the origin of the Homunculi and other apparitions to imagination. His primitive perspectives led him to endow the projection with a reality which, in the light of psychological effects, was far more warranted than is our rationalistic presupposition on the absolute unreality of the projected content."[30]

Paracelsus was not a mystic in the true sense of the word. He mystifies us today, but that is largely because our culture has lost the essential skill for dealing with the problems of being in the encompassing manner that was common to his age, and of which he was a master. And here it is pertinent to observe that Paracelsus was not a psychiatrist in the definitive sense of the term. Indeed he probably would have considered such specialization a degradation both of the physician's position and of his obligations. He dealt with mental illness. He studied experience and evolved a classification of the disorders and a rationale of psychopathology. It is proper, therefore, to speak of the psychiatry of Paracelsus. But he nowhere

---

29 "Ehe die Welt untergeht, müssen noch viele Künste, die man sonst der Wirkung des Teufels zuschrieb, offenbar, und man wird alsdann einsehen, dass die meisten dieser Wirkungen von natürlichen Kraften abhängen." (Quoted in M. B. Lessing, *Handbuch der Geschichte der Medizin*, Berlin, 1938, p. 366.)

30 "Seine Homunculi, Trarames, Durdales, Nymphen, Melusinen usw. sind zwar zunächst krassester Aberglaube für uns sogenannt Moderne, für seine Zeit aber keineswegs. Diese Figuren lebten und wirkten noch in jenen Zeiten. Es waren zwar Projektionen; aber auch davon hatte er eine Ahnung, indem er, wie aus zahlreichen Stellen hervorgeht, um die Entstehung der Homunculi und sonstigem Spuk aus der Imagination wuuste. Seine primitivere Anschauung schrieb den Projektionen eine Realität zu, welche deren psychologischer Wirkung um vieles gerechter wurde als unsere rationalistische Voraussetzung der absoluten Unwirklichkeit projizierter Inhalte." (C. G. Jung, *loc. cit.*, pp. 128, 129.)

appears to have visualized the specialty of psychiatry. This observation is pertinent to the fact that much of his best psychiatric insight and understanding is revealed in those of his works which do not deal by title or otherwise with psychiatric disorders. It is, for example, most interesting to see how much psychiatric wisdom enters into his writings on "the female." "Darumb so ist Frau ein ander *Subjectum* denn der Mann.[31] Denn ihr Wurzen dienet zu der Nahrung: Des Mannes stehet still im Mann." "Therefore, is woman a different subject from man. For her roots serve to nourish; the man's remain fixed in man." Woman is the "smallest world" and is quite different from the microcosm-man, she "has a different anatomy, *Theoricam, Causas, Rationes, Curas*. And no matter how much like man in many illnesses, yet it is for the physician to distinguish from the other, that is, from man, for she is a different world."[32]

Paracelsus evaluates quite fully the role of the procreative function in shaping the physical, the psychological, the nosological, and the psychopathological, constitution of the female. But there was nothing of the misogynist in Paracelsus; on the contrary, he prized the "female of the species." "Wer kann einer Frauen Feind sein, sie sei gleich wie sie woll?" "Who can be an enemy of woman, be she as she will? For it is with her fruits that the world is settled, therefore God grants her long life, even though she were a shrew."[33]

Jung, in his account of the inner personality of Paracelsus, lays much weight upon the fact that Paracelsus was bereft of his mother at the age of nine. This traumatic experience, together with the fact that his father never remarried and remained for many years his son's teacher and companion, undoubtedly did have a profound influence upon Paracelsus' attitude toward womankind.

Perhaps the richest psychiatric yield is to be derived from those of Paracelsus' writings which are concerned with the immortal, the cosmic, the godly, phases of the human being. Here we are confronted not only with the equivalent of the *Super-ego* of modern psychiatry, but we witness also

[31] J. Huser, *loc. cit.*, vol. I, pp. 194, 195.

[32] "Die Frau hat im selbigen ein Gebresten, sie ist die kleineste Welt, und ist ein anders dann der Mann, und hat seine andere Anatomey, *Theoricam, Causas, Rationes, Curas*. Und aber, wiewohl gleich in viel Krankheiten mit dem Mann, das ist aber dem Arzt zu unterscheiden von einander, das ist, vom Mann, denn sie ist ein andere Welt." (*Ibid.*, vol. I, p. 1900.)

[33] "Wer kann einer Frauen Feind sein, sie sei gleich wie sie woll? Denn mit ihren Früchten wird die Welt besetzt, darumb Sie Gott lang leben lässt, ob sie gleich gar ein Gall wäre." (*Ibid.*, vol. I, p. 309.)

the appreciation which Paracelsus had of the Unconscious, and what in present-day terms is called the phylogenetic components of the psyche.

All of this was not known to Paracelsus, nor yet was it mysterious. It was logically deduced by Paracelsus from his cosmological premises (the relations of macro- to microcosm), and intuitively appreciated. There was a deep impulsion operative in Paracelsus to be concerned with such unsettled and undetermined matters, an impulsion which the present generation can well appreciate. "The physician should talk of (treat and be concerned with) the invisible (imperceptible) and know the perceptible."[34] "He who knows the imperceptible is a physician, the imperceptible that which has no name, that which is without substance (insubstantial) and yet has effect."[35] Paracelsus is deeply concerned with the double nature of man, with his temporality and with his timeless ties to all the universe, with his substantiality and with his immaterial effects upon the universe. He experienced no difficulties in visualizing in what manner this double nature of man could serve to account for health and for illness. In all this he was neither slavish nor fatalistic. The macrocosm rules the microcosm, but the relation is reciprocal. As the Greeks taught that "character is destiny," so Paracelsus taught "Der Charakter des Menschen meistert das Gestern."—("The character of man masters the stars").

The whole of Paracelsus' teachings sums up to an effort to perceive and understand man in his physiological and psychological functions, within the framework of nature and the universe, from which he is not set apart, but of which he is rather a component.

Of the Paracelsian treatment of psychic disorders, there is little that needs to be said. His therapy is founded on and conforms to his understanding of the etiology of the disorders. Some have stressed the odd and the bizarre in the Parcelsian therapy, but it can be easily demonstrated that such writers either fail to understand or misconstrue the intent of the treatment they criticize. Bloodletting seems barbaric to us, yet in the instance of mania with much agitation is it any less "barbaric" to achieve sedation by means of the barbiturates than by bloodletting? Paracelsus advised drilling holes in the patient's skull to let out mania. Is prefrontal leucotomy any less or more rational a procedure? It is, however, not the gross and violent therapeutic procedures advocated by

---

[34] "Von dem nun, das unsichtbar ist, soll der Arzt reden, un das sichtbar ist, soll ihm in Wissen stehen. . . ." (*Ibid.*, vol. II, p. 138.)

[35] "Der ist ein Arzt, der das unsichtbare weiss, das kein Namen hat, das kein Materie hat, und hat doch sein Wirkung." (*Ibid.*)

Paracelsus, but his more sedate, basic, common ones that deserve notice. Paracelsus believed in psychotherapy, in the manner practiced today. He believed in persuasion, exhortation, instruction, fasting, and prayer. He set great value on the therapeutic effects of sleep and advised the use of somnifacients. He believed in the self-healing powers of the soul, *die Heilkraft der Seele.* The violent and hopelessly insane he advised should be incarcerated. In relation to this, it should be borne in mind that Paracelsus firmly believed that every disease was curable, and also that compassion was the physician's crowning gift and virtue. *"Barmherzigkeit ist ein Schulmeister der Artzten."*

Coming to the end of this brief sketch on the psychiatry of Parcelsus, I can attest to the validity of Jung's words. "Man ist mit der eigenen Bemühung, wenigstens einen Teil seines Wesens genügend zu erfassen, stets unzufrieden." How can one be satisfied when the subject is so vast and the man unfathomable, *unerschöpflich,* inexhaustible? Then, too, there is the tantalizing problem of one's interest in Paracelsus, which is never academic, but always freighted with emotions and barbed with psychological implications. My own interest is never in the direction of modernizing Paracelsus. He was, is, and ever will remain, man of the Sixteenth Century. Nor would I be a follower of that fatuous sport that scans the past for precursors of Freud. To that motley crew of historical scavengers, someone, somehow, should make clear that all the past and all the past holds of men, things, and thought are precursors to every man that follows in the chain of unfolding generations. My interest in Paracelsus has different roots. It arises out of the appreciation that in his *Anschauung,* in the embrace of his thoughts, there is much that has meaning and inspiration for us today. We have come around the bend and completed the circle. Once again we can contemplate heaven and earth, man and the firmaments, within one intelligible framework.

Yet there are those who will not agree. On that score only this need be said. Many among us, confronted with the eternity that is within us, (that which Paracelsus termed *unsichtbar*), are frightened, and in their fear, deny what they beheld, and berate those who lifted the curtain.

Finally, I have dealt with the psychiatry of Paracelsus because it is psychiatry which, I believe, has taught us and will continue to teach us to understand and to prize the eternal, the unfathomable, and *das Unsichtbare* in man.

30

Descartes and Modern Psychiatric Thought

THOSE WHO HAVE been nurtured in the Anglo-Saxon traditions, by the very condition of their upbringing, look upon Francis Bacon as the initiator of the scientific Renaissance.

Bacon's fame, however, at least among the English peoples, is greater than is warranted by the ponderable results of his writings. It stems rather from the rare and superior quality of his style than from the enlightenment he offered. The enchantment of his eloquent pen, the ring of his fine framed sentences intoxicate our judgment. In this intoxication we have failed to recognize the superior claims and merits of Bacon's contemporary, René Descartes, who upon more valid ground can be regarded as the true initiator of the scientific Renaissance. Descartes not only gave to the young scientific movement of his age his *Méthode*—which in essence is applied even in the science of today—and valuable instrumentalities in the form of his mathematical discoveries, but he also propounded a number of fundamental problems which ever since have occupied the best intelligences and which still engage our interest and our efforts.

It is to Descartes that we can trace many of the disputed problems of modern science, finding that they had been formulated by him in one or another of his writings, and that the partisan sides owe the framework of their differing theories to the thoughts that were engendered by Descartes' fertile intellect. Descartes was as stimulating by his errors as by his truth, and as much has come from those who have undertaken to refute and controvert his errors as from those who defend and continue to labor in his traditions.

Descartes was a profoundly original thinker, but also the child of his

Age. He crystallized the intellectual challenge of his Age, and to it he imparted the singular bias of his unique personality.

It is not relevant to our thesis to review the whole of Descartes' philosophy, or to recite in detail the particular contributions he made to mathematics, to physics, and to optics. We must rather confine our review to those elements of his philosophy which have a significant bearing on modern psychiatric thought. Among these we need to include the following: his foundation premise, the famous dictum *"Cogito ergo sum"*; his *Méthode*, or procedures for the analysis of scientific problems; his conception of the body as a self-regulating mechanism; and, the complete and absolute dichotomy of body and soul. Each of these has profoundly influenced our thinking and to a larger extent than most of us realize still moulds our thought. Thus, while few today subscribe to the Cartesian dictum *Cogito ergo sum* as the primary demonstration of our existence, we still operate in the absolutist intellectual tradition inspired by that dictum. *Cogitatio* is the rock bottom foundation of our intellectual security, and only that is held to be valid which will pass the critical scrutiny of our thought and that proves projectable in thought patterns. We maintain that that which is not thinkable is not real, and paradoxically insist that that which does not conform to the logistic patterns of our thought-function and to our rational knowledge cannot be.

In the dictum *Cogito ergo sum,* the individual was abstracted from his social matrix and set out in splendid isolation, and in that splendid isolation he has been largely viewed, studied and anatomized ever since.

In the Cartesian *Méthode,* Descartes advanced the proposition that the solution of every intricate problem can be achieved by the division of the problem into its simplest elements, by the solution of those simple elements, and by the subsequent summation of the elemental solutions; in other words that an understanding of the whole can be gained in the summation of the resultants of the study of its parts.

The mechanistic concept of the universe and of man, advanced by Descartes, has been accepted by the world of science as an "article of faith."

Only the Cartesian dichotomy, the complete separation of body and soul, has proved unacceptable to modern science.

The effects of the Cartesian philosophy are patent in the thought and science of the last three hundred years. Its influence permeates all of our intellectual life. Every specialized division of knowledge, whether it be sociology, economics, physiology, or psychology, has drawn its tangents from Cartesianism. This is largely so because in Descartes the temper and intellectual potentialities of his Age came to a burning sharp focus.

In the study of the influence of Cartesianism upon modern scientific thought it would, however, be a mistake to neglect or to underestimate the effects of Descartes' personality upon Descartes' philosophy. To do so would be to blunder as so many historians of thought have blundered, who seemingly believe that a man's thought and his work are but little affected by his psychology. Here I must permit myself a divergent excursion.

It is rather interesting to observe that practically all histories of philosophy, of psychology, and of psychiatry present their respective data in the pattern of progressive systems of thought, with little or no reference or regard to the personalities of those who did the thinking. There is in this manner of exposition a sort of naive animism which assumes that "systems of thought" are self-engendered and that the person of the thinker is an accidental and indifferent, though necessary, agent to the propagation of thought. Some histories do sketch the biographies of the men whose systems of thought they elaborate, but the biographical data they offer are of the most elementary significance, and practically never afford any insight into the possible experiential and psychological motivations for the system of thought created by the thinker. Yet assuredly what the man *is* must deeply influence what he thinks. And what he *has* thought, and to a lesser but still significant degree *why* he thought so, could be better appreciated and understood in the light of the thinker's experiences and their psychological resultants.

The lack of pertinent biographical data and the difficulties faced in drawing sound deductions from those available may in part account for the neglect of the "personality factor" in the histories of thought, but a much more significant cause for the neglect is the historian's failure to understand how deeply the thinking of the person is influenced by his psychology—as this is determined by constitutional factors and by experience. The philosophers in particular are too prone to regard the history of their discipline as a history of pure thought, as if Kant's punctiliousness had no relation to his Categoric Imperatives, or Schopenhauer's conflict with his mother had no bearing on his philosophy of the Will to Power, on the pessimism, and on his misogynism. It is not contended that the psychology of a philosopher is the *sole* determinant of his philosophy. Philosophy as a social culture has a dynamism of its own. Schopenhauer could not escape the influence of Kant and of Hegel, nor Nietzsche that of Schopenhauer. Yet both Schopenhauer and Nietzsche could not but leave their singular imprints upon philosophic thought, and the singularity of the imprint was manifestly the homologue of the thinker's psychology.

From time to time there has been shown some rather vague and sporadic appreciation of the bearing which the philosopher's psychology has to his philosophy. Nietzsche in his *"Jenseits von Gut und Böse"* wrote, "Hinter aller Logik un ihrer anscheinenden Selbstherrlichkeit der Bewegung stehen Wertschätzungen deutlicher geredet, physiologische Forderungen zur Erhaltung einer bestimmten Art von Leben."[1]

Freud in his fascinating study of Leonardo da Vinci was the first to show the deep insight into the character of the artist's work that can be gained by an appreciation of the artist's personality.

A noteworthy example of this application of psychiatric knowledge is also to be seen in Dr. Alf. Frh. von Winterstein's contribution, *Psychoanalytische Anmerkung zur Geschichte der Philosophie* (Imago, Band II, 1913, pp. 175-237). Winterstein, however, devotes far more attention to the psychoanalytical connotations of philosophical concepts and criteria than to the psychic dynamism of the philosophers. He endeavors rather to interpret the psychoanalytic implications—of, say, Platonic love—than to fathom the psychological motivations that prompted Plato to advance such a love ideal.

Other psychoanalytic writers too have analyzed the personalities of well-known authors and philosophers, and have traced the effects of "personality upon the work."[2] Despite this, however, it is not commonly appreciated that fully to understand the work of an artist, author, or philosopher, it is essential to know the psychological components of his personality. This is particularly necessary when the work considered presents obscure and paradoxical elements.

With this "apologia" we can return to Descartes. Descartes was born on March 31, 1596, at LaHaye in Touraine. His mother died shortly after his birth,[3] and he was raised by a nurse, to whom Descartes remained deeply attached throughout his life. Descartes was a sickly child, and for a time it was feared that he would not survive his infancy. However, he gained in health and grew to be a robust individual.

---

[1] Behind all logic and its seeming independent momentum stand conceptual evaluations, or more clearly expressed, physiological requirements essential to the maintenance of a given mode of life.

[2] Noteworthy contributions in this direction have been made by Alexander Herzberg, Eduard Hitschmann, Heinrich Gomperz, and Siegried Placzek.

[3] It is stated by some (Sirven) that she lived long enough to have another infant, and that she died shortly thereafter.

At the age of eight Descartes entered the recently founded Jesuit Collège de la Flèche, and there he remained for eight years. At the age of 17, Descartes left La Flèche, went to Paris and was there drawn into the sportive life of the capital city. He evidently did not savour it, for in 1614, when he was in his eighteenth year, he renounced all worldly pleasures to return to his studies. Save for four years which he spent in military service, Descartes devoted the remainder of his life to his intellectual pursuits. However, he was not a complete recluse, for he traveled widely over the European continent, and during his long stay in Holland moved many times from place to place. Descartes maintained, as was the practice among learned men, an extensive correspondence, and thus sustained contact with a fairly large group of friends.

Descartes' first published work, the *Discours de la Méthode*, appeared in Leyden in 1637, when he was 41 years of age. Four years later, Descartes' father died, and in the same year Descartes recorded the death of his daughter Francine, born five years previously of a woman to whom he was not married and about whom we know nothing else. In 1641 there was published Descartes' second work, *Méditations touchant la première Philosophie, où l'on démontre l'existence de Dieu, & l'immortalité de l'âme*. His *Principes de Philosophie* was published in Latin in 1644; and his *Traité des Passions de L'Ame* in 1649, when he was 53 years old. This was the last of his works published during his lifetime. Two works appeared posthumously: *De L'Homme*, and *Traité de la Formation du Foetus*.

Descartes died in Stockholm, where he had gone on invitation of Christina, Queen of Sweden, on February 11, 1650.

These are the bare facts of Descartes' "outer life," and were they the only facts known about his life, we would hardly be in a position to acquire any insight into Descartes' personality. Fortunately, however, Descartes wrote into his works much psychobiographical material and this enables us to appraise, in a diagnostic manner, the psychological qualities of his being. From a scrutiny of these data, we believe, it is possible to understand the psychological *vis-a-tergo* of Descartes' philosophical bias.

We shall not attempt to deal with all of the available psychobiographical data, for they are too numerous to be encompassed in a short treatise. We will be obliged rather to restrict ourselves to those data which appear to have a major bearing on his philosophy.

In his *Méthode*, published when he was 41 years of age, Descartes gives his version of the genesis of his philosophy.

"I have been nourished on letters from my infancy," wrote Descartes, and because people persuaded me that by their means a man could acquire a clear and certain knowledge of all that is useful in life, I had a great desire to become acquainted with them. But as soon as I had finished all the course of study at the termination of which a man is usually received into the ranks of the learned, I entirely altered my opinion, for I found myself hampered by so many doubts and errors that it seemed that I reaped no benefit from my effort to instruct myself, except that I discovered more and more my own ignorance. And yet I was in one of the most celebrated schools in Europe, where I thought learned men would be found if such existed anywhere. I learned there all that the others learned, and even being dissatisfied with what we were taught, I went through all the books I could get hold of which treated of those sciences which are esteemed the most curious and most rare; moreover, I knew the opinions that the others formed concerning me, and I did not see that they held me inferior to my fellow students. (*Discourse On Method And Metaphysical Meditations of René Descartes*. Translated by Gertrude Burtford Rawlings. London, Walter Scott, pp. 5 & 6).

"This is why," Descartes continued, "as soon as I was old enough to quit the authority of my preceptors, I entirely gave up the study of letters, and resolving to seek only that knowledge which could be found within myself, or rather in the great book of the world, I employed the remainder of my youth in travelling, in observing courts and armies, in associating with persons of divers tempers and conditions, in gathering various experiences, in testing myself under such conditions as fortune offered me, and above all in reflecting upon the things which came before me in such wise that I might draw some profit from them" (*Op. cit.*, p. 11).

It is pertinent to observe that from all that Descartes had learned and later rejected, he retained only mathematics, not because of a love for the science of numbers, but rather because of his esteem for its methodologies. Mathematics appealed to Descartes even when he was a youth. "Above all," he wrote in the first part of his *Discourse*, "I took pleasure in mathematics, because of the certainty and evidence of their reasons." (*Op. cit.*, p. 9.) Later he tells us (second part of *Discourse*) that when doubt had swept away all the "errors" he had learned, and he was set upon the discovery and the recreation of truth, he "was not put to much trouble to find out which (method) it was necessary to begin with." (*Op. cit.*, p. 23.) *That method* was the one applied by the mathematicians —by the geometers in particular. "The long chains of perfectly simple and easy reasons," wrote Descartes, "which geometers are accustomed to employ in order to arrive at their most difficult demonstrations, had given me reason to believe that all things which can fall under the knowledge of man succeed each other in the same way (*Op. cit.*, pp. 22-23).

On the basis of such reasonings Descartes formulated his *Méthode*—which, in essence, consists of the following provisions: Never to accept anything to be true which is not upon critical mental scrutiny recognized to be true; to divide each difficulty confronted into as many segments as is possible, and as may be required for its better solution; to conduct one's thoughts in order, by beginning with the simplest objects, and to progress thus to the most complex knowledge; to make everywhere enumerations so complete and surveys so wide as to preclude the omission of anything.

To recapitulate, Descartes informs us that upon issuing from the Collège de la Flèche he discovered that what he had learned was honey-combed with error; that he despaired of finding truth either in the lives or the works of other men; that he therefore determined to discover truth in and through his own person; that the prime faculty for such a task was his mind and its thinking; and the best procedures to follow were those of the geometers who "of all those who have heretofore sought truth in the sciences—alone—have been able to find demonstrations, that is to say, clear and certain reasons" (*Op. cit.*, p. 23).

Such is the exposé of the origin and substance of his *Méthode,* given to us by Descartes in his autobiographical recitation.

All of the aforegoing is taken from the *Discourse on Method,* which, it needs to be remembered, was published when Descartes was 41 years of age. The biographical experiences recited in this work, however, refer to Descartes' very early manhood. Descartes would have us understand that his intellectual disaffections began with his graduation from La Flèche and that the basic inspiration or the discovery of his *Méthode* "came upon him" at a certain time, on the night of November 10, 1619, when Descartes was 23 years of age. But the story of the events then initiated was written 18 years later.

Time and the inborn tendency to rationalize experience conspired to distort and corrupt the reality and to foist upon us a grossly fictional picture of the genesis of Descartes' philosophy.

The known events of Descartes' life do not harmonize with his version of the genesis of his philosophy. They lead us rather to quite different conclusions.

Descartes informs us that at the age of 17, having issued from La Flèche, he discovered that what he had learned was full of error. On this score it is pertinent to inquire how a young man, 17 years of age, so very promptly discovered the errors of his previous eight years of learning. What had he learned? What in his learning was erroneous? How was it he had no misgivings during the very process of learning? Descartes points to no specific errors. It was not that, for example, he had been taught that the earth was flat and stationary, and then had been persuaded to see it round and moving about the sun. The sole fault he found with his learning was that it did not provide him with *certainty,* with *certain knowledge.* His learning, in other words, did not afford him *security.*

This deficiency in his learning he discovered when after finishing "all the course of study at the termination of which a man is usually received into the ranks of the learned" he went to Paris and there took part in the gay social life of the capital ("Dans cette ville Descartes se laissa entraîner par l'amour du jeu et des plaisirs." J. Sirven: *Les Années d'Apprentissage de Descartes.* Paris, 1928, p. 53).

It is more reasonable to assume that release from the monastic restraint of La Flèche served to accentuate Descartes' erotic conflict, and that this conflict was then displaced into the realm of the philosophic and the abstract.

J. Sirven, in his scholarly work cited above, catalogues the courses followed by Descartes when he was a student at La Flèche. The Jesuit instructors followed the *Ratio Studiorum* of 1603 which included instruction in literature, in philosophy, arithmetic, geometry, Aristotelian physics, morals, metaphysics, music and astronomy.[4]

It seems hardly possible that upon issuing from La Flèche, the errors in what he had learned of mathematics, philosophy, and literature were suddenly revealed to him, even while he was steeped in gaming and in the pleasure-laden life of Paris. That which led Descartes, after one year in Paris, to give up his gay life and to determine, henceforth, to devote himself entirely to study and to meditation was unrelated to the discovery of errors in scholastic learning.

Descartes, upon coming out of the cloistered life at La Flèche, experienced the first of two major "moral crises" known to have occurred in his life. The fable of the "discovery of error" must be considered as Descartes' latter-day rationalization of a purely psychological experience.

Descartes, at the age of 18, underwent a sudden conversion and indulged in a fugue. He disappeared from the circle of his friends and remained hidden for almost two years. Not even his parents knew of his whereabout. During his retirement, Descartes devoted himself to mathematical studies.

The nature and quality of this psychological experience is not difficult

---

4 Descartes also took, not at La Flèche but at the Faculté de Poitiers, some courses in law and in medicine, 1615-1616.

to evaluate. The moral crisis likely to confront a young man of 18, a social fledgling late out of the Jesuit nest, is more likely to be of an erotic, than of a philosophical nature. The quest for certainty, the urgent want of security, which Descartes records for those years, reflects the state of his emotional insecurity and conflict rather than of his purely intellectual disaffection. This presumption is clearly validated by the circumstances and nature of Descartes' second "moral crisis"—that of November 10, 1619. But before turning to the events of that day we need to review the intervening years.

Descartes' first fugue, as we saw, occurred in 1614 and lasted until 1616. Thereafter he went to Holland and joined the army of Prince Maurice of Nassau. He remained in service for two years, but took no part in any active fighting. In July 1619 he left Prince Maurice's army and joined that of the Duke of Bavaria. This army was garrisoned in Neuberg on the banks of the Danube. This brings us to October, 1619. In the following month Descartes experienced his second "moral crisis," and to this crisis he specifically assigns the origin of his philosophy and of his *Méthode*. In his *Discourse* (second part) Descartes makes but passing reference to his experiences on the night of November 10, 1619, but elsewhere (*Olympica*) they are described in full detail.

The moral crisis, or, as Gaston Milhaud terms it, the *Crise Mystique* (*Descartes Savant*. Paris, 1921. Chap. II, pp. 47-52) of Descartes, is mirrored in three dreams which Descartes had during the night of November 10, 1619.

The first of the three dreams was characterized by marked anxiety. He was walking along the street and was frightened by several phantoms. In order to reach a certain place, he was obliged to lean on the left side for he felt a great weakness on the right side, so that he could not stand upright. In this attitude he was caught by a whirling wind, which turned him about three or four times on his left foot. This anxiety continued to the extent that he was afraid of falling with each step.

He then perceived an open college into which he entered, in order to find shelter and alleviation. It seemed to him that he tried to get into the church of this college in order to pray. As he walked, he passed an acquaintance without greeting him, and in his effort to retrace his steps to correct the incivility, he was violently pushed back by the wind, which blew against the church. At the same time he saw another person who called him by name in civil and obliging terms, saying to him that a Mr. N. had something to give him. The dreamer thought that that something was a melon from some strange land. He was very much surprised to note that the persons about him stood firmly and upright on their legs while he stood stooped and tottering on the same ground, although the wind had now considerably abated.

At this point he awoke and felt that a certain evil spirit strove to corrupt him. He turned from the left to the right side, and prayed for protection against the evil influences of his dream and his sins, realizing at the same time that he had not always led a sufficiently irreproachable life. After about two hours of contemplation on the good and evil in this world, he fell asleep.

In his second dream Descartes heard a sharp and loud noise which he perceived as a clap of thunder. This anxiety awakened him, and on opening his eyes, he thought that his room was filled with many bright sparks of fire. This did not surprise him for he had perceived similar photisms on previous occasions. This time, however, his thoughts turned to the logical bases of philosophy, and the conclusions he drew harmonized with his spirit. After alternately opening and closing his eyes, his fear was dissipated and he fell asleep again in a great calm.

The third dream was without any terror. There was a book on the table; it was a dictionary which he thought would be very useful to him. There was another book, the *Corpus Poetarum,* a collection of poetry by different authors. On opening the book, he read the verse: *"Quod vitae sectabor iter"* (Which way of life will I choose?). There was an unknown man, who presented him with an excellent piece of verse, which began with *"Est et Non"* (It is and it is not). The dreamer told the man that this line was found in the *Idyls of Ausonius,* in the volume of collected poems lying on the table.

The next part of the dream deals with the difficulty in finding this verse in the book, which the dreamer thought he could easily locate. The book disappeared and reappeared. The dreamer then found Ausonius' collection of poetry, but he could not find the part which began, *"Est et Non."* He then told the man that he knew a more beautiful poem by the same author, which began with *"Quod vitae sectabor iter."* On being asked to point it out, the dreamer in searching for it found a number of different little portraits engraved on copper plates (*Gravez en taille douce*). Suddenly the books and the man disappeared completely from his imagination without awakening him. Descartes then had some doubt whether that which he had seen was a dream or an actual experience, but while still sleeping decided that it was a dream and proceeded to interpret it before awakening.

These dreams attracted considerable attention before the advent of

Freud's dream interpretation. Descartes, himself, interpreted the first two dreams as a heaven-sent admonition to mend his life; and the third as an apparition of the Spirit of Truth, whose wish it was to show him the treasures of all the sciences. It was in gratitude for this revelation that Descartes vowed right there and then to make a pilgrimage to the shrine of Our Lady of Loreto.

The twelve-page manuscript carrying the title *Olympica,* in which Descartes recorded his dreams, begins with the notation—"X *novembe 1619 cum plenus forem Enthousiasmo, et mirabilis scientiae fundamenta reperirem, etc."* By these tokens and the professions of Descartes, notably in his *Discourse,* it has been assumed by most who have considered his dreams that they did in fact concern the *fundamenta scientiae.* The larger part of the discussion about these dreams has centered about the nature of the *fundamenta;* did they really embrace the whole of the *Méthode,* or were they confined merely to some mathematical discoveries? Gaston Milhaud in his book, *Descartes Savant* (Paris, 1921), competently criticizes the many disputations as to the significance of Descartes' dreams, and gives it as his opinion that all of them are inexact. But the best interpretation he can offer is that the dreams were inspired by Descartes' want of self-confidence, and that in his dreams he sought and found heavenly sanction for his life's mission. Milhaud describes Descartes as "une âme naïvement religieuse, plus simple, moins compliquée qu'on n'est généralement disposé à le croire" (*Op. cit.,* p. 62).

Maxim Leroy[5] asked Freud to interpret these dreams, and we cannot do better than quote what he thought of them. Professor Freud starts by saying that one can tell very little about the details of a dream without the cooperation of the dreamer, and then makes a few remarks on the general features of the dreams insofar as they resemble certain type-dreams. Such dreams according to Freud belong to "dreams from above" (not to be construed in the mystical sense), that is, dreams whose content could just as well have been formed in the waking state as during sleep, and only certain parts of them draw their substance from the deepest part of the psyche. Moreover, such dreams are often expressed in abstruse, poetic, or symbolic form.

The analysis of this type of dream gives us no real understanding of the dream, but the dreamer himself can usually interpret them without any effort. This shows that the content of the dream is very near the

---

[5] Freud: *Brief an Maxim Leroy über einen Traum des Cartesius* (1929). **Gesammelte Schriften**, Bd. XII, p. 403.

conscious level. Those parts which the dreamer cannot interpret invariably belong to the unconscious and represent the most interesting part of the dream, but they can only be interpreted with the help of the dreamer. What Descartes himself thought of the dreams fully agrees with the rules of dream interpretation, but he only gave one part of the dreams. Freud then goes on to say that the inhibitions in the dream which impeded Descartes' freedom of locomotion are well known; they represent an inner conflict. The left side represents evil and sin, and the wind the "evil genius" (animus). The various persons of the dream could only have been identified by Descartes. As to the bizarre and almost absurd elements in the dreams, such as "the melon from a strange land," and the little portraits, all these must remain unexplained. Freud does not agree with Descartes' interpretation that the melon represents "the charms of solitude present by purely human solicitation." He thinks that by correlating it with his feeling of sin, this association might have led to some sexual ideas which have absorbed the solicitary young man.

Stephen Schönberger, another psychoanalyst, did venture to interpret Descartes' dreams but most of his deductions are too general to throw any definite light on the problem (Stephen Schönberger: *A Dream of Descartes: Reflections on the Unconscious Determinants of the Sciences.* The Int. Jl. of Psychoanalysis. Vol. XX, Part I, Jan. 1939, pp. 43-57). Schönberger thinks that the first dream centers round masturbation and homosexuality (p. 43) and that the photisms in the second dream represent "psychic equivalents of the sight of the performance of a sexual act" (p. 44).

It would seem to us that the *scientia mirabilis,* which filled the spirit of Descartes, did not refer to science, but rather to a "way of life," which was opened to Descartes, as he believed, by heavenly inspiration, and in all probability this represented a resolution of Descartes' emotional conflicts centering about sexuality. One could say that the inner resolution, as it seems to be reflected in his dreams, represented figuratively a castration, or a renouncement of sexuality, or more broadly, a decision to dedicate himself to the discovery of truth and of knowledge. His vow to make a pilgrimage to the shrine of Our Lady of Loreto could be interpreted as the unconscious desire to remain loyal to his mother.

The poems included in his dreams, "Quod vitae sectabor iter" and "Est et Non" (D.M. Ausonius) pointed to the uncertainties of life and the difficulties experienced in making the right choice. They mirrored Descartes' inner insecurity which he consciously perceived as doubts in the whole structure of science. The relief which he experienced in his *"Cogito ergo sum,"* points to a regression to the infantile omnipotence of thought.

The second moral crisis which Descartes experienced, at the age of 23, was rooted in the same psychological conditions which gave rise to his first crisis at the age of 18. These conditions were Descartes' incompetence to meet the demands of adult life, notably those of heterosexual relations. There was evidently a strong latent component of homosexuality in Descartes, of which he was probably aware, and with which he was in vigorous conflict. These difficulties which in another person might have produced homosexuality or paranoia, resulted in Descartes' case in new philosophical and scientific orientations.

This latent homosexuality showed itself throughout Descartes' life. Thus, Baillet describes Descartes' relations to his subordinates in the following terms: "On his part he treated them (his valets and secretaries) with a gentleness and indulgence that bound them to him with love. Those of the first rank who came in intimate contact with him, in the capacity of valet de chambre—or secretary, he considered so little beneath him, that they could have been taken for his equal." Descartes not only took charge of their instruction, but advanced their fortunes as well (Adrien Baillet: *La Vie de M*^r*. Des-cartes.* Réduite en abrégé. Paris, M.DC.-XCII, pp. 341-342).

Other phases of his behavior, which point to infantile fixations, were his habit of staying in bed during a great part of the day and his addiction to day dreaming.

In the light of these psychobiographical data, we can appreciate the fictional, rationalized character of Descartes' version of the genesis of his philosophy. By the same illumination we can appreciate the origin of the bias which characterizes Cartesianism, its intellectualistic foundation, its universal mathematics, its analytical fragmentation of problems, and its simplifying, mechanistic version of man and the universe.

The psychic insecurity of Descartes, the emotional conflict and confusion he suffered, he *"resolved"* in his philosophy. This was his projected solution to his inner difficulties: security through mathematical patterns of thought and procedures, applied to a world, rendered orderly and simple in an all-embracing mechanical scheme. The above does not imply that Descartes' conflicts gave origin *de novo* to the mathematical or mechanistic concepts involved in his philosophy. These concepts were not entirely original with Descartes; they were the heritage of his age. What *is* intended is that Descartes took the knowledge that was to hand, added to it out of his own genius, employed it in the resolution of his emotional difficulties and thus fashioned his unique philosophy. By implication, it is proper to argue that were Descartes of a different psychological constitution, with the same matter at hand he would have fashioned a different philosophy—one akin, say, to the pantheism of Spinoza.

Before sketching the influence of Cartesianism on modern psychological thought, it is desirable to evaluate more discretely certain aspects of Descartes' philosophy. The foundation dictum of his philosophy is *Cogito ergo sum*. In philosophy this dictum is labeled subjectivism. Psychiatrically, however, it is to be recognized as the quintessence of autistic thinking. The dictum characterizes the whole of Cartesianism in that it proclaims the sovereignty of thought. This corresponds to what Freud labeled the Allmacht der Gedanken, the omnipotence of thought. This belief in the omnipotence of thought is characteristic of the infantile, primitive and regressed personalities.[6] It is the refuge of the personality that finds itself threatened by its incompetence to fulfill the affect relations involved in adult existence.

Descartes' effort to develop a universal mathematics, which really implied a mathematical formula to sum up the universe, stems from the same emotional conflict. It represents striving for absolute security. We must not miss its psychiatric significance, merely because it led to the discovery of analytical geometry.

In this connection it is pertinent to quote from Freud's observations on the function of mathematics in the repression of sexuality. "Mathematics," Freud wrote on *Gradiva*,[7] "enjoys the greatest reputation as a diversion from sexuality; J. J. Rousseau had to submit to the counsel proffered by a woman dissatisfied with him—to 'leave women alone and study mathematics instead' (Lascia le donne e studia la matematica)."

"Refuge in mathematics" was ably portrayed in a book of fiction published some years ago. The book, written by Maurice Samuel, was interestingly enough entitled "Beyond Woman."[8]

---

[6] Sigmund Freud: *Über einige Übereinstimmungen im Seelenleben der Wilden und der Neurotiker*. III. Animismus, Magie und Allmacht der Gedanken. (Imago, Band II, 1913, pp. 12, 13.)

[7] Sigmund Frud: *Der Wahn und die Träume in W. Jensens "Gradiva"* (Schriften zur angewandten Seelenkunde, 1. Heft, 3. Auflage, 1924, p. 30.)

[8] H. v. Hug-Hellmuth: *Einige Berziehungen zwischen Erotik und Mathematik* (Imago, Band IV, p. 68, 1916).
Der geheimnisvolle Zusammenhang zwischen Sexualtrieb und mathematischer Forschung ist auch der Gegenwart nicht fremd. In Multatulis Briefen findet sich folgende Stelle: "Ich hoffe, ich hoffe, eine vereinfachte Methode für die Trigonometrie zu finden. Alle Schüler werden mir dankbar sein. Ich habe noch viele andere Dinge von dieser Art zu untersuchen. Es ist herrliche Poesie, das Aufheben des keuschen Gewandes der Natur, das Suchen nach ihren Formen, das Forschen nach ihren Verhältnissen, das Betasten ihrer Gestalt, das Eindringen in die Gebärmutter der Wahrheit, Siehe da die Wollust der Mathematik!"

The concept of the "closed universe," though common to science, in the case of Descartes' philosophy likewise represents the resultant of his quest for certainty. The completed circle offers security. The open universe is too disturbing, precisely because it is open.

In surveying the psychiatric development and experiences of Descartes, we are persuaded that the two moral crises which he suffered were of a schizoid nature, and that his total personality was of like quality. His personality improved somewhat when he reached the fifth decennium of his life. Descartes had a very superior intelligence which readily absorbed and utilized the scientific and philosophical knowledge new sprung in his age. This competence exposed him to the charge of plagiarism. We know too how promptly he accepted the discoveries of Galileo and of Harvey. By virtue of his great intelligence Descartes was able to make numerous and very valuable contributions to science and to philosophy, but because of his psychological handicap he imparted to scientific thinking a peculiar bias from which we are only now beginning to recover.

Descartes is credited with being the father of modern psychology. To Descartes can be traced the initiation of the major concepts which have framed psychological thinking during the last three hundred years. He advanced the notion, later to be substantiated by the neuroanatomists and the neurophysiologists, that the brain is the organ of the mind. He projected the pattern of the basic mechanism in neurophysiology—that of the reflex action. The greater portion of the energies of the neurologists and physiologists, ever since the time of Descartes, have been devoted to the elaboration of both these notions and to the revelations of their structural and functional equivalents. He, to a no lesser degree, shaped and affected the thought of the following centuries in what is called philosophical psychology.

It is not necessary, since the data are both well established and well known, to trace the concrete manifestations of the impulsions given to psychologic thought by Descartes' work. The histories of neuroanatomy, of neurophysiology, and of experimental psychology fully reflect them. However, Descartes not only charted the paths of future studies, he also dictated and imposed the viewpoint, we might say the mentation method, in which the studies were to be conducted. This he effected through his *Méthode*—with its intellectualistic criteria—its fragmentation of complex problems into their simpler components, and its persuasion that the solution of complex problems may be achieved by the summation of the solutions of the simpler elements of the problem. Descartes, too, set the pattern for the study of man—torn from his social matrix.

How deeply these *mentation methods* have become fixed upon science and upon psychiatric thinking is reflected in an address made by Adolf Meyer[9] in 1921.

"The great mistake," said Meyer, "of an overambitious science has been the desire to study man altogether as a mere sum of parts, if possible of atoms, or now of electrons, and as a machine, detached, by itself, because at least some points in the simpler sciences could be studied to the best advantage with this method of the so-called elementalist. It was a long time before willingness to see the large groups of facts, in their broad relations as well as in their inner structure, finally gave us the concept and vision of integration which now fits man as a live unit and transformer of energy into the world of fact and makes him frankly a consciously integrated psychobiological individual and member of a social group." The overambitious science to which Meyer refers is the legitimate progeny and true descendant of Cartesianism.

But *overambitious science* is not the only progeny of Descartes' fertile intellect. There is in that family a Cinderella—some even would say a bastard member, identified with the Cartesian dichotomy of the body and soul. This Cartesian element has been far too long neglected. It merits our consideration.

Descartes' "dichotomy" is the most distinctive feature of his psychology. Others before Descartes had recognized that the brain is the organ of the mind, and the idea of reflex action is to be found current among the Greek philosophers. But no one had propounded so complete a separation between body and soul as did Descartes.

Many, as La Mettrie, dismiss Descartes' dichotomy and his works on the soul, saying that Descartes merely tacked a soul on to the human body in order not to offend the clergy. This is a false and superficial judgment. It is true that Descartes was eager to avoid conflict with the church. When Galileo was condemned, Descartes suppressed the publication of his own work, *Le Monde,* in which he espoused the Galilean astronomy. But Descartes was no craven coward, as can be seen by his conflict with the Jesuits. Furthermore, the soul and its relation to the body was the preoccupation of Descartes' mature years. The work embracing his most definitive thoughts on these matters, *Les Passions de L'Ame,* was the last to be published during his lifetime.

Descartes made numerous references to the soul in his *Discourse* and in his *Meditations,* but they were secondary considerations devoted to

9 Adolf Meyer: *The Contribuiotns of Psychiatry to the Understanding of Life Problems.* Psychiatric Milestone. Bloomingdale Hosp. Cent. 1821-1921, p. 24.

the demonstration of the existence of God. In his work on Man, he likewise deals with the soul, but here again, the subject is secondary to his exposition of the automaton-like operations of the body. Only in his work *The Passions of The Soul* does he fully amplify his thesis on the separateness of the body and soul. This work has an interesting and significant history. Descartes was for many years the intimate of Princess Elizabeth of Bohemia, who was an enthusiastic student of his philosophy. To her Descartes dedicated his work *The Principles of Philosophy,* published in 1644. In the same year, the Princess Elizabeth was obliged to remove from Holland to Germany, and she maintained her contact with Descartes by correspondence. In 1645 Descartes composed a short essay on *The Passions of The Soul.* In this unpublished work he merely attemped to establish certain foundations for morality. In the following year (1646), Princes Elizabeth asked Descartes to review critically Seneca's Morals. He did so, and the ensuing correspondence ranged widely over many questions. Out of this correspondence issued the substance of Descartes' published work *The Passions of The Soul.* Herein he most clearly defined the separateness of body and soul (Article II) and he examined minutely the varieties of passions to which the soul is subject. The word "passions" as employed by Descartes, be it noted, is not to be equated in meaning to "passions" in English, but rather to "affects."

It is no easy matter to translate Descartes' thoughts on the affects of the soul into the vernacular or criteria of modern psychological thought. Those who are interested, will find such a rendition very ably given in an article in the *Journal de Psychologie* (July 15, 1924, No. 7) by P. Quercy, entitled *Remarques sur le "Traité des Passions" de Descartes.* That which is of significance to us in *Les Passions de L'Ame,* is not Descartes' conceptions of the affects of the soul, but rather his exposition on the *bearing* which the soul has upon the actions of the body. The soul, according to Descartes, is independent and distinctly different from the body. It, however, makes contact with the body through the pineal gland. Furthermore, the soul permeates and extends through the body. The soul does not set the body in motion, but the soul can influence the vital spirits already set in motion, and thereby alter the direction of the body's motion—or behavior. The soul, in its relation to the body, may thus he compared to that of a rider on a horse, who directs what are really the movements of the horse.

Princess Elizabeth, to whom Descartes expounded these thoughts, complained that she could not grasp them entirely. What troubled her particularly was how the soul, being so very separate from the body, could yet be united with the body and act and suffer with it. To this Descartes responded with the completely baffling observation, "I do not think that the mind of man is capable of forming a clear and simultaneous conception of the distinction between the soul and the body, and also of their union; for to that end, one must think of them as a single thing, and at the same time as two things, which is contradictory" (Quoted by Cardinal Mercier: *Origins of Contemporary Psychology*. New York, 1918, p. 53).

We must take Descartes' words to mean "I know it, but I cannot explain it." He really could not. He was too hemmed in by his own scientific and philosophical restrictions. The formulation of a "clear and simultaneous conception of the distinction between the soul and the body and also of their union," had to wait on the advance of science, and on the advent of psychoanalytic psychiatry.

This may appear to be, as no doubt it is, a somewhat odd linkage, for by implication it postulates that Descartes' dichotomy is substantiated, and at that by psychoanalytical psychiatry. Precisely that is intended.

There is no evidence that Freud ever concerned himself with Descartes' philosophy or psychology. Yet, in Freud's teachings, in his basic hypothesis, he has corrected most of the major deficiencies of Cartesianism. Freud has taught science, though I will not say the lesson has been well learned, the errors of its intellectualistic interpretations and evaluations of the acts and motives of man. He has shown the artifact elements that creep into, distort and invalidate the data obtained in the study of man torn from his social matrix. He has defined the psyche, the soul of Descartes, in its genetic, structural, and experiential origins, and components. The control which Descartes pictured in terms of "rider and horse," Freud has demonstrated in the inhibitions exercised by the ego on the instinctual drives. The counterpart of much that is in Descartes' *Les Passions de L'Ame*, can be found in psychoanalytic theory and in its clinically demonstrated experience.

The psyche with its three component elements: the Id, the Ego, and the Super-ego, is, as Freud has stated in many connections, rooted in the antiquity of man. There is no difficulty in recognizing that the Id contains phylogenetic components, notably the instinctual and primitive drives of man. It is however somewhat difficult to visualize that the Super-ego too contains phylogenetically derived components. Yet Freud and a number of his disciples are very clear on this score.

Freud with his characteristic scientific exactitude is cautious but clear on this matter. In *Moses and Monotheism*[10] he wrote:

[10] Sigmund Freud: *Moses and Monotheism*, translated by Katherine Jones, published by the Hogarth Press and the Institute of Psycho-Analysis, 1939, p. 157.

There probably exists in the mental life of the individual not only what he has experienced himself, but also what he brought with him at birth, fragments of phylogenetic origin, an archaic heritage.

Again, Freud calls in witness the evidence produced by analytic research to support the existence of archaic and phylogenetically derived elements in the psyche.[11]

In studying reactions to early traumata, we often find to our surprise that they do not keep strictly to what the individual himself has experienced, but deviate from this in a way that would accord much better with their being reactions to genetic events and in general can be explained only through the influence of such . . . such reactions which seem unreasonable in the individual . . . can only be understood phylogenetically, in relation to the experiences of earlier generations.

Franz Alexander corroborates Freud, and describes the Super-ego as a "faculty which reflects certain phylogenetic echoes of primitive man."

Jung, too, has expounded similar views. In his essay on *The Conception of The Unconscious* Jung[12] wrote, "In the same way as the individual is not only an isolated and separate, but also a social being, so also the human mind is not only something isolated and absolutely individual, but also a collective function. And just as certain social functions or impulses are, so to speak, opposed to the egocentric interests of the individual, so also the human mind has certain functions or tendencies which, on account of their collective nature, are to some extent opposed to the personal mental functions. This is due to the fact that every human being is born with a highly differentiated brain, which gives him the possibility of attaining a rich mental function that he has neither acquired ontogenetically nor developed."

It is in the *phylo*genetically derived, dominant element of the human mind and the human psyche, revealed to us by psychoanalytic psychiatry, that we find intelligent illumination of Descartes' meaning when he propounded the complete dichotomy of body and soul and at the same time considered both of them bound in inseparable union througout life.

We can understand, too, why Descartes, though steeped in his insight, could not frame it in communicable and in intelligible terms, why, indeed, he despaired that the human mind might ever grasp it. Descartes was wanting in that knowledge and ideology which our age gained in the

---

[11] *Op. cit.*, p. 159.

[12] C. G. Jung, *Collected Papers on Analytical Psychology*, 2nd Edition, London, 1922, p. 451.

concept of evolution. This concept has linked the universe in a continuous chain of progressions and relationships. Embryology has revealed to us the processes by which hereditary forces shape individual structure and function. It has demonstrated how phylogeny is reflected in ontogeny. It has made conceivable how forces which antecede the origin of the individual may operate in him, for ends that transcend his consciousness or his volition. These facts are most clearly revealed in the inherited neural reflex mechanisms and in the instinctual drives that motivate and guide so many of the activities of living things. In a more subtle fashion they are reflected in the architectonics of postnatal development, in differential growth, and in the dramatic sequence of endocrine dominance and regression. The psyche, as Freud demonstrated, has its phylogenetic history, reflected in its ontogenetic development, and in its everyday functions.

Among the determinants of human personality must be counted the Super-ego,—the *Cartesian soul*. It is as immortal and as dominant as the germ plasm. It is, no doubt, in part conveyed by the germ plasm, but also by the whole of the milieu in which the individual is born and lives. In this sense, a sense deep and profound, the Super-ego phylogenetically derived is distinctly apart from the body. There *is* as Descartes maintained a complete dichotomy between body and soul.

Viewed purely in the light of his biological and social functions, the human being appears to be a time, space, and energy bound congelation of matter, largely moved by force-determinants which antecede his formation, toward ends which largely transcend the grasp of his consciousness and which in many instances during his life cut across his own volitional directions. From these conditions of his individual being arise most of the psychiatric ills from which the individual suffers.

The foregoing interpretation of Descartes' ideas on the soul, and on its separateness from the body, in the terms and theories of modern psychiatric thought is offered as a prospectus for study and research rather than as a fully-proved rendition.

It does, however, illustrate the fertily of Descartes genius which not only shaped and influenced modern psychiatric thought at the time of its inception, but even today affords us rich matter for speculation and study.

31

Psychopathia Intellectualis

THE INTELLECTUAL is much discussed and little defined. But this is not for want of effort. It is rather that the intellectual, viewed as a specimen of *homo sapiens,* is so annoyingly without any definitive qualities by which he might be distinguished from the rest of mankind. Yet there is no doubt that he does exist and that many among his kind are, to put mildly, in one hell of a fix. All this adds up to an odd paradox. But only seemingly so. The intellectual cannot be defined save in terms of his *modus operandi,* and that only in a special sense. Thus, as Russell Kirk has so ably shown, the intellectual cannot be described operationally as the thinking, the philosophizing, the scholarly man. The intellectual is not "a man who is notably devoted to and uniquely skilled in the uses of the intellect." Such a definition is too general and too sweeping in its embrace. It is also rather embarrassing, for it is obviously as applicable to those who criticize the intellectual as to the intellectual criticized.*

It is, therefore, not the operations of the intellectual per se, but rather the framework of faiths and basic assumptions within which he operates that distinguishes the intellectual from the rest of his thinking brethren. It is this framework that marks him as a man apart. To his faiths and

---

* For this reason the egghead intellectual can best be described as an intellectualist, that is, "a compulsive character who substitutes formal pseudo-cold thinking for understanding and feeling." The intellectual was a term dear to the Russian, but this term did not refer to the intellectualistic psychopath but to the representative of the intelligentsia. The Marxists and the anti-Marxists fought about the concept. The Marxists recognized no intelligentsia but considered them merely the representatives of the bourgeois class gone liberal. The Populists thought of the intellectual as "a critically thinking individual whose social and ideological position was outside and above any economic class."

410

basic assumptions can be traced much of what I call the *"psychopathia intellectualis."*

The unique framework of the intellectual—I'd rather say of the egg-head among intellectuals*—is easily described: it is an extrapolated framework projected upon the propositions of Baconian, Cartesian, Hegelian, and Marxian "science." Its orientation points include unwavering faith in evolution, in specific causality, in materialism, and in Pavlovian psychology. It is logical and logistic in quality, but of that order best labeled as logical positivism. It is inimical to the avowedly irrational, and to everything that is not translatable into the vernacular of science. It is nonecological, and nonholistic. It posits man outside and above all nature. Such being the case, the intellectual—*qua* egghead—is an enthusiastic planner, an unconscionable manipulator of man, society, and the universe, and a gullible sucker for everything that carries the label of science.

The intellectual's framework of operations is a derivative of the intellectual bias developed in and by eighteenth-century science. It remains unaffected and uncorrected by all that we have learned since, in both science and philosophy, that bears on that bias. Indeed the intellectual is in that respect a reactionary, a conservative, a staunch defender of vested knowledge. He cannot, nor will he trouble to study or to understand, say, Whitehead, or Schoedinger, or Cassirer. He is likely to prefer Bertrand Russell's "clear, objective, and rational philosophy." The former are encyclical and acutely perceive and appreciate the relatedness of man to the universe. They teach a modern version of "microcosm and macrocosm." But Russell sets man free to rule the world.**

It is to this illusory belief in the "freedom of man," in his independence from and his mastery over his environment—that is, over nature—that the *psychopathia intellectualis* can be traced.

---

* A word on the use of the term "egghead." I employ it reluctantly, and only because I know of no better term by which to designate this particular member of the intellectual confraternity. Literary and critical tradition offers some precedents and warrants in the use of such designations. There come to mind von Chamisso's shadowless Peter Schlemihl, Voltaire's obtuse Candide, and Carlyle's Prof. Teufelsdröckh. I cannot trace the Alsops' derivation of the expression "egghead" but I suspect it may have been suggested by the phrase "addlebrain" or "addlehead."

** "The universe as known to science is not in itself either friendly or hostile to man, but it can be made to act as a friend if approached with patient knowledge. Where the universe is concerned, knowledge is the one thing needful. Man, alone of living things, has shown himself capable of the knowledge required to give him a certain mastery over his environment." Bertrand Russell, *An Outline of Philosophy* (London: G. Allen & Unwin, Ltd., 1927), p. 312.

The intellectual is at best prone to disparage, and at worst likely to deny emphatically that he is a creature of the universe and bound to it by a variety of exacting requirements. He will perforce grant that he cannot evade certain vital physiological requisites such as eating, sleeping, and evacuating. But even these he is most likely to fulfill at his own, and not at nature's discretion. He is by consequence and mental disposition a great believer in the utility and efficacy of drugs, operations, and psychoanalysis. Parenthetically it should be added that he seldom proves a good analysand. He is too resistant, and too much of a doctrinaire intellectual to be able to appreciate or to act upon the insights proffered by analysis. Hence many intellectuals are the "victims" of unsuccessful and/or interminable analyses.

The egghead intellectual is seldom a good lover, an effective husband or wife, a successful parent, or a rewarded and rewarding grandparent.

The composite clinical psychiatric history of the intellectual, given in brief, sums up to the following. He (or she), even when young, overinvests in his intellectual acquisitions and exercises. In psychiatric terms—he eroticizes his intellect. In effect, he talks a good line, but performs rarely and badly when circumstances call for emotional and erotic interrelations. He is likely to suffer from *ejaculatio praecox*, and from the precipitous and periodic loss of virility. His relations with the opposite sex are prone to be "companionable," with the emphasis on equality. This is a neat rationalization by which *he* manages to evade the role of the aggressive male, and *she* that of the submissive (masochistic) female. He is not likely to fall in love at the age and in the way others do. He explains this to himself and to others by saying that he hasn't found the right person. He is not, however, averse to having sexual relations with likely prospects. Indeed, since sexual intercourse is one of those necessary functions which a culturally and scientifically backward society has surrounded with innumerable obstacles and taboos, he sees no reason why an exploration of prospects should not begin in bed. He thus severs love from sex, and reverses that sequence by which erotic play in most of the higher animal world is paced. When he marries it is by deliberate decision and not as a romantic achievement. He *chooses* to marry, and he either marries brains and personality or else a "cute thing." The latter is the better and more promising marriage. But in essence it is a marriage of condescension, not so much to the "cute thing" as to the pesty prurience of concupiscence. The "cute thing" is generally from the other side of the social, cultural, or religious track. The "brains and personality" marriage is likely to prove more trying, and not infrequently ends in a late divorce.

Both partners are too narcissistically involved to team up for the serious and exacting business of marriage. Both, and the female more pre-eminently so, are bent on fulfilling themselves *in and by themselves.* In time they each come to feel, with full warrant but with little or no discernment as to how or why, that the other has failed them. The general complaint is that the other is "not giving." They see the beam but not the mote.

Since the marriage was entered upon in cool premeditation, it is not readily dissolved. That were too great an admission of reason's fallibility. Hence if and when divorce does take place it is generally after ten or fifteen years of marital travail. The intellectuals do bear children, but generally somewhat late in life, that is, when the male is past thirty. They seldom have more than three children, generally only two. The children are spaced from three to four years apart. The third child is likely to be the product of an irrational impulse, and is not infrequently explained as "an accident." The intellectual eagerly and readily farms out his (her) children. They are sent to a variety of schools beginning almost from the time that they can toddle and babble. The persuasion, i.e., the rationalization, is that they need to be with other children "to socialize." The need to be with mother, and with father too, is not recognized or esteemed. In summertime when school is out the youngsters are exiled to camp, there "to learn nature."

When the intellectual's children show, as they so frequently do, the stigmata of their upbringing in a variety of emotional, behavioral, and learning disabilities, they are again delegated to a motley of so-called therapists, many of whom are trained laymen. They are then treated for years. The intellectual's children, natively gifted, but starved in affection and otherwise emotionally deprived, are thus started early on the compensatory overinvestment in intellect. They are good-to-excellent scholars, quickly maturing eggheads, and promising candidates for the analyst's couch.

Meanwhile the aging intellectual begins to suffer from a variety of psychosomatic illnesses. These may include precocious impotence, and a variety of psychosexual complaints. In the female, dyspareunia, pruritus vulvae, dysmenorrhea, migraine, and hyperthyroidism are not uncommon. Insomnia, chronic obstipation, gastrointestinal disorders, hypochrondiasis, and what Abraham Meyerson so aptly termed anhedonia—a loss of relish for life and living—are some of the later complaints common among intellectuals. These are some of the quittance claims which Eros exacts from those deluded souls who hope to dissipate his sovereignty in the sway of their rationality.

The intellectual ages but does not grow old. He is against it on principle. Hence he is an abiding pal to all ages. His children refer to him and call him by his first name, and almost never "father" or "dad." He in return is a *Duzbruder* to everyman. When grown old, calendar-wise, he is especially prone to favor the company and the companionship of the very young and to share in their exercises (hiking, for example) with an ingenuous enthusiasm. Not for him the wisdom and dignity *de senectute*. He prefers to be, as indeed he remains, *juvenilis* in mind and spirit.

Though he suffers many psychosomatic illnesses, he seldom becomes psychotic and rarely exhibits any of the classical forms of neurosis. His are chiefly those psychological disorders which can best be described as due to faulty character formation—that is, as character disorders. Among his children, however, schizophrenia and suicide do occur rather frequently. A distinctive feature of the egghead intellectual's psychic operations is its pseudo emotionality. The intellectual of this order is effusive in his avowals of friendly interest and sympathy—and conversely as shallow and ephemeral in their exercise. This is true not alone of his relations with his friends, but also and equally of his affect relations with his family, marriage partner, and children. For this reason he can be, and frequently is, sadistically cruel, and betraying. Furthermore his affections and interests are more likely to extend to masses and groups than to given individuals. He will enthuse about India and its people, or Negroes, or the Chinese, or be incensed by the abuses and injustices suffered, say, by Arab refugees, or Koreans, but will not always sense the plight nor render a Good Samaritan's service to one in his immediate sphere.

I have written of the intellectual in the masculine, intending of course both male and female. But the "female of the species" deserves a special note. As she is a creature more proximate to the primal upsurgings of life, any psychic corruptions which she may suffer are bound to have multiple and far-reaching effects on her own person and on those with whom she is associated. Psychoanalysts have had a good deal of sport with this specimen of womankind. Their fancies have been both riotous and prolific, and their theories ingenuous. Thus she allegedly suffers from a castration complex, i.e., she believes she had had a phallus but lost it by castration; she is supposed to suffer penis envy—wanting to be "like a man"; she is said to rejoice in castrating the male, to square things, so to say. Taken in earnest and literally, these hypotheses engender much nonsense, but understood in their symbolic implications they cast a revealing light upon the psychopathology of the female intellectual. In the persuasions of the "science"-oriented intellectual, she rejects and seeks to negate her femininity. She resents her biological primacy. She does not envy man, she rather disparages femininity. Yet paradoxically the female intellectual is not infrequently also an obstreperous feminist. Her feminism, however, is animated primarily by the desire to wipe out "the differences." Her aim is not feminism, i.e., the flowering of womanhood and of womankind, but rather asexual egalitarianism. The effects of these persuasions on her own life and functions as a female are not difficult to envisage. More complicated and grievous are their effects upon her family and notably upon her children. Her sons are likely to grow up "intimidated, dependent males," who either marry older women, as aggressive as the mother, or else exist as intersex creatures floating between hetero- and homosexuality. Her daughters, on the other hand, not infrequently "avenge" their upbringing in riotous promiscuity.

For all these features of his psychic being, the intellectual can advance many justifications. He can explain them all and find nothing wrong in or about them. If and when, as frequently it does happen, he finds himself troubled and unhappy, he is "at a loss" to understand why. Under these circumstances he treats himself to a mild paranoia. He reifies the evil which afflicts him in the pattern of a "reactionary government," or "vested interests," or "social Darwinism." In other words, he resolves his puzzlement in the conviction that he is a misunderstood, opposed, and abused man. Should he seek psychotherapy it will be in order to gain help in overcoming "his enemies." One of the prize understatements to be found in Fenichel's classical work on the neurosis reads as follows: "Analytic therapy in the case of character disorders meets with specific difficulties." The specific difficulties are mainly these: the patient has no insight into, nor does he recognize his pathological attitudes; he does not appreciate that "the chief part of the conflicting energies the analysis aims to release is tonically bound in the attitudes," nor can he grasp that these very attitudes interfere with the process of analysis. (Otto Fenichel, *The Psychoanalytic Theory of Neurosis*, New York, W. W. Norton & Co., 1945, p. 537.)

The psychotherapy of the intellectual is extremely difficult, but not impossible of success. The yield is better with the younger than with the older. The most trying feature in the treatment of the intellectual is his persevering efforts to entice his therapist into a longwinded and involved intellectual *analysis* of the analysis. Pathetically and naïvely he will protest that he doesn't understand, that it all seems so contradictory, that the therapist isn't consistent, that the time before he said *that* and now he says *this*. It is all very taxing, but when the intellectual does "break through," the results are most rewarding, and not infrequently of much social consequence. Koestler comes to mind in this connection.

The composite picture given above, and one must bear in mind that it *is* a composite picture and not a typical case history, is not very pleasant to contemplate. It does proffer a valid index to *psychopathia intellectualis* but it doesn't quite do justice to the intellectual as a creature. In person, that is, as one beholds him in the flesh, the intellectual (egghead) isn't bad at all. Indeed he can be quite nice, that is, until he begins to go off on the tangent of his bias. Then he is akin to the "monomaniac" of ancient psychiatry. The amphoteric quality of his being, his seemingly benign charm and his potential as well as real malignity account for the bitterness with which he is condemned when discovered. The egghead intellectual is passionately hated, as a betrayer of the intellect. Yet in full justice, and in psychiatric objectivity, he cannot be held "a traitor." He is rather a victim. He is a denatured man, a man *déraciné*. And the fault, if any, is a truly collective guilt, the fault of us all who have been so uncritical in the acceptance of the dicta and the pretensions of modern science.

Writing this brief excursion into the psychopathology of the intellectual, I became aware that at the very end I must add this: Of whomsoever this tale is told, dear reader, it is told also of me and thee, for in this age none of us but suffers from a touch of that madness which in full measure sums up to the *Psychopathia Intellectualis*.

32

Psychiatry and Religion

ANYONE WHO UNDERTAKES to treat of psychiatry and religion at once comes upon a problem of great complexity, namely how to define what he intends and understands by the term "religion." Psychiatry has some commonality of meaning for most people—but religion has not. Yet unless the term "religion" be clearly defined, there is little likelihood that any effective interpersonal communication on that score will be achieved.

Many men have endeavored to define "religion," and it is possible to run the "gamut of definements" from Marx's dictum that "religion is the opium of the people" to William Penn's somewhat humanistic definition of religion as "nothing else but love to God and man."

An exhibit of the definitions advanced in time by different men, though it might prove entertaining, would yet profit us little. For in the end we would come out not unlike the youthful Omar, who—"when young did eagerly frequent Doctor and Saint, and heard great argument about it and about: but ever more came out by the same door wherein"—he went.

For our ends we require not an historical nor yet an epistemologic definition of "religion," but rather one derived analytically. To achieve this we need to dismember, to consider and to evaluate the complex of factors embraced in the term "religion." Subject to such a critique it becomes readily evident that the term "religion" embraces three factors. These are: the corporate church, its doxy or dogma, and what I chose to term the psychologic substratum of religion. I will not at this point elaborate on the third of the three factors embraced in the term "religion," but will rather underscore its differences from the first two enumerated. Thus it is to be appreciated that the corporate church and its dogma are in effect specific concretizations of the psychologic substratum

417

of religion. Also, and this is most important, of the three factors given, only the psychologic substratum is universal; the other two are accidental and parochial. To paraphrase this last affirmation it needs to be appreciated that all peoples are disposed to be religious, but the specific pattern in which this disposition is effected and realized varies not only from one group to another but may vary within the same group, even when that group numbers not more than two individuals.

There are no fewer than 105 distinctly separate religious bodies in the United States, that is to say, 105 separate corporate churches, with 105 separate, distinctive and all too frequently antagonistic dogmas. This variety of religious denominations both illustrates the meaning and substantiates the validity of the affirmation that the psychologic substratum of religion is universal, while the corporate church and its dogma are accidental, variable and parochial. All worshipful souls worship God, but they worship Him in different churches and in differing ways.

This catalogue of religious denominations both illustrates the meaning and substantiates the validity of the affirmation that the psychologic substratum of religion is universal, while the corporate church and its dogma are accidental, variable and parochial. All of the 2,275,000,000 worshipful souls worship God, but they worship Him in different churches and in differing ways.

It is to be granted that our analysis of religion by which it is made to yield its three component factors, the corporate church, its dogma and its psychologic substratum, does violence, as most dismembering analyses do, to reality and to experience. That much the Gestalt School has taught us, and taught us well. In real life we confront religion as religion. At different times, it is true, we may be made particularly and acutely aware of its psychologic or spiritual qualities, as in the celebration of the Eucharist, or when the sound of the ram's horn calls the faithful Jew to repentance on the Day of Atonement; at other times we may become aware of its all too corporate nature, as when we are dunned for our tithes, or the collection plate is passed—a second time. Still again we may be chafed by the rub we suffer when some alien church seeks to yoke our unwilling neck to its galling dogma. But these are generally accents in experience, instances in which some one of the three components of religion intrudes upon our awareness, overshadows but does not obliterate the other two. In actual experience we seldom if ever confront "religion in the abstract." We ordinarily confront believing, or (the difference is little) disbelieving, Jews, Protestants, or Catholics.

Yet in the effort to define the relation of religion to psychiatry we are obliged, at least when attempting to deal with the fundamentals of that relationship, to exclude the accidental factors of religion, that is, the corporate church and its dogma, and to restrict our consideration to the universal factor, namely to the psychologic substratum of religion. Failure to do this invariably results in mental confusion, and at times also in a foamy churning up of emotions.

Agreeable to this exclusion of the accidental, variable and parochial factors of religion, we are nonetheless obliged to inquire into the validity of the alleged universal factor, the so-termed psychologic substratum of religion. To allege the existence of this factor is not of course tantamount to proving its existence. Before we go on to consider its bearing to psychiatry, we needs must first demonstrate to our own satisfaction that it actually exists, that it is indeed a psychologic dynamism, concretized in the corporate church and in its dogma.

This is indeed the greater part of the issue, for if it can be demonstrated that mankind is possessed of an impulsion toward religion—that the psychologic substratum of religion is indeed an actual psychologic dynamism, and not, as some contend, a delusion, an illusion, a by-product of fear and of ignorance, or the end result of the clever machinations of vested interests—if that can be demonstrated then the bearing of religion on psychiatry must prove little short of obvious.

Our analysis of religion thus far has therefore yielded us not a final definition, but rather a delimitation of the field within which the issue may be contested. And the issue at this time centers about the validity of the affirmation that man is predisposed to religion; that the psychologic substratum of religion of which the corporate church and its dogma are concretizations, is a valid, normal and, let me add, salutary component of the individual's and of the group's psychologic dynamism.

There are many among our psychiatric leaders who would dispute and deny this affirmation. Some few are likely to agree. I myself not only subscribe to the existence and to the operation of the psycholoigc substratum of religion, but further contend that the most crystal-clear demonstration of its being and operation is to be found in the theoretical framework and in the clinical and other achievements of modern dynamic psychiatry, the psychiatry of Freud, Jung, and Meyer.

The issue, of course, is a very old one. In the long span of known history, it has come to the fore again and again, each time to be passionately contested; each time presumably to be finally and decisively resolved—yet no solution quite conforms to the preceding ones, and some are entirely opposite to their antecedents. The writings of the ancient authors show that they were much concerned with the meaning and significance of religion. It is not difficult to find evidence among these authors to prove that some were deeply convinced of man's religious nature; that they appreciated the existence and understood the operations of what I have termed the psychologic substratum of religion. It is, I believe, somewhat easier to prove that some of the ancient authors held the opposite beliefs.

"It was fear," wrote Petronius Arbiter, "that first brought gods into the world." And Lucretius exclaims with passion: "How many evils have flowed from religion!" Heraclitus opined that religion was a "disease, albeit a noble disease." And Polybius, with an air of superior wisdom, explained religion thuswise: "Since the masses of the people are inconstant, full of unruly desires, passionate, and reckless of consequence, they must be filled with fears to keep them in order. The ancients did well, therefore, to invent gods, and the belief in punishment after death. It is rather the moderns, who seek to extirpate such beliefs, who are to be accused of folly."

The deep religious spirit of the ancient Greek authors, on the other hand, is very beautifully demonstrated and expounded in Gilbert Murray's *Four Stages of Greek Religion* (1).

We cannot, at this time, trace the vicissitudes of the issue down the long stretch of time. We need to begin somewhere close to our own period. For us the issue of whether or not there actually exists a psychologic substratum of religion may be dated with the Age of Enlightenment, *at which time it was most decisively resolved in the negative.* No matter what the particular professions and practices of the individual men of science might have been, there is no doubt but that the trend of the science, initiated in the Age of Enlightenment, was inimical to the belief in a psychologic substratum of religion *as a normal and wholesome component of the individual's psyche.* Indeed, the very existence of the psyche was doubted. Modern science was, and largely still is, mechanistic. Galileo no less than Descartes envisaged the operations of the universe and all that is in it in terms of matter and force. No phenomenon of experience but could be ultimately explained as the interplay of the two: force and matter.

In the early years of the New Science, the subject of religion was not at issue, at least not too patently, nor was it raised by the scientists. Yet the corporate church was not unaware of how great was the challenge of these new Alchemists, these new Astrologers, and these new Men of Physic. Galileo was forced to retract; Spinoza was excomunicated; Servetus was burned at the stake!

I think it well to interrupt at this point the flow of the argument in order that we might complete our orientation both as to where the argument is leading as well as to who and what is involved in it. Let me deal with the last matters first. Who and what are involved? The people, that is the great masses, are deeply concerned with religion, but they seldom if ever become aware of such matters as the corporate church, doxies and dogmas, or the psychologic mainspring of religion. To them religion is an irrefragable something into which they are born, and in whose grace they hope to die. The issue, therefore, of whether or not there exists and operates a psychologic substratum of religion, concerns not the people as such, but only some few men of learning. And it is these men of learning, not individually but sequentially, who have raised the issue again and again, and who fought it through each time, but each time to a different end. These battles were not fought for a laurel crown, but for the world itself. These men of learning, though they seldom were, or are, politicians or men of arms, yet manage to influence the affairs of the world. What they think, the faith they support, ultimately affects "the sparrow in its fall." Bearing this in mind we can better visualize the double aspect of real experience—wherein we are confronted with the spectacle of a few men agitated by some esoteric problem that is neither known to, nor concerns, the masses, and, off in time, a mass phenomenon of seemingly unexplained momentum, which in effect is the late end result of the "agitations of the learned men."

This orientation as to who and what are involved should help us to pursue the argument further. Until the Renaissance, and more particularly until the Age of Enlightenment, for close to a thousand years, the Catholic church held sway over our Western civilization. The church, in more learned ways than is now commonly appreciated, taught the lesson that man is essentially a religious creature. It credited him with a distinction not shared by any other living creature, namely the possession of a soul. To the preservation of the soul, and about it, the church built its vast, its intricate, its all-embracing edifice. It was this very soul that the Age of Enlightenment denied. It said that the soul was nonexistent. And, of course, if the soul be nonexistent, then there is no need for a church to foster and preserve it, and if there be no need for a church, then what remains there for religion? Relative to our own consideration, the denial of the soul by the Age of Enlightenment is tantamount to the denial of the existence and operation of a psychologic substratum of religion.

It is noteworthy and significant that the person who formulated the theoretical basis of modern scientific research was also the man who launched the most violent and telling assault on the concept of, and credence in, the human soul. René Descartes accomplished both. In his *Méthode* he provided modern science with an intellectual technique. In his postulation of "reflex action" he initiated a line of reasoning and of research which yielded the picture of the "reasonable automaton," the soulless, intellectual mechanism, man.

I cannot here dilate on the significance of Descartes' well known preoccupations with the human soul, nor defend him against the calumny of scientific apostasy. These matters I have treated in another essay. It is sufficient here to recognize that modern neurology and a great deal of modern psychiatry (excluding, of course, dynamic psychiatry) descended in a straight line from the Cartesian postulates on reflex action and on the rational automaton. Incidentally we are now witnessing a reviviscence of Cartesian neurology and psychiatry in the wave of chemical, electrical and surgical techniques developed in recent years for the treatment of mental disorders.

It is proper to speak of a reviviscence of Cartesian neurology and psychiatry because, after having held sway for more than two and a half centuries, it was overshadowed, and I would add, greatly discredited, by the dynamic psychiatry of Freud. Actually Cartesian psychology never held an indisputed sway. It was at all times subject to some criticism and to some contest. Yet undeniably it was the predominant school and it engaged the interest and labors of the best scientists. Its chief virtue, and that which proved so irresistibly attractive, was its great tangibility. In a literal sense it was easy to grasp, materially, in the structure pattern of the nervous system, and functionally, as a pyramiding hierarchy of reflex actions and reflex centers. In contrast to the Cartesians all those who dwelt upon the soul, the animists and the vitalists, appeared like so many vapid sophists and metaphysicians, who spent their time in spinning fine webs of gossamer arguments wherein to trap and entangle the ignorant and the simple-witted.

We know the dismal history of Mesmer and of mesmerism. The world of science would have nothing to do with animal magnetism, not even when Esdail and John Elliotson demonstrated that under hypnosis a subject could be rendered insensible to the pain of a surgical operation. It was quite different when anesthesia was achieved by means of chloroform or ether. Then the world of science could see that *that* was no humbug! Both, ether and chloroform, even though they evaporate rapidly, are really tangible. If nothing else, one can at least smell them. But how is one to touch, smell or otherwise make certain that animal magnetism, hypnosis or suggestion is not a humbug, but is indeed real?

History has given the answer to this riddle. But I am not sure that the answer is always and everywhere appreciated. I must, therefore, indulge in an excursion which I am sure is pertinent, and which I hope will also prove illuminating.

The ancient Greeks were not the very paragon among peoples, but they were certainly very wise and subtle in their understanding of men and of life. They were as original and as refreshing as a bright and as yet unsophisticated young child. The Greeks, as is well known, distinguished between *sophia* and *techné,* between wisdom, or pure knowledge, and the knowledge of the technique. They carried this distinction to the point of prizing their philosophers and teachers and disparaging their technicians and craftsmen. They particularly held in contempt the laborer who worked with his hands, considering such pursuits to be worthy only of slaves. This odd attitude of the ancient Greek, odd at least in our light, has puzzled me for a long time, and only recently have I been able to see into its rationale. I confess I gained this insight not by analyzing the Greeks, but rather by analyzing my own emotional reactions to some of our own techné, and to some of our contemporary technologists.

There is this which is characteristic of the technician, and of the craftsman: his horizon is likely to be limited by his immediate task, and his knowledge and wisdom are likely to be bound up with, and to be restricted by, his matériel. Craftsmen are notorious for thinking and talking in the vernacular of their crafts, and our language has been enriched with scores of "wise saws" that had their origin in and drew their inspiration from the workshops: "Beat the iron while it's hot"; "too many irons in the fire"; "a stitch in time saves nine"; and so on. The technician is likely to project his easy facility with the matter of his craft to beyond the affairs of his shop, into the spacious world. He is subject to an unconscious self-deception, a kind of delusion of grandeur, which persuades him to believe that after all there is little difference between cobbling and running the world, and hence that he could well instruct those whose hands are upon the helm. One of the wise saws that did *not* issue from the shop, but was rather turned against it, is "Shoemaker—stick to your last!"

The vision of the technician is sharp but entirely central. He is not prone to look nor to see out of the corners of his eyes. He misses the margins, peopled with shadowy objects, and animated with peripheral motions, which though seemingly irrelevant yet make the picture complete, and provide both wisdom and safety to the mind's motions no less than to the body's.

Despite all this, technicians and craftsmen are likely to be rather contented with their lot. This perhaps would be all to the good; for the contented are good workers. However, technicians and craftsmen are generally not content to be content, but are rather impelled to try and convert others to their blissful state. They are particularly impatient of those who do not share their simple and obvious understanding of things and life; of those who, in other words, trouble the heavens' and the mind's peace with seemingly impertinent and vain questionings. It was of course just these impertinent and vain questionings that the learned among the ancient Greeks found most enchanting. Hence their contempt for the technician and the craftsman.

The relevance of this brief excursion and the illumination which I hope it will afford lie precisely in this: modern science is mainly a techné—and its workers mainly technicians. If I should lean upon Aristotle rather than Plato, I would be obliged to say that modern science is an *episteme* even more than a techné, for the latter term in Plato's usage still carried some connotation of art. Modern science being furthermore a practical pursuit, learns chiefly by experience. Modern science is not anticipatory, save in the working out of its own "work projects." It follows, in other words, its own logical tangents until experience either proves their merits or blocks all further progress. In the latter instance science may shift its line of attack and may even follow a tangent heretofore rejected. Such procedure represents a process of development that could properly be described as *"progress by bankruptcy and despair."*

Here, we find the answer to the riddle of how modern science finally convinced itself that hypnosis and suggestion are not humbug, but are indeed potent realities.

Cartesian psychology, particularly as applied in the treatment of mental disease, proved wanting in many instances, and incompetent in the most protean and widespread of the psychologic disorders, the psychoneuroses. *Volens nolens,* modern science was compelled to recognize the phenomena of hypnosis and of suggestion. Once that was achieved, a long chain of consequences followed which finally yielded, at the turn of this century, psychoanalysis and modern dynamic psychiatry. With the advent of psychoanalysis the psyche once again was brought to the fore, and with it, according to *my persuasion,* the psychologic substratum of religion; for I hold the latter to be an inherent component of the psyche.

We now come to full grips with the issue of our thesis. Psychoanalysis has been descriptively termed "the psychology of the unconscious" and also "ego psychology." The warrant for such designations lies in Freud's uncovering of the unconscious, and his further derivation therefrom of the three components of the psyche, the Id, the Super-ego and the Ego. The rationale of that derivation is simple and obvious. Within the unconscious of all so-called normal persons, and particularly within that of the psychoneurotic, Freud found a great deal of repressed material. Obviously what is repressed must *have been* repressed by a repressing agent and in the ultimate Freud identified this repressing agent as the Super-ego.

Before launching on a consideration of the Super-ego, a subject loaded with passionate charges, it is certainly appropriate to recall Freud's own words: "concerning the origin and function of the Super-ego a good deal remains insufficiently elucidated."

There is universal agreement as to the existence and operations of the Super-ego. The great controversy rages about its derivation. I am convinced that on this rock foundered the friendship of Freud and Jung. In defense of *his* side of the controversy Freud wrote *The Future of an Illusion,* and also his *Moses and Monotheism.* Yet Freud was always a bit diffuse, and somewhat ambivalent when treating of the derivation of the Super-ego. Precisely why Freud so dealt with this most important factor in the theory of psychoanalysis is too involved a theme to treat here. We need to consider Freud's derivation of the Super-ego as *he* developed it, without going behind the scene for his motivations.

Freud derives the Super-ego from the child's identification with parental authority, particularly with that of the father. The prohibitions and taboos emanating from the parental authority are introjected and incorporated within the individual, giving rise thereby to the Super-ego. Later the injunctions and prohibitions of other authorities, such as teachers, are adsorbed to the Super-ego, the whole forming and acting as censor and conscience. Freud therefore derives the Super-ego from the father, that is, the father, father substitute or father equivalent, in imposing prohibitions upon the primitive and instinctual drives of the child and, parenthetically, in offering libidinal rewards for conformity, engender the child's Super-ego. So far, so good. But now the question may be asked, who taught the father to approve of some actions and to condemn others? Or, to paraphrase it, how did the father gain his Super-ego, which, as is plainly to be seen, he actively seeks to impose upon or to cultivate in his offspring? Freud's answer to this question seemingly is as follows, "The father got it from his father, and so on down the line." But I say *seemingly* advisedly, for in fact, such was not Freud's *unreserved* answer. Every so often, Freud lifted the curtain and looked behind the seeming order ot the Super-ego's descent. Then he would allow that the Super-ego had a great many contacts with the phylogenetic endowments of the individual, that is, with his *archaic inheritance.* In *Moses and Monotheism,* Freud wrote: ". . . there probably exists in the mental life of the individual not only what he experienced himself, but also what he brought with him at birth, fragments of phylogenetic origin, an archaic heritage" (2). This is a grudging recognition of a large subject. The facts are that the individual brings with him not mere fragments but the whole of his phylogenetic share of experience—he brings with him "the engrams of his descent."

Jung has done much better with this subject. He maintains that every individual shares in what he terms the collective unconscious, which he defines as "the sediment of all the experience of the universe of all time, and . . . also an image of the universe that has been in process of formation for untold ages (3). Again Jung affirms: "In the same way as the individual is not only an isolated and separate, but also a social being, so also the human mind is not only something isolated and absolutely individual, but also a collective function. And just as certain social functions or impulses are, so to speak, opposed to the egocentric interests of the individual, so also the human mind has certain functions or tendencies which, on account of their collective nature, are to some extent opposed to the personal mental functions. This is due to the fact that every human being is born with a highly differentiated brain, which gives him the possibility of attaining a rich mental function that he has neither acquired ontogenetically nor developed." (4)

One will, of course, recognize the relationship between Jung's formulations on the collective unconscious, and my own postulations on the psychologic substratum of religion. They are not do be equated but implied in both is the idea that the Super-ego is rooted in the experience of the human race and is derived phylogenetically; that it is inborn in the individual, and is part of that *élan vital* which, initiated in the conjunction of two gametes, guides and directs all the subsequent evolvement of the creature in accordance with the pattern common to humankind. That *élan* is to be witnessed no less in the postnatal than in the prenatal existence of the individual.

Seen in this light, the derivation of the Super-ego is not dependent on the fortuitous transmission of prohibitions and taboos from man to man, from father to son, but is rather a something which each man brings with him into this world.

Care must here be taken not to misread the meaning of this last statement. Its sense is not that each man is born with a pre-established *code of morals,* but only that each person is born with the *psychologic impulsion to religion.* How that impulsion becomes concretized is a matter of accident. However, and this too is important, in the last analysis, the psychologic substratum of religion is always expressed in *altruism,* in *jenseits des Egoismus.* Even the "moral code" of cannibalism and the injunction to kill one's decrepit parents, gross and cruel as they may appear to us to be, are still motivated by an *altruism* stemming from the psychologic substratum of religion. Let me phrase it otherwise: It is conceivable that a Robinson Crusoe, shipwrecked as an infant, and by some miracle growing into adulthood, even without the man Friday for a companion, would yet have a Super-ego. This fantasy, incidentally, has been developed with fine psychologic insight by Gerhart Hauptmann in his novel *Die Insel der gross mutter.*

We need not, however, rest our case on psychological hypothesis. There are two additional orders of proof which are available to us. One is biologic and the other clinical. With the presentation of these, I expect to end my argument. First as to the biologic: Man, in this category, is at one with all other living things, that is, a converter of energy. The human organism, in the language of the physicist, degrades matter, and thereby draws for its own use energies invested in matter by preceding upgrading experiences, such as photosynthesis. The human organism as an energy converter has a limited span of operation. Like all converters it wears out. At a certain point it fails to function—and death ensues. We commonly speak of energy conversion as metabolism and we know that reproduction is in the strictly biologic sense a phase of metabolism. In all this, I repeat, man is at one with all other living things. But there is one respect in which man differs from all other living things, and that is in his capacity to reflect on, and to appreciate, his experiences. By virtue of this competence man is subject to powerful antipodal stresses, which, unless they are culturally interpreted for him, he seldom understands, rarely reconciles but only senses and suffers. Somehow even a dull man, if he but experiences adult love, must sense that he is caught between two eternities, and he will be troubled as to his linkage with both the past and the future. He will recognize that the individual is a time, space, and energy-bound congelation of matter; that he is largely moved by force determinants which antecede his formation, toward ends which largely transcend the grasp of his consciousness, and which in so many instances cut across his volitional direction. Man stands in need of reconciliation of his mortal self with his immortal end. For unless reconciliation between the antipodal forces is achieved, man cannot be healthy or happy. Man needs must render to the Id what is the Id's and to the Super-ego what is the Super-ego's.

Here I turn to the final proof which I would present in support of my thesis. Clinical experiences show that a weak or lacking Super-ego is a very frequent source of psychopathy. We are accustomed to think more often of the obverse, of the neurosis engendered by the too severe and exacting Super-ego. That is an historical accident, due largely to the type of case which came to the attention of Freud and his early co-workers. The neurotic suffering from the aggressions of his Super-ego is likely to be more noticeable. He is likely to be compulsive, exacting, rigid, or else deeply melancholic. In any case he is palpably sick and engaging. But the individual with a deficient Super-ego is generally "unattractive." We are inclined to consider him "no good." He belongs to the category of the so-called psychopathic or psychopathic inferior personality. These persons do not symbolize their conflicts in delusions, hallucinations, hypochondriasis, compulsions, obsessions, and the like. They rather "act out" their difficulties in antisocial or in socially nonacceptable patterns. The more severe type sooner or later is entangled with the law. The less severe we see in our clinics and in private practice. They are personalities who in different degrees have failed in life, who are ineffective and unhappy. If you seek for a specific traumatic experience in their background, something to be abreacted, you are not likely to find anything of importance. If you explore their unconscious for repressed material which needs to be brought forth and reintegrated you will not be rewarded by a flood of matter. You will find rather that they have functioned and are functioning on the level of the narcissistic child, but without the child's full satisfaction. The one distinguishing characteristic of their common history is that the development of their Super-ego was thwarted and corrupted. Their homes and the sociocultural milieu in which they grew up were wanting in that respect. Such patients are not helped unless their Super-ego is strengthened, and the therapist is thus frequently obliged to be "censorious."

Something akin to this is affirmed in Jung's dictum: "Ultimately it is infallibly the moral factor that decides between health and disease" (5).

The subject of religion and psychiatry is of vast and fundamental importance and deserves the most earnest study. It must not be allowed to become the tilting ground of bigoted interests and of intellectual nihilism. It must be lifted above that level to the preeminence it deserves, for it concerns "the health of the people." I believe that, as the psycho-neurotics outnumber the psychotics, so do the psychopathic personalities outnumber the psychoneurotics. I believe that a great deal of the social and individual unrest which we witness today is due to the fact that our culture has not provided us with the moral equivalent of the religions which it has helped to discredit.

I must end with a *caveat*. No one I trust will mistake anything in the aforegoing as a plea for the corporate church in any of its multiple forms, nor for any of its doxies! I have endeavored only to throw some light on what I chose to call the psychologic substratum of religion, to relate it to known and accepted psychologic forces and mechanisms and to estab-lish its significance in psychopathy and psychotherapy. I am mindful how vast the theme is, and how much of it still remains obscure and uncertain.

As my apology for the shortcomings of my presentation, patent and undiscovered, I can only plead that I have endeavored to follow the injunctions of Gilbert Murray, who in his *Four Stages of Greek Religion* wrote:

> The uncharted surrounds us on every side and we must needs have some relation towards it, a relation which will depend on the general discipline of man's mind and the bias of his whole character. As far as knowledge and conscious reason will go, we should follow reso-lutely their austere guidance. When they cease, as cease they must, we must use as best we can those fainter powers of apprehension and surmise and sensitiveness by which, after all, most high truth has been reached as well as most high art and poetry: careful always really to seek for truth and not for our own emotional satisfaction, careful not to neglect the real needs of men and women through basing our life on dreams; and remembering above all to walk gently in a world where the lights are dim and the very stars wander.

REFERENCES

1. MURRAY, G.: *Four Stages of Greek Religion*. New York, Columbia University Press, 1912, pp. 152-153.
2. FREUD, S.: *Moses and Monotheism*. Trans. by Katherine Jones. London: Hogarth Press and the Institute of Psychoanalysis, 1939, p. 157.
3. JUNG, C. G.: *Collected Papers on Analytical Psychiatry*. 2nd Ed. London, 1922, p. 432.
4. *Ibid.*, p. 451.
5. *Ibid.*, p. 470.

33

Man and the Immortal

MAN, PLAGUED BY HIS MORTALITY, puzzles the immortal. For of all the creatures in the animal kingdom, man alone acquires an awareness of death long before death is upon him. This early and lifelong cognizance of death goads man to query not only about death but also about life itself. To this inquisitive search for knowledge and understanding we can trace the origins both of philosophy and religion, for truth is a basic dimension of life and death is a crucial factor in religion.

Man's search for understanding, begun in remote historical time, has been a long, groping process, and no doubt will continue as such to the end of time.

The first concern of man was with death. Life he largely took for granted, at least initially, for as Rohde observes in *Psyche,* "To the immediate understanding nothing seems so self-evident, nothing so little in need of explanation, as the phenomena of Life itself, the fact of man's own existence" (1). On the other hand, the cessation of this so self- evident existence, whenever it obtrudes itself upon his notice, arouses man's ever renewed astonishment. But Life itself, standing as it does on the threshold of all sensation and experience, began, in time, to appear no less mysterious than Death, and the poets then articulated the common man's bewilderment, asking the perplexing question, "Who knows whether what we here call Life be not Death, and what we here call Death be not called Life there below?"

This discontinuity of his own existence is in effect inconceivable to man, for *he needs must be existent* to attempt this impossible concept. All he can achieve is the knowledge and awareness that at some point in time he will die, and then he will be dead, that is, no longer existing.

430

This knowledge, this awareness, however, has never really contented any large portion of mankind anywhere in the world. It afforded no answer to the troubling query, "If Life, why Death, and if Death, why Life?" It reconciles man neither to Life nor to Death. It carries the stigma of an unbalanced equation.

Life of and by itself, Life bracketed within a span of limited time, Life terminating in total non-being seemed to mankind a ghoulish jest played upon man by a malign and evil power. It is this perplexing frustration that moved the Gnostic pleader to ask of the Creator, "Why hast thou created this world, why hast thou ordered the tribes (of Life eternal) into it, out of thy midst?" For this world, the Gnostic pleader laments, is "A World of Turbulence Without Steadfastness, a World of Darkness Without Light . . . A World of Death Without Eternal Life, A World In Which The Good Things Perish and Plans Come To Naught" (2).

This is an elaboration on the original puzzlement, "Why Must Life Terminate in Death?" That in itself is a grief and would be such even were Life sweet and rewarding. But the world is *not* good and Life is *not* sweet and rewarding. To the Gnostic both birth and death were insults inflicted upon hapless man. But the Gnostic was in effect only reaffirming the dictum of Sophocles: "Not to be born is best" (3).

Somewhere in time the issue of injustice was added to that of mortality. Man, it was patent, must not only die, but while living must also suffer gross injustice and grave misfortune. In the Book of Genesis, it is recorded that at the very beginning of civilization man's innate evil was made manifest. Cain, tiller of the soil, in a fit of jealousy slew his brother Abel, a keeper of sheep. "And when Jehovah said unto Cain, 'Where is Abel, thy brother'? he said, 'I do not know; am I my brother's keeper?' " (4).

Death and injustice are the essence of what has been aptly termed Man's Tragic Vision of Life, a clear vision that has long darkened man's existence and has impelled him to fancy many versions of rectification and compensations on the other side of Life, in the beyond and in the hereafter. What inspired man to a belief in the Life beyond Life, in immortality, was not only the wish for continued existence, hopefully among those dear to him *in* life, but, no less, the compelling need to win for Life a rationality not manifest in common experience. Part of this faith in immortality derived from man's sense of his double self. There was the wakeful, active, sensating self, and the *other* self that "migrated" during sleep and moved miraculously in dreams. What happened to the other self, the transcendent one, when death quieted the sensating self? Where did it migrate? How did it thrive?

It is not possible here to trace or even to merely sketch the numerous ways in which men in different times and diverse cultures conceived the after life of the dead. Erwin Rohde in his masterful work *Psyche* deals amply with the cult of souls and the belief in immortality among the ancient Greeks. Frazer's *Belief in Immortality* is a comprehensive study that embraces the beliefs of numerous people both primitive and advanced (Frazer, H. G. *Belief in Immortality*, London 1913).

Morris Jastrow, Jr. has skillfully and learnedly analyzed and set forth the Hebrew and Babylonian views of life after death in his work *Hebrew and Babylonian Traditions* (Charles Scribner's Sons, New York, 1914, pp. 196-253). I will draw rather freely on his work for it is the Hebrew-Christian version of soul and immortality that has prevailed in western civilization for near to two millennia.

The pre-exilic Hebrews consigned their dead to Sheol, the general gathering place of the dead, a deep hole underneath the earth. Sheol was pictured as in total contrast to life and to everything connected with life. There the dead lie huddled together, conscious but inactive. "It is a land of darkness, of dense darkness, where even light is dark" (Job 10:22). There was no thought of possible redemption from Sheol. The dead were to rest there for all eternity.

But a new spirit and a new hope was engendered by the teachings of the Prophets. "Such was the force of the doctrines of the Prophets," wrote Jastrow, "that righteousness alone exalteth people and that only those who walk in straight paths can obtain favor, that it came to be looked at as inconceivable that the same fate should be measured out to the good and bad alike." A new hope was held out for those who suffered in this world because of their fidelity to higher standards of conduct. The pious and godfearing individual who suffered poverty, humiliation, and apparent failure in his earthly career would find his compensation for clinging to the law of God after his earthly career had closed.

The full realization of what the Prophets meant did not, according to Jastrow, come until the great lesson of the Exile had sunk deep into the minds and hearts of the people (p. 225): that Yahweh demanded loyalty to ethical ideals, and not, like other gods of the nations, a mere observation of ritualistic ordinances (p. 227).

Thus the introduction among the Hebrews of the ethical element led to the doctrine of individual retribution. It reached its culmination in Jewish and Christian teachings of rewards and punishments in future existence, accompanied by such concomitant beliefs as the distinction between Paradise and Hell, as well as the impressive doctrine of the immortality of the soul as the imperishable divine element in man (p. 252).

The Christian doctrinal scheme of salvation commanded the faith of the "Believers" and afforded them consolation as well as an answer to the problems of death and injustice. But there were also some non-believers; these found no consolation, nor did they believe, in the promise of heaven or the threat of hell.

Such disbelief is encountered as far back as the earliest ventures to assuage the dread of death with some promise of immortality. "Do not try and explain away death to me," says Achilles to Odysseus in Hades (Rohde, p. 4). "He that goeth down to Sheol," it is said in the Book of Job (7: Mark 9-10), "shall not come up. He shall return no more to his house, neither shall his place know him anymore." In The Words of Koheleth (The Book of Ecclesiastes) it is said, "For The Fate of the Children of Men and the Fate of the Beasts is The Same. As this one dies, so is the death of that, and there is the same spirit to all. Man has no advantage over the beast, for all is vanity. All go to one place. All are dust and all return to dust." (3:16-22). In the first century. A.D. Lucretius, the Roman poet, mocked the promise of heaven and the menace of hell in his De Rerum Natura.

However, despite the cynicism of the skeptics and the criticism of the sophisticated, the masses of Christiandom accepted in faith and with fervor the promise of a life after death, be it as Dante pictured it, in Inferno, Purgatorio, or Paradiso.

The Christian doctrinal scheme of salvation was soundly and firmly entrenched in the minds and hearts of the Faithful. It encountered no telling challenge until—may we phrase it dramatically—until June 1633 when Galileo Galilei, then 70 years of age, was forced to kneel before the Inquisitorial Tribunal of Rome to renounce the Copernican theory of the universe. It is said (Ortega y Gasset, p. 9) that this humiliation of Galileo was due more to the intrigues of private groups than to any dogmatic reservations of the Church. But, if such was indeed the case, it was because the Church did not fully appreciate the implications of the theory that decentralized the earth and dislodged both the heavenly Paradise and the terrestrial Hell.

Ortega y Gasset (5), writing on Galileo's effect on history, states: "The greatest crisis through which European destiny ever passed ends with Galileo and Descartes, a crisis which began at the end of the 14th century and did not taper off until the early years of the 17th century. The figure of Galileo appears at the end of this crisis like a peak between two ages, like a divide that parts the waters. With him man enters into the modern age" (Ortega y Gasset, p. 11).

The modern age is the age of reality, the age of science. Under Pristine Christianity man lived with his back to this life and his face toward the life beyond. Man despaired of himself and for that reason went to God. Then man despaired of the church; he detached himself from God, and he remains alone with things. Man has faith in himself; he has a feeling that he is going to find within himself a new instrument to resolve his struggle with his environment, a new reason, a new science, the *nuova scienza* of Galileo (Ortega y Gasset, p. 174).

The *nuova scienza* has flourished ever since and coincidentally has involved mankind in a new crisis, possibly the most grievous and menacing it has encountered in its long history. In essence this is a moral, and not, as in commonly believed, a technological crisis—though technology as the product of science in many ways concretizes the moral issues that comprise the crisis. The crisis does not at this time revolve around the issue of a life after death or the ultimate retribution of injustices suffered on earth. It is clearly more fundamental, more basic. For what has emerged as the challenging problem of the times is "the meaning of life." Has life any meaning at all, any that is comprehensible to man? Is there any real warrant for the numerous, onerous exactions imposed upon the individual by society? Is the so-called moral code of the so-called civilized man anything more than an imposition by the powerful upon the weak? Why should not every human being "do his own thing in his own way?"

There is something familiar in this challenging, desperate, questioning. It is reminiscent of Ecclesiastes and the Words of Koheleth. But to the Gentle Cynic life was a parade of vanities. To many today life is a madness, a many faceted incomprehensibility. Koheleth could yet nurture a doubt about an after-life existence, but today certainty is against the story of Heaven and Hell.

Darwinian evolution, the findings of archeology and of cultural anthropology, the studies in comparative religion have tamed the biblical version of Heaven and Hell, and rendered it a classical myth. But the rejection, the mythologizing of the Christian schema of immortality and salvation does not provide an alternate answer to the puzzlement of death and injustice. There are some today who attempt to dispose of the puzzlement by simply denying its validity. It is, they say, unreal; it is merely the vapid agitations of a disturbed and misdirected intelligence. Life itself, as B. F. Skinner argues, is "Beyond Freedom and Dignity." Meaning, justice, injustice, it is argued, are not innate qualities of life and experience, but only the artifacts of arbitrary definition, conditioned by circumstances.

But of course the attempts to dispose of the puzzlement of death and injustice by simple denial is neither convincing nor satisfying. It reminds one of the child's naïve attempt to make things disappear by covering its eyes.

Fortunately for the inquisitive mind and the troubled spirit, the very sciences that unwittingly discredited the Judeo-Christian schema of Heaven and Hell now afford one the data, and inspire the comprehension, wherewith to forge a much more sophisticated and more realistic answer to the problems of immortality, of death, and of individual injustice. The sciences have not undone individual death, nor have they eliminated injustice, but they have made it possible to view immortality in a way that does not violate reason, nor even transcend individual experience. It is to the exposition of this comprehension of immortality that I will devote the rest of my presentation.

To begin with, we need to appreciate that the living individual is a congelation of pre-existing matter. Whatever is material in the individual was in existence for "endless time" before *he* came into being. Also, the individual, each individual, is both time bound and space bound. These are unique features of man's individuation. And furthermore, this individual, this congelation of pre-existing matter, this space- and time-bound being, lives suspended between two eternities, the Eternity of the past and the Eternity of the future.

These eternities are open ended. Their extensions, the one into the past and the other into the future, are indeterminate and, for the present, inconceivable. They do, however, meet at the given instant in the given individual, *for it is he who serves to bind them together.*

Were there no person on earth, no being existing, there would be no Eternities to bind.

By derivation it is patent that the Eternity of the past into which the individual emerges, first at conception and effectively at birth, *that* Eternity is the repository of man's living past. It is his inheritance. We understand that clearly now on the material plane, in the sciences of human embryology and human genetics. But man also has a cultural inheritance, into which, so to say, he is born.

It is his cultural inheritance that distinguishes man from all other living creatures. Only man has a cultural history and it is for him the living witness of the Eternity of the past.

It is here that a moral injunction enters into man's existence: that he guard and cherish his cultural inheritance, that he foster and advance it, enrich it if he can, and that he pass it on through his being.

This is the meaning of the formulation, "Man is suspended between two Eternities, that of the past and that of the future, and serves to bind them together."

Insofar as the individual achieves this linkage, to that extent does he enter into Eternity, to that extent does he share in immortality. In this realization it is easy to find "meaning" to life, for life with all its tribulations, its trials, its suffered injustices, is thus justified in the opportunities and privileges provided in being.

I referred above to a moral injunction that enters into man's existence, namely, to guard, to cherish, to foster and if possible to advance his cultural inheritance. It may be asked: whence does this moral injunction emerge? Where is its origin? The answer is: it emerges from the same sources that gave origin to culture. It is in effect an innate dynamic in culture. When this is denied, then man's humanity is itself denied.

But this moral injunction does not emerge in or for every man. Goethe counseled: to possess one's inheritance one must earn it. "Was du ererbt von deinen Vätern hast, erwirb es, un es zu besitzen."

Alas, there are far too many who are unaware of the inheritance their Fathers left them, and as many who will not labor to gain it. It is this that, for me, makes understandable the Calvinist concept of the Elect.

Man, in general, has the potential to achieve four echelons of being. These are: the biological, the societal, the aesthetic and the moral. The biological and the societal, man shares with all orders of complex creatures, those above the mono-cellular level. But the aesthetic and the moral are uniquely human achievements. Yet it is precisely these last two echelons of being that relatively few are able to achieve to any appreciable degree. Nor is it to be assumed that mankind does very much better in the biological or societal echelons. Many lower creatures, the higher apes for example, do better in these categories than does mankind.

But the pursuit of this theme would carry us far afield. I must confine myself to the echelons of the aesthetic and the moral.

Man is the only creature that is capable of aesthetic creativity. Birds can sport beautiful feathers, insects exhibit intricate patterns of color and design, spiders weave superbly complex webs. But admirable as these are and inviting of aesthetic appreciation, they are not in effect aesthetic *creations*. They are genetically determined products realized in, but not by, the creatures concerned. But man creates his aesthetic products, deliberately and for a reason, the latter not always definable or even known.

Primarily, or primitively, man's aesthetic creativity was linked with magic and religion. In a measure it still retains this linkage. This bind is not difficult to fathom, for in creating that which as such has no exact counterpart in reality, man shares in the "potenzia" of the Creator; he is a piece of the Godhead.

Cicero considered those men to resemble the gods most who brought health to men ("Homines ad Deos Nulla re propius accedunt quam salutem hominibus dando"). I would replace the healer with the aesthetically creative individual. And let me add—I do not intend merely the maker of the traditionally beautiful. In my aesthetic realm there is room too for the proverbially ugly and irrational.

It is my persuasion that in the evolvement of man the aesthetic preceded the moral, but be that as it may, the moral is the highest of man's four echelons of beings. The "moral" is not primarily preoccupied with what has been fittingly termed moralisms—that is, with injunctions concerning what may and what may not be done—but rather with the transcending meaning of life. And that question of what *is* the transcending meaning of life materialized, I posit, as mankind came to grips with the experience of death. Is it not recorded in the Old Testament that the first biblical death—Cain's homicide—led to that question so basic to morality: "Am I my brother's keeper?" It could indeed be said, even though the affirmation is much too terse and hence may seem cryptic, that all men share in the immortal, even the evil ones; but those have the greatest share who are in the higher sense generous and loving keepers of their brothers.

Thus my vision of man is as a congelation of pre-existing matter, time- and space-bound, suspended between two open-ended eternities, the Eternity of the past and the Eternity of the future, and serving to bind them. The "immortality" of man derives from this condition, from this position, and from this function.

REFERENCES

1. ROHDE, ERWIN: *Psyche, The Cult of Souls and Belief in Immortality Among the Greeks.* Translated by W. B. Hillis. New York, Harper Torch Books, 1966, p. 3.
2. JONAS, HANS: *The Gnostic Religion.* Boston, Beacon Press, 1966, pp. 56-57.
3. SOPHOCLES: *Oedipus Coloneus,* 1225.
4. GENESIS, 4-1216a.
5. ORTEGA Y GASSET, J.: *Man and Crisis,* translated from the Spanish by Mildred Adams, New York, W. W. Norton & Co., 1958.

ACKNOWLEDGMENTS

CHAPTER 1. *The Anatomy of a Psychosis.* Reprinted from THE PSYCHOANALYTIC REVIEW, Vol. 33, No. 1, January 1946.

CHAPTER 2. *The Psychopathology of Paternal Deprivation.* Reprinted from SCIENCE AND PSYCHOANALYSIS, Vol. XIV. Copyright by Grune & Stratton, Inc., 1969.

CHAPTER 3. *The Psychodynamics of the Triad: Alcoholism, Gambling and Superstition.* Reprinted from MENTAL HYGIENE, Vol. XXXV, No. 4, October 1951.

CHAPTER 4. *The Gambler and His Love.* Reprinted from THE AMERICAN JOURNAL OF PSYCHIATRY, Vol. 117, No. 6, December 1960.

CHAPTER 5. *On the Etiology of Depersonalization.* Reprinted from THE JOURNAL OF NERVOUS AND MENTAL DISEASE, Vol. 105, No. 1, January 1947.

CHAPTER 6. *Prophylactic Psychopathology: The Rationality of the Irrational in Psychodynamics.* Reprinted from THE PSYCHOANALYTIC REVIEW, Vol. XL, No. 4, October 1953.

CHAPTER 7. *Psychiatry and the Maverick.* Reprinted from THE DYNAMICS OF DISSENT. Jules Masserman, Ed. Copyright by Grune & Stratton, Inc., 1968.

CHAPTER 8. *Dream Morphology: Its Diagnostic and Prognostic Significance.* Reprinted from THE AMERICAN JOURNAL OF PSYCHIATRY, Vol. 109, No. 4, October 1952.

CHAPTER 9. *Dynamics of the Cure in Psychiatry.* Reprinted from ARCHIVES OF NEUROLOGY AND PSYCHIATRY, Vol. 70, September 1953. Copyright by the American Medical Association.

CHAPTER 10. *Psychosomatic Medicine.* Reprinted from ARCHIVES OF NEUROLOGY AND PSYCHIATRY, Vol. 74, October 1955. Copyright by the American Medical Association.

CHAPTER 11. *The Place of Psychoanalysis in Modern Medicine.* Reprinted from CANADIAN PSYCHIATRIC JOURNAL, Vol. 1, No. 2, April 1956.

CHAPTER 12. *Psychiatry without Freud.* Reprinted from ARCHIVES OF NEUROLOGY AND PSYCHIATRY, Vol. 66, July 1951. Copyright by the American Medical Association.

CHAPTER 13. *Freud and Romantic Medicine.* Reprinted from BULLETIN OF THE HISTORY OF MEDICINE, Vol. XXX, No. 6, November-December, 1956.

CHAPTER 14. *Freud's Influence on Contemporary Culture.* Reprinted from the BULLETIN OF THE NEW YORK ACADEMY OF MEDICINE, Vol. 32, No. 12, December 1956.

CHAPTER 15. *A Midcentury Assessment of the Residuum of Freud's Psychoanalytic Theory.* Reprinted from AMERICAN JOURNAL OF PSYCHOTHERAPY, Vol. XI, No. 3, July 1957.

CHAPTER 16. *Psychoanalysis in 1959.* Reprinted from the BULLETIN OF THE NEW YORK ACADEMY OF MEDICINE, Vol. 36, No. 10, October 1960.

CHAPTER 17. *Eros and Thanatos: A Critique and Elaboration of Freud's Death Wish.* Reprinted from THE AMERICAN JOURNAL OF PSYCHOANALYSIS, Vol. XV, No. 2, 1955.

CHAPTER 19. *Job, Jung and Freud: An Essay on the Meaning of Life.* Reprinted from BULLETIN OF THE NEW YORK ACADEMY OF MEDICINE, Vol. 34, No. 12, December 1958.

CHAPTER 20. *The American Family in Crisis.* Reprinted from MENTAL HYGIENE, Vol. 42, No. 2, April 1958.

CHAPTER 21. *The Rise and Decline of Fatherhood.* Presented at the 49th Annual Fall Clinical Conference of the Kansas City Southwest Clinical Society, October 30, 1971. Reprinted from PSYCHIATRIC ANNALS, Vol. 2, No. 2, February 1972.

CHAPTER 22. *Our One-Generation Culture.* Reprinted from Proceedings of the Governors' Conference on Aging, Hartford, Connecticut, May 7, 1958.

CHAPTER 23. *The Addictive Personality.* Reprinted from GEIGY SYMPOSIA SERIES, November 1972.

CHAPTER 24. *Community Psychiatry: Its Social and Historic Derivations.* Reprinted from CANADIAN PSYCHIATRIC ASSOCIATION JOURNAL, Vol. 10. No. 6, December 1965.

CHAPTER 25. *Psychiatry for the Millions.* Presented at a meeting of the American Academy of Psychoanalysis, May 10, 1970.

CHAPTER 26. *Existentialism and Psychiatry.* Reprinted from BULLETIN OF THE NEW YORK ACADEMY OF MEDICINE, Vol. 37, No. 12, December 1961.

CHAPTER 27. *An Existential Clinical Exposition of the Ontogenic Thrust.* Reprinted from the AMERICAN JOURNAL OF PSYCHOANALYSIS, Vol. XXIV, No. 2.

CHAPTER 28. Reprinted from EXISTENTIAL PSYCHIATRY, 1963.

CHAPTER 29. *The Psychiatry of Paracelsus.* Reprinted from BULLETIN OF THE HISTORY OF MEDICINE, Vol. XXIV, No. 3, May-June 1950.

CHAPTER 30. *Descartes and Modern Psychiatric Thought.* Reprinted from Isis, Vol. XXXV, Part 2, No. 100, Spring 1944.

CHAPTER 31. *Psychopathia Intellectualis.* Reprinted from THE PACIFIC SPECTATOR, Vol. X, No. 2, Spring 1956.

CHAPTER 32. *Psychiatry and Religion.* Reprinted from THE JOURNAL OF NERVOUS AND MENTAL DISEASE, Vol. 112, No. 1, July 1950.

CHAPTER 33. *Man and the Immortal.* Reprinted from ENDLICHES AND UNENDLICHES IN MENSCHEN, Editio Academica Zurich, 1972.

Index

441